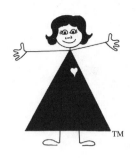

Taking Charge of
FIBROMYALGIA

Fifth Edition

Everything You Need to Know to Manage Fibromyalgia

Julie Kelly, M.S., R.N.
Rosalie Devonshire, M.S.W., LCSW

with contributions by
Jorge Flechas, M.D., M.P.H.
Jenny Fransen, R.N.
Michael McNett, M.D.
Thomas J. Romano, M.D., Ph.D., FACP, FACR
Jacob Teitelbaum, M.D.

Edited by
Thomas J. Romano, M.D., Ph.D., FACP, FACR

Fibromyalgia Educational Systems, Inc.
326 Broadway Ave. South, #206 • Wayzata, MN 55391-17
Phone: 847-480-7479 or 952-224-4413

www.fibrobook.com or *www.fmsedsys.com*

Medical Disclaimer

The treatments and therapies discussed in this handbook are intended for educational purposes only and are not to replace the services of a trained health professional. Consult your physician or healthcare provider before beginning any medication, treatment, or therapy as you may require specific precautions or modifications. The authors and editor do not accept liability in the event of negative consequences incurred as a result of information presented in this handbook.

Fibromyalgia Educational Systems, Inc.
326 Broadway Ave. South, #206 • Wayzata, MN 55391-1712
Phone: 847-480-7479 or 952-224-4413

www.fibrobook.com or *www.fmsedsys.com*

Please call or check the Web site for ordering information.
The Web site has prices for bulk quantities, shipping rates, and instructions for orders outside of the U.S.

Does this sound like your day? If it does, then you need to read this book!

A day in the life of a person with fibromyalgia.

After not sleeping half the night, you wake up feeling so stiff you can barely get out of bed. You feel like the tin man from the Wizard of Oz. At least he can get his joints oiled! You feel more tired and achy in the morning than before you went to bed the previous night! As you get out of bed, you notice that you feel a little spacey or lightheaded. You may even feel faint.

You go to the bathroom to brush your teeth and comb your hair. You have trouble lifting your arms to comb your hair, because of the pain and stiffness. You take a long, hot shower because the warm water helps soothe your muscles. You know you are supposed to stretch, but you are in too much pain to stretch, so you don't do it and feel a little guilty. After showering, you must get dressed. You pick the most comfortable and loose-fitting clothes, because if they are too tight, they make your pain worse. So you put on your baggy sweats and maybe you don't put on a bra, because the straps hurt. Also, you have gained 20 pounds from the medication your doctor put you on, so your old clothes don't fit. You feel fat. You could throw the carrot sticks you carry around all the time at your doctor every time she mentions that "you should watch what you eat; eat healthy and nutritious foods. You'll lose the weight," she says. You don't even get on the scale anymore, as it hasn't budged downward no matter what you do. Maybe it's the constipation causing the weight gain, you think.

You start down the stairs and feel your hips ache with every step, so you go slowly, for fear of hurting yourself. Your doctor told you the pain does not mean there is damage going on in your muscles, but you continue to worry. How could it be? No damage! This much pain must be causing damage! You don't really believe what your doctor says. You are sure that every step you take is causing huge tears in your thigh muscles, not to mention what is happening to your knees.

You go to the kitchen to eat breakfast, but skip the coffee because caffeine is out of the question. Then you realize that you forgot to take your medicine, which is upstairs in the bathroom. I should post a note on my mirror, you say to yourself. I'll do that when I go back upstairs. Your breakfast consists of one of those supposedly great-tasting shakes that includes all the necessary nutrients in it for FMS people. You doctor it up with yogurt and a banana. It's not too bad, you think, and it is helping me! You look at all the vitamins in your cabinet and wonder if it is possible to swallow them, as there are so many. Surely, your throat and stomach will not be able to handle all of them. So, you take half of them and hope you won't get an upset stomach.

You try reading the newspaper, but have difficulty comprehending what you read, so you give up. You think, maybe I'll try to exercise because my doctor told me that will help relieve my symptoms. As you get started, you feel so tired that it is difficult to do even simple exercises. After you perform the required exercises, you feel worse than before you started. What is that doctor talking about anyway? How does she know? She doesn't have fibromyalgia! So you wonder how exercise can help when it makes you feel so bad.

Then you have to go to work. You are tired and worn out before the work day has started. You get in your car and hope you remember how to get to your office. Once you manage to find your workplace, you are overwhelmed by the amount of work on your desk. You start feeling a migraine coming on. You search through your desk, looking for the Excedrin migraine medicine. Uh, oh, the bottle is empty. If your job entails computer work, you wonder how your neck, back and arms will feel when the day is over. If you have a job that entails physical labor, such as a grocery checker or factory worker, you know that you will suffer from pain all day long. Your employer does not allow you to take the necessary breaks you need to get control of your pain levels, and you have struggled to make him understand your plight. Your coworkers feel you are just pretending to be sick—because you don't look sick—and talk about you behind your back.

At lunch time, you start to feel even more pain and fatigue, and you tell your coworkers that it is going to rain. They have come to know that you are a potent weather predictor. You can tell whenever a storm is coming and feel you could make some money in marketing yourself as a human barometer. You know you are better at predicting the weather than the weatherman on TV. The day goes on, it starts pouring down rain, and you don't have an umbrella.

As you muddle through the rest of your day, you wonder how you will make it through the day. You mange to muddle on and can't wait for 5 o'clock.

Back in your car, you start thinking about all the household chores you have and all the running around your family wants you to do. You think to yourself, how will I ever get these tasks accomplished? If you are lucky, your family is supportive and helpful. Often, you hate to ask for help and try to do everything, anyway. Maybe you just give up and decide to live in a dirty house. What's wrong with a few dust bunnies? If you are the man of the house, you feel guilty because you haven't been able to do all the carpentry chores around the house, due to the pain. Every time you try to fix things in the house, you are laid up for days afterwards. You don't feel much like a man anymore.

After dinner, you collapse on the couch and use one of those electric massaging devices which heats up. You want to use it for hours because it does seem to help. Your family may think you are just being lazy and become critical of you. You try to explain how you feel to them, and you may even give them an article on FMS you found on the Internet. They don't read it. You may begin to doubt yourself and think that maybe those who say, "You're just crazy," are right! You go into your kitchen and see the bag of candy in the cupboard, and even though you know you shouldn't eat it, you reach for one and it tastes so good, you eat five candy bars! Then you feel guilty. Maybe you should turn into a purger, you think.

When you go to take your nightly warm bath, which does help, you notice your morning medication lying on your bathroom counter. You can't believe you forgot to take it. So now, you wonder, do I take both morning and night medication at the same time? If I do that, what will happen to me? Your doctor didn't explain that to you and you try to call the office. You get the answering service and feel bad about bothering your doctor, so you hang up. You don't think the medications are helping anyway and wonder if your doctor really knows what she is doing. You wonder if you can't think clearly because of the medications, or is it the fibromyalgia? Your doctor seems to be in such a hurry during your appointment time that you never get to ask her all the questions you had written down. It makes you angry. Maybe you will look for another doctor, but you've already seen five. So, being afraid to take too much medicine, you take your evening dose and leave out the morning dose to take tomorrow.

You get into bed and lie down on the magnetic pad you paid a small fortune for, which the manufacturer guarantees will make you feel better. When your spouse gets into bed, you realize you have stopped having sex, because you haven't felt sexual in a long time (due to side-effects of your medication) and it is painful when you do try to engage in intimate relations. You both feel lonely.

Your spouse falls asleep in two minutes and you lie there, wide awake, tossing and turning due to pain. You start to worry because you can't fall asleep and may be afraid to take the sleeping medication your doctor prescribed for you, because you are concerned you will become addicted to it. Your legs are jerking around, and you can't keep them still. You forgot to tell your doctor about this symptom. You get up to write a note to yourself to remember to tell the doctor. Oh, but you forgot to put a notepad next to your bed, and you don't have the energy to get one. You finally fall asleep at 2:00 A.M., but wake up often, sometimes to go to the bathroom, other times for no reason. You *want* to sleep. It's now 4:00 A.M. and you know you have to get up in two hours to go to work. You *know* you will feel bad when you do wake up and think that maybe you will try that sleeping medication tomorrow night. You can't wait for the weekend so you can sleep in.

A new day! You wonder when you will feel better, if ever. You worry about the FMS getting progressively worse and worry how you will manage. Will you have to quit your job? Will your family leave you? Maybe your friends have already stopped calling you. Why did this happen to me? Maybe you worry that you have been a bad person and God is punishing you. Will there ever be a cure? Will this be with you for the rest of your life? Will you end up in a wheelchair like the one other person who attended your local support group meeting last month? No wonder you feel depressed. Maybe you should go to see a psychiatrist. Maybe it is all in your head.

If you can recognize yourself in any parts of this, then you may find this book helpful. Our book has been helping fibromyalgia patients take charge of their illness for over a decade. Julie and I know how you feel, because we used to feel like this, too.

Acknowledgments

Many patients diagnosed with fibromyalgia have limited resources for educating themselves about their condition. We have developed a six-hour, self-help class called *Taking Charge of Fibromyalgia*, which we have been teaching at Abbott Northwestern Hospital in Minneapolis, Minnesota, and other locations, since the fall of 1991. The purpose of the class is to educate people with the most up-to-date information on their condition, enabling them to become the primary movers in the management of their fibromyalgia syndrome.

We especially want to recognize Jenny Fransen, R.N., as the originator and contributing author of the *Taking Charge of Fibromyalgia* course. Her vision, contributions, and support were critical for the creation of this course, and we owe her our deepest thanks.

Many thanks to Shelly Wesolowski, who coordinated the production of our most recent edition. We value her expertise and the many contributions she made to this handbook. We'd also like to remember the late Donald G. Kocina, who coordinated the production of our earlier editions. His vision and mentoring were invaluable. Many thanks to Faith Brynie who was responsible for proofreading. Her competence and attention to the details have helped make our handbook what it is today. We'd like to thank Dr. Thomas Romano and Dr. Karen Kindervater for their professional advice and input. It would have been very difficult to write this new edition without their contributions.

Many thanks to the national FMS organizational leaders Rae Gleason, Tamara Liller, Lynne Matalano, Mary Anne Saathoff, Margy and David Squires, and FMS physicians and activists for their invaluable contributions. We cannot thank them enough for their continued encouragement and support. The tireless dedication of the FMS community has provided a wealth of research, educational tools, and improved treatment options for the patient. With the continued cooperation of all of these people and organizations, we will certainly see better treatments in the future.

This handbook is not designed to take the place of your regular medical doctor's advice. You will want to discuss this information with your doctor and decide with him or her what is appropriate treatment for you.

We have created this handbook and educational program with loving care, and we dedicate it to all of you who live with this condition. Our deepest thanks to those of you who gave us encouragement to continue with our efforts and to those who provided us with personal experiences of living with fibromyalgia. Your comments were validating and invaluable.

Julie Kelly, M.S., R.N. and Rosalie Devonshire, M.S.W., LCSW

About the Authors

Julie Kelly, M.S., R.N., is a fibromyalgia nurse clinician and co-owner of Rheumatology Nurse Associates, LLC in Minneapolis, Minnesota. She works with fibromyalgia patients and their family members and educates health professionals on the diagnosis and treatment of this condition. She codeveloped the materials for the *Taking Charge of Fibromyalgia* educational program and is a cofounder of the first fibromyalgia support group in Minnesota. She is married and has two children.

Rosalie Devonshire, M.S.W., LCSW, is a former teacher, business owner, former FMS and CFIDS patient, and mother. She works clinically with individuals and families facing nonmedical difficulties and provides stress management, biofeedback and psychotherapy treatment to those with physical illnesses. She co-developed the materials for the *Taking Charge of Fibromyalgia* educational program, was a co-founder of the first fibromyalgia support group in Minnesota, and is a former board member of the Fibromyalgia Alliance of America. She is currently working with FMS patients at the Fibromyalgia Treatment Centers of America in Chicago, Illinois.

Julie and Rosalie have lectured extensively on the topic of fibromyalgia and bring a personal understanding to their audiences, because they, too, live with fibromyalgia.

Editor

Thomas Romano, M.D., Ph.D., FACP, FACR. We thank him for editing our handbook and offering us advice and guidance. His knowledge and expertise have helped us tremendously in putting this edition together. Dr. Romano is a compassionate and dedicated rheumatologist and a tireless supporter and advocate for fibromyalgia patients.

Contributing Authors

Jorge Flechas, M.D. M.P.H., is a family practitioner in North Carolina who works with many patients who have fibromyalgia (FMS) and patients with chronic fatigue and immune dysfunction syndrome (CFIDS). He has developed a new protocol for treatment of these illnesses using oxytocin (OT), dehydroepiandrosterone (DHEA), and some natural nutrients. His treatment protocol is discussed in the Appendix.

Jenny Fransen, R.N., is a rheumatology nurse clinician at Abbott Northwestern Hospital in Minneapolis, Minnesota. She is the originator of the *Taking Charge of Fibromyalgia* educational program and coauthor of *The Fibromyalgia Help Book*.

Michael McNett, M.D., is the Medical Director of Fibromyalgia Treatment Centers of America. He is board certified in family practice with additional training in emergency medicine, psychology, addiction medicine, pharmaceutical research, and integrative medicine. He studied under Dr. Muhammad Yunus, one of the world's most influential fibromyalgia researchers. Dr. McNett is committed to treating patients compassionately, researching new treatments for fibromyalgia, and educating both professionals and the public in the fact that there is a great deal that can be done to help fibromyalgia patients.

Thomas Romano, M.D., Ph.D., FACP, FACR, is in the private practice of rheumatology and pain management in Martins Ferry, Ohio. He is a board certified internist and rheumatologist and is a diplomate of the American Academy of Pain Management. He is a fellow of the American College of Physicians and the American College of Rheumatology as well as serving on the Board of Advisors and Board of Directors of the AAPM. He is past president of AAPM Board of Directors as well as chairman of its Examination Committee. He has authored numerous scientific and medical articles and book chapters regarding rheumatology in general and fibromyalgia syndrome in particular. His treatment protocol for fibromyalgia patients is discussed in the Appendix.

Jacob Teitelbaum, M.D., is a board certified physician in internal medicine who practices in Annapolis, Maryland. He has experienced fibromyalgia and chronic fatigue syndrome and also treats patients with these conditions. He is author of *From Fatigued to Fantastic!* An overview of his treatment protocol is discussed in the Appendix. Dr. Teitelbaum educates physicians and other health professionals throughout the United States on how to treat FMS.

Margy and David Squires, of To Your Health, a nutrition and supplement company, have provided quality nutritional supplements for FMS patients for many years. They have been active in the fibromyalgia community and have developed *Get with the Program*, a nutritional program designed specifically for FMS patients. Their program is outlined in our "Diet and Nutritional Supplements" chapter.

TABLE OF CONTENTS

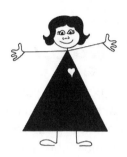

DEAR FIBROMYALGIA

Dear Fibromyalgia,

If you and I are to be constant companions for the rest of my life, I think we should be on speaking terms. First, I must let you know that you will never be able to possess me. You may at times have control of my body, but never my mind or my faith. Also, I am not a quitter. There will always be a battle going on between us. Sometimes you think you are going to win, but it is I who will win the war. For you see, my other companion is God.

Peggy J. Donahue

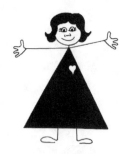

A FIBROMYALGIA JOURNAL

We feel it is very important to keep a record of your progress for your *Taking Charge of Fibromyalgia* program. Often, getting better is a slow and laborious task, and it becomes difficult to remember all the details of your program and of your progress. We've designed specific journal pages for this purpose that can be found at the end of the appropriate sections in your handbook. We suggest that you copy these pages, put them in a three-ring binder or folder, and start keeping a fibromyalgia journal. Keep your journal in a convenient place and please use it! You will be amazed at how useful it is when you go to your doctor and have an accurate record of your sleep, medications, and exercise—and so will your doctor! It's also very rewarding to keep track of your progress and to see how much better you're getting. It's the best incentive we know to keep up with all the components of your *Taking Charge of Fibromyalgia* program. It may be helpful to delegate some pages in your journal for "worry time," those 10 to 20 minutes a day when you write down all your worries. You might even sleep better!

Make your journal work for you. It can be an important component of taking charge of your fibromyalgia.

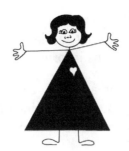

HISTORY OF FIBROMYALGIA

Jenny Fransen, R.N.

Muscular rheumatism was first described over 150 years ago. In fact, some believe that even the biblical sufferings of Job were those of a fibromyalgia patient: "The night racks my bones, and the pain that gnaws me takes no rest" (Job 30:17). In 1904, Gowers first used the term *fibrositis* to describe the muscle pain syndrome that we know today as fibromyalgia. Fibrositis described what was believed at that time to be an inflammation of the soft tissue and muscular fibrous tissue.

During the 1950s and 1960s, fibrositis was considered to have a psychological origin. Since that time, research has been inconclusive in proving that inflammation or abnormality of the muscle tissue exists. For that reason, fibrositis does not accurately describe the condition.

Travell defined myofascial pain syndrome as a condition of tenderness and pain in the muscles that is related to trigger points, which are sometimes associated with a taut muscle band that can be palpated, or felt, with the hand. Trigger points are defined as tenderness or pain in the muscle that usually cause referred pain. Referred pain is pain or deep aching that is made worse by palpating this abnormality in the muscle, the taut band, which spreads or radiates beyond the muscle area that is palpated. Myofascial pain syndrome is usually limited to a certain group or several groups of muscles. Fibromyalgia commonly can create muscle pain that is more widespread, affecting more of the body, as well as having more of a chronic nature.

There has been confusion between the two conditions of fibromyalgia and myofascial pain syndrome, and often the terms *trigger point* and *tender point* are used interchangeably even though they may not be the same.

In the 1970s, Smythe began defining the problem as widespread pain and aching with local tenderness, accompanying fatigue, morning stiffness, and a worsening of pain with activity. He began to propose its underlying causes, as well as standardized criteria to diagnose patients with fibromyalgia.

Later, during the 1970s, rheumatologists began to develop the diagnostic criteria, or standard set of symptoms that must be met in order for the diagnosis to be made.

In 1981, Yunus and Katz renamed the condition fibromyalgia or fibromyalgia syndrome, because a number of symptoms other than muscle pain and tenderness were found to exist together as a syndrome. Yunus was responsible for further defining the symptoms and tender points. It was during this period that the foundation of today's comprehensive treatment approach was begun, which utilizes different types of treatments and therapies together to bring about an improvement in symptoms.

Kellgren observed that in fibromyalgia, the pain came from deep below the surface of the muscle. His research showed that there was irritation of fascia, tendon, and muscle producing pain that radiated, leading to more research that gave us information on trigger points and trigger areas.

Smythe defined the problem as widespread pain and aching with local tenderness with accompanying fatigue, morning stiffness, and a worsening of pain with activity, without apparent cause. He offered a hypothesis about the cause of this condition, as well as criteria to help with more accurate diagnoses.

Over the past 15 years, there has been an explosion of research into the pathogenesis, or origin, of fibromyalgia; yet there remains much to be learned.

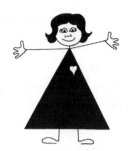

DIAGNOSIS AND SYMPTOMS

Fibromyalgia syndrome (FMS) is characterized by widespread musculoskeletal pain, aching, and stiffness with associated sleep disturbances and fatigue. It is seen in all age groups from young children to the elderly, with many patients experiencing their initial symptoms in their 20s and 30s. The majority of adult patients are women, experiencing this condition seven to eight times more often than men. In school age children, boys and girls are affected about equally. The symptoms and treatment are generally the same among men, women, and children.

The prevalence of fibromyalgia syndrome in the general population was studied by Fred Wolfe, M.D., and found to be approximately 2%. Other findings by Wolfe, et al. were that 3.4% of women and 0.5% of men in the communities studied met the American College of Rheumatology criteria for the diagnosis of fibromyalgia. Similar prevalence rates have been found worldwide.

Among individuals with fibromyalgia syndrome, there is a variable onset of symptoms. Some individuals recall a specific triggering event associated with an abrupt onset of symptoms. The triggering event could be

▲ **Physical trauma**	▲ **Sudden hormonal change**
▲ **Emotional trauma**	▲ **Steroid withdrawal**
▲ **Flu or other viral illness**	▲ **Hypothyroidism**
▲ **Nonviral infection**	▲ **Extended disruption of sleep**

Some individuals report that their symptoms began for no obvious reason. Others describe a very gradual onset of their symptoms over many years.

Some individuals experience musculoskeletal pain and tender points only in one particular region of their body and may have what some researchers call regional fibromyalgia (RF). A subgroup of these individuals report that, over time, their pain "grows" to gradually affect many areas of their body, developing the widespread pain of fibromyalgia syndrome (FMS). In a recent study of regional fibromyalgia patients by Yunus, et al., a majority of RF patients felt better after a mean follow-up period of 5.8 years, but about 40% developed widespread pain. This finding suggests an overlap between regional fibromyalgia and fibromyalgia syndrome.

The course of fibromyalgia for many is characterized by periods of remission and flare-ups which vary in length and severity. It is a condition that is invisible to others and is not life threatening. Many individuals with FMS learn to manage their symptoms quite well, especially after learning about FMS and actively participating in the appropriate treatment. Unfortunately, there are some who experience more persistent symptoms. These individuals may have another illness or injury that contributes to the complexity of their treatment, making management of their symptoms more difficult.

The diagnosis of fibromyalgia is made from your history and a detailed musculoskeletal exam. The absence of certain symptoms and signs is just as important as the presence of certain characteristics.

Positive and Negative Diagnostic Features of Fibromyalgia

	Positive	Negative
History	Patient complains of chronic diffuse pain, paresthesias	Normal history in respects other than pain, e.g., no joint swelling, no redness
Constitutional symptoms	Fatigue, sleep disturbance	No fever or major weight loss
Joint examination	Pain on full motion may be present	No joint effusions or deformities
Muscle examination	Tenderness at certain muscle-tendon junctions and muscle bellies, muscle tightness	No muscle weakness or atrophy
Neurologic examination	No characteristic positive findings	No sensory or motor abnormalities
Laboratory studies	No characteristic positive findings with routine testing	Normal complete blood count, erythrocyte sedimentation rate, muscle enzymes, thyroid function

Goldenberg, D. L., M.D. Diagnostic and therapeutic challenges of fibromyalgia. *Hospital Practice*, 1989, September 30.

The American College of Rheumatology 1990 Criteria for the Classification of Fibromyalgia*

▲ History of widespread pain for at least three months

Definition. Pain is considered widespread when all of the following are present: pain on the left side of the body, pain on the right side of the body, pain above the waist, and pain below the waist. In addition, axial skeletal pain (cervical spine or anterior chest or thoracic spine or low back) must be present. In this definition, shoulder and buttock pain is considered as pain for each involved side. "Low back" pain is considered lower segment pain.

▲ Pain in 11 of 18 tender point sites on digital palpation

Definition. Pain, on digital palpation, must be present in at least 11 of the following 18 tender point sites:

Occiput: bilateral, at the suboccipital muscle insertions.

Low cervical: bilateral, at the anterior aspects of the intertransverse spaces at C5-C7.

Trapezius: bilateral, at the midpoint of the upper border.

Supraspinatus: bilateral, at origins, above the scapula spine near the medial border.

Second rib: bilateral, at the second costochondral junctions, just lateral to the junctions on upper surfaces.

Lateral epicondyle: bilateral, 2 cm distal to the epicondyles.

Gluteal: bilateral, in upper outer quadrants of buttocks in anterior fold of muscle.

Greater trochanter: bilateral, posterior to the trochanteric prominence.

Knee: bilateral, at the medial fat pad proximal to the joint line.

Illustration of Tender Points

Arthritis Foundation, Atlanta, Georgia, 30326.
Fibromyalgia (Fibrositis), 1992.

Digital palpation should be performed with an approximate force of 4 kg.

For a tender point to be considered positive, the subject must state that the palpation was painful. "Tender" is not to be considered "painful."

* For classification purposes, patients will be said to have fibromyalgia if both criteria are satisfied. Widespread pain must have been present for at least three months. The presence of a second clinical disorder does not exclude the diagnosis of fibromyalgia. The American College of Rheumatology. Criteria for the classification of fibromyalgia. *Arthritis and Rheumatism*, 33 (2), 1990, February.

Symptoms of Fibromyalgia Syndrome

There are a number of symptoms associated with fibromyalgia syndrome. You may or may not experience all of the symptoms listed below, but will likely experience the more common symptoms:

- ▲ **Muscle pain**
- ▲ **Tender points**
- ▲ **Sleep disturbance**

Other symptoms associated with FMS are

- ▲ **Fatigue**
- ▲ **Subjective swelling**
- ▲ **Joint pain**
- ▲ **Neurological symptoms**
- ▲ **Headache**

- ▲ **Irritable bowel syndrome**
- ▲ **Irritable bladder**
- ▲ **Morning stiffness**
- ▲ **Raynaud's phenomenon**
- ▲ **Memory problems**

Symptoms of fibromyalgia vary considerably among people.

Additional Reported Symptoms

In recent years, a number of research findings have broadened the understanding of fibromyalgia and have included a greater array of symptoms now thought to be associated with this condition. Research suggests that individuals with FMS are not just tender in specific tender point areas, but are more sensitive to painful stimuli throughout the body. The comment that "I hurt all over" certainly makes sense when viewed in this context.

In a 1992 study of 554 individuals with FMS compared with a group of 169 controls, Waylonis and Heck also reported a number of additional symptoms that appeared to be associated with fibromyalgia. "Individuals with fibromyalgia self report a greater incidence of bursitis, chondromalacia, constipation, diarrhea, temporomandibular joint dysfunction, vertigo, sinus and thyroid problems. Symptomatic complaints found statistically more prevalent in fibromyalgia patients included concentration problems, sensory symptoms, swollen glands and tinnitus. Other associations occurring with significant increased frequency were chronic cough, coccygeal and pelvic pain, tachycardia and weakness." Twelve percent of the participants reported that they had children with symptoms of fibromyalgia, and 25% reported that they had symptomatic parents. Of the participants, 70% noted that their symptoms were aggravated by noise, lights, stress, posture, and weather.

The following table by Daniel Clauw, M.D., illustrates the wide variety of additional symptoms and syndromes now linked to fibromyalgia.

Symptoms & Syndromes
Now Linked to Fibromyalgia

Neurological
- Paresthesia: numbness or tingling (nondermatomal).
- Headaches: tension and migraine.
- Neurogenic inflammation: inflammatory sensation (rashes, itching, inflammation) initiated by nerves. A discrete, localized inflammatory response which does not activate the immune system or show up on tests.
- Cognitive: difficulty with concentration and short-term memory.

Sensory
- Auditory: low frequency, sensorineural hearing loss; decreased painful sound threshold.[1]
- Vestibular: exaggerated nystagmus (involuntary rapid movement of the eyeball), dizziness, vertigo.[1]
- Ocular: impaired function of smooth muscles used for focus as well as skeletal muscles used for tracking.[2]

Cardiac Pulmonary
- Mitral valve prolapse–a benign cardiac condition; 75% incidence in fibromyalgia patients according to one study.[3] Disorder may be due to neurological hyperactivity rather than a defect in the heart valve.
- Heart palpitations.
- Non-cardiac chest pain which may simulate cardiac disorder.
- Abnormal smooth muscle tone in muscles surrounding the bronchi of the lungs.[4]

Gastrointestinal[5]
- Heartburn.
- Irritable bowel syndrome.
- Esophageal dysmotility: objective abnormalities in smooth muscle functioning and tone in the esophagus; 40-70% incidence according to one study.

Genitourinary
- Painful menstruation.
- Increased urinary frequency and urgency.[6]
- Increased incidence of interstitial cystitis.[7]
- Vulvar vestibulitis or vulvodynia: characterized by a painful vulvar region and painful sexual intercourse.[8]

Miscellaneous
- Joint hypermobility.
- Temporomandibular joint disorder. In many fibromyalgia patients, problems are encountered because of the abnormal tone in muscles around the joint, not because of abnormalities in the joint itself.
- Plantar arch or heel pain.

References

(1) Gerster, J. and A. HadjDjilani, Hearing and Vestibular Abnormalities in Primary Fibrositis Syndrome. *J. Rheumatol*, 1984. 11: p. 678-80.

(2) Rosenhall, U., G. Johansson, and G. Orndahl, Eye Motility Dysfunction in Primary Fibromyalgia with Dysesthesia. *Scand J Rehab Med*, 1987. 19: p. 139-45.

(3) Pellegrino, M., D. Van Fossen, C. Gordon, J. Ryan, G. Waylonis, Prevalence of Mitral Valve Prolapse in Primary Fibromyalgia: A Pilot Investigation. *Arch Phys Med Rehabil*, 1989. 70: p. 541-3.

(4) Lurie, M., K. Caidahl, G. Johansson, B. Bake, Respiratory Function in Chronic Primary Fibromyalgia. *Scand J. Rehabil Med*, 1990. 22: p. 151-5.

(5) Hiltz, R., P. Gupta, K. Maher, et al., Low Threshold of Visceral Nociception and Significant Upper Gastrointestinal Pathology in Patients with Fibromyalgia Syndrome. *Arthritis Rheum*, 1993. 36(9S): p. C93.

(6) Wallace, D., Genitourinary Manifestations of Fibrositis: An Increased Association with the Female Urethral Syndrome. *J. Rheumatol*, 1990. 17: p. 238-9.

(7) Koziol, J., D. Clark, R. Gittes, E. Tan, The Natural History of Interstitial Cystitis. *J. Urology*, 1993. 149: p. 465-9.

(8) Friedrich, E., Vulvar Vestibulitis Syndrome. *J Reproduct Med*, 1987. 32(2): p. 110-4.

(9) Cleveland, C. Jr., R. Fisher, E. Brestel, J. Esinhart, W. Metzger, Chronic Rhinitis: An Under-recognized Association with Fibromyalgia. *Allergy Proc*, 1992. 13: p. 263-7.

DIAGNOSIS

Table and references are printed with permission from an article entitled "New Insights into Fibromyalgia" by Daniel Clauw, M.D. Article was published in *Fibromyalgia Frontiers*, 2(4), Fall 1994.

Postraumatic Fibromyalgia

▲ **Most common injury is a whiplash.**

▲ **Twenty percent of people who had whiplash developed FMS in one study.**

▲ **It may take two months to two years to develop FMS after an injury.**

FMS has been shown in numerous studies to occur following a traumatic injury, such as an automobile accident, surgery, or fall. Dr. Dan Buskila of Israel found that over 20% of people who sustained injuries developed FMS symptoms.

People who experience a whiplash from an auto accident may take from two months to two years to develop the symptoms of FMS. This author developed FMS after a whiplash injury and shoulder surgery within one year. The pain began in my neck area and "grew" to envelop my whole body. This same experience is often expressed by patients who attend our workshop or clinic.

Dr. Mark Pelligrino feels that many physicians neglect to look for more serious physical abnormalities such as chiari malformations, or spinal compression, which are treated by neurosurgery. Dr. Pelligrino and others, such as Dr. Romano, firmly believe many patients go on to develop FMS after a whiplash or traumatic injury. Pelligrino has authored a book called *Understanding Post-Traumatic Fibromyalgia*. It is available from Anadem Publishing and is listed in the "Resources" section in the back of this book.

Some individuals file for disability or may sue the person or institution they feel caused their injury. There are a few doctors who will work with you in this area. Dr. Thomas Romano is a tireless supporter of patients who have lost their ability to work due to postraumatic fibromyalgia. There are many who do not support this and do not want to become involved in litigation, even if a patient was perfectly well prior to the accident or surgery. See our information on disability in this book.

Modulating Factors

Modulating factors are those which influence the symptoms of your fibromyalgia. Some modulating factors are as follows:

▲ **Lack of, or too much, physical activity** ▲ **Postural strain**
▲ **Weather changes** ▲ **Anxiety**
▲ **Depression** ▲ **Repetitive and mechanical stress**
▲ **Major stressful events** ▲ **Interrupted sleep**
▲ **PMS** ▲ **Illness**

Fibromyalgia in Children and Adolescents

▲ **It affects school age boys and girls about equally.**

▲ **The majority of adolescent patients are female.**

▲ **Symptoms are comparable to those in adults with FMS.**

▲ **Treatment is generally the same as with adults.**

▲ **It is important to distinguish from juvenile rheumatoid arthritis.**

In recent years, juvenile primary fibromyalgia syndrome (JPFS) has become an increasingly recognized chronic syndrome. While it is known to affect younger school age boys and girls about equally, once they are adolescents, the majority of patients are female. In a study by David Siegel, M.D., M.P.H., fibromyalgia symptoms in children and adolescents were found to be similar to those in adults. Sleep disturbance was reported by 96% of the pediatric patients and diffuse pain by 93% of these children and

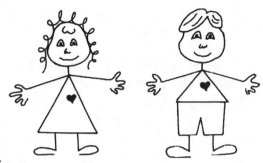

adolescents. Headaches (71%), general fatigue (62%), and morning stiffness (53%), were the symptoms reported as the next most frequent. While these symptoms are similar to those in adults, this study noted two important exceptions: 1) a higher prevalence of sleep disturbance in children and adolescents and 2) frequent finding of fewer than 11 tender points on physical examination. C. E. Tayag-Kier, M.D., et al. studied the sleep of patients with JPFS and noted a number of abnormalities. Not only did they present with prolonged sleep latency, shortened total sleep time, decreased sleep efficiency, and increased wakefulness during sleep, they also had excessive movement activity during sleep, with 38% exhibiting periodic limb movements in sleep (PLMS). An explanation for the fewer areas of tenderness in these younger patients is not clear, but may be because they are often seen at an earlier stage in the progression of their illness than are patients identified in adulthood. As the lower tender point count has been documented over the years, M. Yunus, M.D., and others have used the criteria of widespread diffuse pain and five or more tender points for the diagnosis of JPFS. Another interesting finding in the Siegel study was that 40% of the children and adolescents also had a diagnosis of hypermobility syndrome. In yet another study, T. J. Romano, M.D., noted that all of the children reported diffuse musculoskeletal pain, 67% noted the presence of muscle stiffness, and 33% had complaints of soft tissue swelling. Other frequently reported symptoms were fatigue (100%), poor sleep or waking up tired (73%), and headaches (53%). A physical examination revealed typical tender points, no joint swelling, nodules or fluid in a joint, and an absence of neurological findings. Standard laboratory tests were normal. Similar results were found in studies by Yunus and Masi and by Calabro. The most aggravating factors were cold or humid weather, physical overactivity or inactivity, anxiety or stress, and poor sleep.

Children's and adolescents' complaints of pain and fatigue need to be taken seriously. In order for an accurate diagnosis to be made and proper treatment prescribed, physicians need to be familiar with the symptoms and diagnostic criteria of fibromyalgia and to listen carefully to their young patients and their parents. Does the child complain of awakening frequently during the night? Is the child a restless sleeper? Does the child change positions often, kick bedcovers off, or jerk or twitch during the night?

Does the child complain of sleeping very lightly most of the night or of having a difficult time getting up in the morning? Is fatigue interfering with getting to school on time, participating in extracurricular activities, or having fun with friends? Is the child able to concentrate in school and complete homework on time? Is memorization becoming more difficult? Sleep problems and fatigue when coupled with aches and pain should not be ignored, especially if one of the child's parents has fibromyalgia. Does the young person complain of deep aching pain, shooting pains, burning sensations or muscle stiffness? Is the pain interfering in the classroom or making it difficult to participate in physical education? Is a previously active child now avoiding activity or feeling weak and exhausted after minimal exertion? Does the child experience increased pain if sitting or standing for long periods of time? Sometimes children squirm and fidget in class to keep themselves awake and to cope with the increased discomfort.

As in adults, symptoms of JPFS may begin after a specific triggering event such as a sports injury, car accident, illness, or major stressful event. Sometimes they may come on gradually, without any obvious precipitating event. If you suspect that your child may be developing juvenile primary fibromyalgia syndrome, it's important to have him or her evaluated by a physician in your community who is very familiar with this condition. Sometimes the symptoms of fibromyalgia are confused with other conditions, such as juvenile rheumatoid arthritis. In order to avoid unwarranted testing and investigation and possibly improper management, an assessment by a knowledgeable physician is essential in order for an accurate diagnosis to be made and the appropriate treatment to be suggested.

Education of both the parents and child should follow the diagnosis. Children and adolescents can be taught and given many tools to help them decrease their symptoms and to cope with the daily challenges of FMS. They need to be encouraged to develop skills in problem solving that will help them manage their condition day-to-day and assist them in feeling some control in their life, despite fibromyalgia. Their active role in self-management is paramount! Age and intellectual and emotional development are important parameters to consider when helping children understand fibromyalgia and what they can do to better control it. This educational process is often very helpful in allaying many of their fears, helping them to understand that no one is "at fault," and eliciting their participation in the subsequent treatment program.

Treatment is similar to the treatment for adults and often begins with treating their sleep disorder(s). Relaxation training with abdominal breathing, biofeedback, pacing, stress management, medication, ways to conserve energy and manage fatigue, gradual conditioning and exercise program, good nutrition, heat, ice and acupressure, massage, postural retraining, and instruction on reasonable accommodations at school can all be helpful. Students may also benefit from planning their study time and activities to correspond to times of the day when they typically experience more energy. Cognitive behavioral therapy can help modify the thoughts of those students who feel that their pain controls and hinders all aspects of their lives. Nurses, physical therapists, occupational therapists, and psychologists who are knowledgeable in FMS can individualize the treatment and guide each young person in the appropriate activities.

A child or adolescent's fibromyalgia can significantly impact his or her personal and social development, ability to attend and succeed in school, and life at home with family. These children and teens can feel very different than their peers who are not living with an invisible illness. It may be difficult to attend school on a regular basis and to continue friendships due to a lack of energy, chronic pain, and inability to participate in an array of activities. They may lack self-confidence as they struggle with performance at school and uncertainty regarding what they might be able to do tomorrow, next week, or next year. Older teens may wonder how fibromyalgia might impact their future options for education and employment. Classmates, teachers, administrators, family members, and healthcare professionals who lack an adequate understanding of FMS and are not empowering to the student can compound their challenges.

Parents and health professionals frequently become advocates for these students within the school setting. They educate teachers, school nurses, guidance counselors and coaches about JPFS and seek appropriate school-related accommodations. These may include providing the student with two sets of books, a flexible class schedule, an option of lying down midday in the nurse's office to listen to a relaxation tape or to do biofeedback, use of a tape recorder for note taking, and the opportunity to change position frequently in class. Teachers need to know that the student cannot predict symptoms from day-to-day, that some days are simply worse than others, and that the student will usually look better than he or she feels. A special needs assessment and individualized learning plan may be very helpful in assuring the appropriate accommodations for the student with JPFS. While students may find it difficult to attend school regularly and may require home tutoring for a period of time, every effort needs to be made for the student to be in school. Participation in the classroom and extracurricular activities, when possible, helps balance the need to feel normal and accomplish age-appropriate life tasks with the need to self-manage fibromyalgia.

Many children and adolescents with JPFS can expect to improve over time and maintain a reasonable level of function at home, in school, and in their leisure activities, even with the periodic exacerbation of symptoms. As these young people are able to integrate the important components of treatment that have been suggested and learn to self-manage their symptoms, they will feel increased confidence in coping with daily challenges.

Excellent resources for children and adolescents and their parents are *The Pediatric Network* at www.pediatricnetwork.org and a packet, *Fibromyalgia in Young People,* which can be ordered for $10.00 at the National Fibromyalgia Partnership's online store (www.fmpartnership.org). This packet may also be ordered by mail: NFP, Inc., P.O. Box 160, Linden, VA 22642-0160.

Fibromyalgia in Men

▲ **About 10% of FMS patients are men.**

▲ **Symptoms are similar to those in women.**

▲ **Men may be reluctant to seek medical attention.**

▲ **It may be difficult to find other men for support.**

Fibromyalgia syndrome is uncommon in men—occurring in about 10% of patients—and data on its characteristics and severity are limited. A study in the role of gender in FMS by M. Yunus, M.D., et al. showed that men experienced significantly fewer total number of symptoms, fewer tender points, and less fatigue, and they hurt less all over than women. Pain severity, global severity, physical functioning, and psychological factors (i.e.: anxiety, depression, stress) were not found to be significantly different between the men and women. Conversely, a study by D. Buskila, et al noted that men with FMS reported more severe symptoms, decreased physical functioning, and a lower quality of life when compared with women. A group of researchers in Sweden (M. Paulson, et al.) studied the experience of men as patients living with fibromyalgia-type pain. The men described a life full of limitations, with pain, weakness, muscle stiffness, fatigue, restlessness, and anxiety as frequent symptoms. They were often unable to participate in the same work and leisure activities as when they were in good health, because of their diminished physical strength or incapacity for sedentary work. If this affected their ability to work full-time, increased anxiety was often a consequence. Living day-to-day with pain that fluctuates and that is impossible to predict affected their humor and contributed to their feelings of increased irritability and anger. The men expressed their reluctance to complain unnecessarily and tried to lead as normal a life as possible. Despite the daily challenges of fibromyalgia, they discussed the importance of never losing courage and of continuing to have hope that their situation would improve.

Fibromyalgia has the potential to significantly impact anyone who is diagnosed with it. The impact on males, however, may not be as apparent to others, because men are often reluctant to discuss their symptoms and choose to persevere with their normal activities. This may delay their initial diagnosis or make it challenging for them to incorporate suggested treatment. Due to the fewer numbers of men diagnosed with this disorder, it may be difficult for them to find other men to talk with in a supportive environment. An excellent Web site designed for men with FMS is Men With Fibromyalgia, www.menwithfibro.com. The National Fibromyalgia Partnership, Inc. has compiled a packet of information and new research on FMS and men. To order, call 540-622-2998, fax toll free 866-666-2727, or visit their Web site at www.fmpartnership.org.

While the mechanisms of gender differences in fibromyalgia syndrome are not fully understood, they are likely to involve an interaction between sociocultural factors, biology, and psychology. Continued research in this area will help provide guidelines for health professionals, families, and caregivers that will assist them in providing better care and support to men living with fibromyalgia.

Pregnancy and FMS

Pregnancy can be a challenging time for many women with fibromyalgia. While FMS affects primarily women and is frequently diagnosed during their reproductive years, the relationship of pregnancy and fibromyalgia has had limited research. In a retrospective study by M. Ostensen, FMS was found to have no adverse effects on the outcome of the pregnancy or the health of the newborn infant. While the outcomes were good, all of these women, with one exception, described a progressive worsening of their FMS symptoms throughout their pregnancies. During the postpartum period, also noted was an increase in depression and anxiety.

In my clinical experience, women report a variety of scenarios regarding their symptoms of fibromyalgia and pregnancy. For some, pregnancy played a major role in the onset of their fibromyalgia. Others found that their mild muscle aches and pains before pregnancy seemed to worsen during their pregnancy and eventually led to the diagnosis of fibromyalgia. Some women reported that their symptoms improved. Many of the women who had fibromyalgia before conceiving found that their symptoms flared up throughout their pregnancy, often worsening in the last trimester. Even though many women with FMS experience greater challenges in their pregnancies, they often tell me that the reward of their beautiful baby is worth the additional suffering that they experience.

From a medical perspective, there are no particular contraindications or unusual medical risks involving fibromyalgia and pregnancy that are known at the time of this printing. Obviously, additional research will be helpful in providing us all with further guidelines for women of childbearing age. If you are considering becoming pregnant, it's important to talk with your physician about the medications you are taking to help manage your FMS symptoms and other medical conditions. It may be necessary for you to stop taking these medications before becoming pregnant and to wait to restart them until after you have weaned your baby from breastfeeding. You may be able to stop some medications abruptly, while others may need to be decreased gradually. Prenatal vitamins are often started before a planned conception. Check with your physician before making any adjustments and be sure to discuss ALL of your medications and supplements with your physician in order to receive the appropriate guidance.

Pregnancy is a time to focus on treatments other than medication to help manage symptoms. These may include regular relaxation and biofeedback, a nutritious diet, massage, acupressure, warm baths and showers (avoid hot tubs!), moist heat packs, cold gel packs, naps, proper posture and body mechanics, and anything to decrease stress. A body pillow in bed may help support your growing body and provide some added comfort. Exercise and gentle stretching during pregnancy are helpful for many women and may include walking, swimming, and t'ai chi. It's very important to discuss exercise and stretching options with your physician to receive his or her permission and guidance. This is the time to rediscover the leisure activities that you love to do, the books you love to read, the music you love to listen to, and to make time every day to do something for you. Some activities may be difficult for you while pregnant, but try various accommodations or make the necessary adjustments and discover what works! Remember to elicit the support of family and friends as you do your best to cope with the physical and emotional stresses of pregnancy.

Labor brings its own challenges to women with FMS. Many patients report becoming fatigued easily during labor, so any opportunity to get extra rest late in your pregnancy might be helpful, as well as taking any and all opportunities to rest between contractions while in labor. You may need more pain medication due to central sensitization (as discussed in the research section) and may benefit from using natural methods to help manage pain, such as massage, ice or hot packs, acupressure, soothing music, and biofeedback. Bring your "bag of tricks" to the hospital and use them!

If you've decided to breastfeed your infant, consider having your partner feed a bottle of expressed milk or formula for one nighttime feeding. A nurse or lactation specialist can help guide you through this transition and provide you with additional suggestions on balancing your need for sleep with your desire to breastfeed your infant. Bottle-feeding is the preferable choice for some mothers with FMS. It offers the obvious advantage for others to participate with feedings and can provide you with a longer stretch of "uninterrupted" sleep during the night.

The biggest challenges to new mothers with fibromyalgia is physically caring for their new baby and finding the time to sleep. The physical and emotional demands of their baby can be exhausting and cause increased stress. The increased stress is often expressed in tense muscles, which cause further pain and discomfort. Proper positioning with pillows and good body mechanics are important in limiting the strain to vulnerable muscles. When you carry your baby, remember to always hold him or her close to your own center of gravity. As your child gets older and heavier, encourage him or her to crawl onto your lap and into the car seat, instead of asking to be picked up. Postpartum depression may also occur in some women and can lead to further disrupted sleep, increased fatigue, and pain.

It's no surprise that many women experience a flare-up of their symptoms after their baby is born. It's an important time to ask your family and close friends for help, to discuss serious concerns such as postpartum depression with your physician, and to take every opportunity to rest when your baby is sleeping. Avoid caffeine, practice regular relaxation and meditation, and do what you can to sleep in longer stretches at night. The other nonmedication treatments that you've previously found helpful are important to continue and may include, among others, biofeedback, massage, acupressure, and hot or cold packs. It's also helpful to resume your regular exercise program as directed by your physician, starting with the amount that is easily tolerated and increasing very gradually. The challenge may be how to integrate exercise into your new lifestyle! Some mothers prefer exercise videotapes they can use at home; others prefer a regular stroller walk with their baby. Some may resume a variation of the exercise routine they did before their pregnancy, especially if they are able to arrange consistent childcare.

When you shop for baby equipment, consider items that may help you care for and transport your baby more easily, while limiting the extra strain on you. Examples may include a lighter stroller that would be easy for you to lift in and out of the car, a backpack with padded shoulder straps and wide hip belt to help decrease strain on your upper back and neck muscles, and a high chair that has a removable tray and a restraint system that is easy to use. If your home has several levels with numerous stairs, consider setting up a couple of changing areas for your infant, to help you minimize the extra steps and effort with your already strained energy reserves.

Even though many new mothers with fibromyalgia experience flare-ups of their symptoms, you may be able to minimize their intensity and frequency by incorporating a variety of these suggestions. Try some, adapt them to your individual situation, and above all, enjoy your new baby!

New symptoms may require a visit to your doctor. It is important to report all of your symptoms.

Because there are so many symptoms associated with FMS, patients who develop new or different symptoms may ignore them, presuming the new symptoms are due to FMS. This may not be the case. It is important to understand that it is possible to develop new medical problems or illnesses at anytime after your diagnosis of FMS, and it is important to report these to your physician. Some patients have lived with certain symptoms for so long, they neglect to report them to their physician during their appointments. Failure to point out all of your symptoms could hinder your medical treatment. Treating your underlying medical conditions is important to your overall well-being. Continuing yearly office visits with routine testing is also important for optimal health.

How do you know when to report symptoms to your physician?

If symptoms are new or of an increased intensity, they may indicate another disorder not related to your FMS and should be addressed with your physician. **This is not a total list of all possible new symptoms that could occur. It is important to keep in touch with your physician. Do not assume that all symptoms are related to FMS.**

- ▲ **Hot, inflamed, or swollen joints**
- ▲ **Chest pain of a new type or that radiates to the jaw or down an arm**
- ▲ **Numbness and/or tingling of a new type**
- ▲ **Persistent numbness or weakness in legs**
- ▲ **Headaches unlike those you have previously experienced**
- ▲ **Swollen glands**
- ▲ **Unexplained weight loss**
- ▲ **More frequent urination at night**
- ▲ **Shortness of breath**
- ▲ **Tachycardia or heart palpitations of an increased intensity**
- ▲ **Loud snoring at night, holding your breath**
- ▲ **Dizziness, fainting, lightheadedness when going from sitting or lying down to standing**
- ▲ **Changes in menstrual cycle, increased pain, or blood flow**
- ▲ **Changes in the strength of your muscles**
- ▲ **Extreme fatigue of a new nature**
- ▲ **Fevers**
- ▲ **Skin rashes**
- ▲ **Persistent cough**
- ▲ **Change in bowel habits**
- ▲ **Wheezing**

- ▲ Sores in mouth
- ▲ Visual disturbances
- ▲ Swelling of the ankles
- ▲ Significant increase in cognitive problems
- ▲ Frequently dropping objects

Primary Fibromyalgia Syndrome and Chronic Fatigue Syndrome

Are primary fibromyalgia syndrome and chronic fatigue syndrome the same condition? The many similarities between FMS and CFIDS have presented researchers with the challenge to continue to reassess the criteria for diagnosing both syndromes.

During the 1980s, Don Goldenberg, M.D., and Anthony Komaroff, M.D., showed that there were no significant differences between FMS and CFIDS when symptoms, tender points, and demographics were assessed. In fact, 75% of the patients diagnosed with CFIDS also met the tender point criteria for FMS. Many patients diagnosed with fibromyalgia syndrome could also have been diagnosed as having chronic fatigue syndrome. H. Moldofsky, M.D., has suggested that no differences were found between these two patient groups in several other studies when brain function, sleep physiology, and immunology were compared.

Do CFIDS and FMS anchor the opposite ends of a continuum of symptoms, with those patients diagnosed with CFIDS presenting with a primary symptom of overwhelming fatigue and those patients diagnosed with FMS presenting with a primary symptom of aches and pains? There seems to be little disagreement among many physicians that CFIDS and FMS at the very least share many common symptoms and that their treatment is very similar. Would one's diagnosis of CFIDS or FMS be different depending on which specialist initially assessed the patient?

The following is a case definition for chronic fatigue syndrome (CFIDS) as published in the December 1994 *Annals of Internal Medicine:*

Chronic Fatigue Syndrome

Fatigue

Patients must have otherwise unexplained, relapsing fatigue that is new (not lifelong); not the result of ongoing exertion; not relieved by rest; and that results in substantial decrease in levels of occupational, social, educational, or personal activities.

Symptoms

The patient must have four or more of the following eight symptoms. Symptoms must persist for six months and the patient must not have predated fatigue.

- ▲ Self-reported impairment of memory or concentration that affects occupational, social, educational, or personal activities
- ▲ Sore throat
- ▲ Tender cervical (neck area) or axillary (underarm area) nodes
- ▲ Postexertional malaise, lasting at least 24 hours
- ▲ Arthralgias (pain along the nerve of a joint) – no redness or swelling
- ▲ Headache of a new type
- ▲ Unrefreshing sleep
- ▲ Myalgias (muscle pain)

If you have chronic sore throats, low-grade fevers of unknown origin, or chronic colds, you may want to discuss these symptoms with your physician to rule out an Epstein-Barr viral infection, cytomegaloviral infection, HMV 6, or other infectious agents. Depending on your test results, other types of treatment may be appropriate.

The FMS and CFIDS controversy continues to intrigue researchers and will no doubt be further studied and investigated. While we, as patients, watch with interest for new studies on this subject to be published, we will best spend our energy on treating our symptoms and focusing on getting better. Let's leave this controversy to the researchers!

TIPS *Diagnosis and Symptoms*

▲ Be sure that the physician who diagnosed you with fibromyalgia performed a tender point exam. If he or she did not, ask for one. This is an important diagnostic tool.

▲ If you are seeing a physician or other healthcare professional who is not familiar with fibromyalgia, either provide him or her with some educational materials on fibromyalgia or seek out someone familiar with this condition.

▲ Use our symptom checklist. It is a useful tool to help you keep track of symptoms for yourself as well as for your doctor.

▲ Some people worry about unusual or new symptoms for a long time before they report them to a health professional. Why suffer needless worry? Remember to write down all of your symptoms, including any unusual ones.

Symptom Checklist

We encourage you to write down any symptoms you may be experiencing, no matter how insignificant they may seem to you. This could go a long way toward providing your healthcare team with needed information to help facilitate improvement in your condition. Fill this sheet out and take it with you to your doctor. Take some time to think about your symptoms: a few days or even a week's time. Add new ones as they occur.

My Symptoms:

_____   _____   _____

_____   _____   _____

_____   _____   _____

_____   _____   _____

_____   _____   _____

_____   _____   _____

_____   _____   _____

_____   _____   _____

_____   _____   _____

_____   _____   _____

Diagnostic Laboratory Tests Useful in Assessment of Fibromyalgia Patients

At this time, there is not a single blood test to help determine the diagnosis of FMS.

When you go to a physician to determine whether you have fibromyalgia, the physician will make a diagnosis by taking a careful history, reviewing all medical records, performing a physical examination, which includes a tender point exam, and by the use of certain diagnostic laboratory tests, and by excluding other illnesses.

Laboratory tests used to assess fibromyalgia patients should be viewed as tests done to

▲ **Rule out other problems such as rheumatoid arthritis, lupus, reflex sympathy dystrophy, multiple sclerosis, or other arthritic conditions.**

▲ **Rule out perpetuating factors such as a growth hormone deficiency, hypomagnesemia (low magnesium levels), thyroid dysfunction, vitamin deficiencies, or infections such as Lyme disease or the Epstein-Barr virus.**

▲ **Follow up on previous testing to refine the diagnosis and establish the most effective treatment.**

When you go to a doctor for an initial assessment and evaluation, be sure to bring the results of any prior medical tests with you. If the tests have been recently performed, you may avoid additonal, unnecessary testing.

Some basic tests include

▲ **CBC (count of your blood cells) to check whether you might have a blood disease such as anemia**

▲ **Blood glucose levels — to determine if you have diabetes, or hypoglycemia**

▲ **Erythrocyte sedimentation rate**

▲ **SMA-18 — liver and kidney functioning and electrolytes**

▲ **Free T4, T3, TSH- thyroid functioning tests**

▲ **Red blood cell magnesium levels**

▲ **Antinuclear antibody (Lupus screen, sometimes positive in FMS patients — called a false positive because patients do not actually have the disease)**

▲ **Rheumatoid factor — tests for chronic inflammatory conditions such as rheumatoid arthritis**

Dr. Romano states that often these tests are normal in FMS patients. If there are signs and symptoms to suggest a need for further testing, your doctor might test also for the following:

Growth Hormone Deficiency - If the patient has weight gain around the abdominal area, complains of a low libido (sexual drive), cold intolerance, and emotional lability, the physician may order an IGF-1 level (a byproduct of growth hormone) to obtain a general idea of how vigorous the patient's growth hormone secretion is. This hormone decreases naturally with age. Dr. Romano uses the following formula in determining appropriate levels of IGF-1: He takes the patient's age, subtracts 30, multiplies that number by 3, and then subtracts that number from 280. Thus, a patient who is 30 would have an ideal IGF-1 level of 280, a 40-year-old, 250.

Intravenous Arginine or Insulin Stimulation Test - If growth hormone deficiency is suspected, this test is useful in ascertaining whether the patient's brain can make growth hormone. Often, patients who have low levels of IGF-1 do not make much growth hormone in response to intravenous secretagogue stimulation and require growth hormone injections. (See Research section for more information on growth hormone.) On the other hand, patients who respond to the intravenous secretagogue (any substance that can cause a gland to secrete or emit a hormone) might be able to take oral secretagogues to raise their levels of growth hormone. Such tests are usually performed by an endocrinologist under very controlled conditions, because the purpose of the test is to lower blood sugar, which is then a stimulus for the patient's pituitary to make growth hormone. If a person has very low blood sugar levels, he or she might become weak and woozy during this type of test and should be monitored carefully.

DHEA Sulfate Level - This test may be useful if a patient complains of a low sexual drive, hair loss, or decreased energy and stamina. As this hormone naturally decreases with age, Dr. Romano suggests that a normal level of this hormone for a patient between ages 30 and 40 would be between 200 and 250. If the level is lower than this, he considers supplementation with DHEA.

Vitamin Profile - Dr. Romano often orders a 12-vitamin profile in patients whose standard laboratory tests are normal. Often, subclinical deficiencies of certain vital nutrients such as B12, folate, thiamin, riboflavin and others can be identified with this test.

Brain SPECT (Single Photon Emission Computerized Tomography) Scan - This test can be ordered to assess problems with brain circulation. This may be particularly important if a person has severe cognitive problems or has suffered injuries in a motor vehicle accident or fall. It can alert the physician if there is an imbalance in brain blood flow. If an imbalance is found, the scan can help the doctor determine which medications could be used to help normalize brain circulation. Beta-blockers and calcium channel blockers can be used.

X-Rays - They show abnormalities in the bones and can aid in determining if arthritis, osteoarthritis, diseases of the bone, fractures, or other bone problems exist.

MRI or CAT Scans - These specialized imaging tests show more detail than X-rays. They can help determine problems in the muscles, bones, soft tissues, or organs, depending on the area being scanned. These are ordered depending on the patient's symptoms and whether the pain is localized. If someone has paralysis or weakness of one limb, then a doctor might suspect a slipped disc in the spine causing the paralysis. See our pioneering treatment section for further information on cervical stenosis (narrowing of the cervical spinal canal) and Arnold-Chiari malformation.

EMG and Nerve Conduction Studies - These can be ordered to measure the function of nerves and muscles. They can help identify certain problems such as carpal tunnel syndrome, neuropathy, radiculopathy, or myopathy. They test for nerve damage as well. These are painful tests for most people.

Other tests physicians may order include

Hormone Levels - If a doctor suspects that you have a problem with your adrenal function or estrogen, progesterone or testosterone levels, he or she may order blood levels to be taken. Some physicians use saliva testing to determine levels.

Tilt Table Test - This test is useful if autonomic dysfunction is suspected, when there is dizziness, lightheadedness or fainting complaints. This test is usually performed by a cardiologist. See our research section for a discussion on this problem.

Viral or Infection Tests - They can be performed to determine if a virus or infection is present. See the research section (immune system) for information on how viruses can be a trigger for FMS.

Sleep Study - A sleep study can be ordered to determine physiological problems with sleep, such as sleep apnea (irregular breathing and periods of breathing cessation during sleep), restless legs syndrome, or periodic limb movement disorder. See the sleep section in our book for more information on sleep problems.

Parasite Testing - These are blood tests for yeast or parasites that may be causing symptoms.

Allergy Testing - These are useful if symptoms of allergy are present, such as bronchial congestion, wheezing, nasal congestion, drainage, respiratory infections or rashes.

Heavy Metal Testing - This may be ordered if symptoms of a heavy metal toxicity are present or if you have a number of mercury fillings in your teeth. See our pioneering section for information on this.

This list may sound like a lot of testing. Your physician may not order all of these tests or may recommend other tests that are specific to your individual symptoms and concerns. If you are worried that your insurance will not pay for these tests, discuss these concerns with your doctor. Some patients will pay out of pocket for the lab tests. It is your body and your health, and you should be able to get the tests that you need to make an effective diagnosis and to rule out perpetuating factors.

Do not forget to tell your physician about all your symptoms! If you leave out some, your physician will be limited in what he or she can do for you.

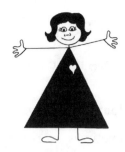

MEDICAL CONDITIONS COMMONLY OCCURRING TOGETHER WITH FIBROMYALGIA

- ▲ Lyme disease
- ▲ Postpolio syndrome
- ▲ HIV infection
- ▲ Rheumatoid arthritis
- ▲ Osteoarthritis
- ▲ Polymyalgia rheumatica
- ▲ Cancer
- ▲ Ankylosing spondylitis
- ▲ Hypothyroidism

- ▲ Endometriosis
- ▲ PMS
- ▲ TMJ dysfunction
- ▲ Cervical and lumbar disc disease
- ▲ Connective tissue diseases
- ▲ Myofascial pain
- ▲ Neurologic disorders
- ▲ Chronic fatigue syndrome
- ▲ Sjogren's syndrome

▲ Raynaud's phenomenon

Many doctors are now diagnosing fibromyalgia more readily, and they may occasionally miss other medical conditions that are frequently present along with fibromyalgia. If you have any of these or any other illness, you'll want it treated, as any illness may make your FMS symptoms worse.

Lyme disease: Following a deer tick bite, a person can develop a bulls-eye rash, fever, fatigue, muscle aches and joint pain. Although there is a blood test for Lyme disease, it is not always conclusive, so a doctor must diagnose it using his or her clinical judgment. Antibiotics are used in its treatment, but will not be effective for fibromyalgia symptoms. Many Lyme patients develop fibromyalgia.

Postpolio syndrome: Muscle weakness rather than pain occurs. A blood test usually shows elevated serum muscle enzyme levels.

HIV Infection: About one-third of HIV patients develop fibromyalgia. A blood test shows if you are HIV-positive.

Rheumatoid arthritis: Generalized stiffness and aching, symptoms usually restricted to joints, not muscles, with swelling, warmth, and tenderness. A blood test is usually positive for rheumatoid factor.

Osteoarthritis: Presents similarly to fibromyalgia; patient will not have tender points. X-rays show degenerative changes of joints.

Polymyalgia rheumatica: A blood test confirms this disease, usually found in people over age 50. Patients respond well to cortisone.

Cancer: Many cancers can cause pain and fatigue, and in certain circumstances, appropriate measures to rule out cancer should be considered. Many cancer patients develop fibromyalgia during the course of their cancer.

Ankylosing spondylitis: X-rays show changes in the spine, and there is limited motion of the spine. There is no cure, but it is treated with NSAIDs.

Hypothyroidism: Can cause symptoms that mimic fibromyalgia. A blood test will confirm the diagnosis.

Endometriosis: Many patients with endometriosis develop fibromyalgia.

PMS: Fibromyalgia symptoms are sometimes worse during the premenstrual phase of the menstrual cycle.

TMJ dysfunction: Many fibromyalgia patients have TMJ dysfunction characterized by locking or clicking of the jaw with associated pain. Your dentist can evaluate this condition and recommend treatment.

Cervical and lumbar disc disease: Can cause pain and is diagnosed by your doctor with a good history, X-rays or MRI.

Connective tissue diseases: These include lupus and Sjogren's syndrome. This is diagnosed with a blood test, although about 10% of healthy women have a low-positive result for this blood test. False positives can also occur in the elderly.

Myofascial pain: Pain of unknown origin usually localized to one area of the body, rather than all over as in fibromyalgia; no fatigue is associated with it.

Neurologic disorders: Multiple sclerosis or Parkinson's Disease can cause neurologic symptoms, such as numbness or tingling, burning and fatigue. Neurologic tests such as an EMG and nerve conduction studies can rule out a neurologic disorder.

Chronic fatigue syndrome (CFIDS): Many doctors think CFIDS and fibromyalgia are the same entity; some think they are different. There seems to be little disagreement that CFIDS and FMS at the very least share many common symptoms, and their treatment is very similar among many physicians. An infectious disease doctor is a specialist who often treats CFIDS.

Sjogren's syndrome: A chronic inflammatory and autoimmune disorder characterized by diminished tears and saliva (dry eyes and mouth).

Raynaud's phenomenon: Characterized by cold hands or feet, with intermittent color changes (red, white, or blue discoloration). Cold temperatures or stress often trigger these neurovascular changes.

If you have any of these conditions, your fibromyalgia symptoms could be exacerbated, so it is important to get the proper diagnoses and treatments.

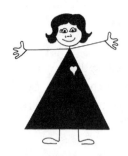

RESEARCH

Putting the Pieces Together

We believe it is important to cover the research aspect of FMS in this handbook and in our seminar, because so many patients have been told their symptoms are all in their heads. Some have also been told that if they would learn to relax and get rid of the stress in their lives, the symptoms of FMS would go away. This has not proven to be the case, and we want you, the FMS patient, to know and be assured that there really is something going on physically in your body.

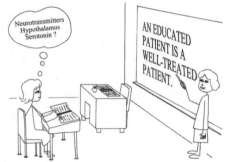

We feel an educated patient is one who will receive quality treatment from his or her medical team and has the best chance of coping effectively with this condition. We have tried to make this information as easy to understand as possible, without leaving out important data. *The Fibromyalgia Network, Fibromyalgia Frontiers, FM Aware,* and others do an excellent job of keeping subscribers informed of new developments in research,

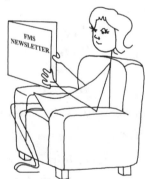

treatments, and medications. Ordering information for these newsletters and other excellent publications is listed in the resource section for your convenience. Other FMS organizations are listed as resources at the end of the book for you to use as well. Please avail yourself of these resources and keep current with advances in research and treatment. You wouldn't want to miss out on any medical discovery which might help you feel better!

Researchers Are Searching for the Key That Will Unlock the FMS Puzzle

Areas of Research

- ▲ Psychological states
- ▲ Central nervous system dysfunction
- ▲ Adrenal-pituitary-hypothalamus axis
- ▲ Neurochemical dysregulation
- ▲ Stress response system
- ▲ Growth hormone deficiency
- ▲ Muscle abnormalities
- ▲ Amino acids
- ▲ Magnesium

- ▲ Abnormal pain processing
- ▲ Wind-up
- ▲ Central sensitization
- ▲ Central sensitization syndromes
- ▲ Autonomic nervous system
- ▲ Limbic system
- ▲ Brain scans
- ▲ Immune system
- ▲ Pain and gender
- ▲ Genetic studies

Abnormalities in Many Systems:
FMS Is a Physical Problem

At this time, no single mechanism has been discovered as the cause of FMS. Researchers have found abnormalities in various systems in the body, but have not been able to tie these together. Much progress has been made in recent years, as more researchers have become interested in FMS and as more funds have become available.

Is This All in Your Head?
Definitely Not!

Many researchers have been searching for a psychological cause for the symptoms of FMS. The studies done in this area are conflicting, as some studies have shown a high incidence of depression in FMS patients, while others show a normal prevalence. Robert Bennett, M.D., is just one of the many physicians who now feel the depression that patients with FMS experience is often due to the pain, fatigue, and stresses of living with an illness that can cause so much disability. The fact that the treatment options are so inadequate can contribute to an anxious, irritable, and depressed patient. It is well known that many chronically ill patients with rheumatoid arthritis, cancer and lupus, develop depression as the result of living with their illness. The FMS patient is no exception. We want you to understand that you are not the cause of your illness, nor are you the cause of your depression. It is very important to have your depression treated if you do become depressed, because it can aggravate your FMS symptoms.

Central Nervous System Dysfunction

Controls

- ▲ Sleep
- ▲ Pain
- ▲ Mood
- ▲ Hunger
- ▲ Memory
- ▲ Emotions
- ▲ Thirst
- ▲ Muscle movement

Central Nervous System Could Be Hyperactive
Sensitive to

- ▲ Bright lights
- ▲ Loud noises
- ▲ Smells
- ▲ Painful stimuli
- ▲ Chemicals
- ▲ Foods
- ▲ Drugs

Robert Bennett, M.D., I. Jon Russell, M.D., and others believe that evidence points to a central nervous system dysfunction in the pathology of FMS. The central nervous system is one of the two main divisions of the nervous system of the body. Through messages sent by chemicals the brain and body manufacture, the central nervous system controls sleep, pain, mood, muscle movement, hunger, and many other functions. It is made up of the brain and spinal cord and is the main network of coordination and control for the entire body. Daniel Clauw, M.D., feels that FMS patients' central nervous systems are hyperactive and overly responsive to stimuli from the environment. This could be why so many patients are sensitive to bright lights, loud noises, noxious smells, drugs, and pain.

Neurotransmitters

Chemical Link between Brain and Rest of the Body

Neurotransmitters are chemicals released from nerve endings which transmit impulses across the gaps between nerve cells. The neurotransmitters function as the chemical link between your brain and the rest of your body. Through messages sent by the neurotransmitters, the central nervous system controls sleep, pain, mood, muscle movement, hunger, and many other important functions. When the levels of these chemicals are abnormal in the body, they can create havoc.

↓ Serotonin ↓

- ▲ **Depression**
- ▲ **Anxiety**
- ▲ **Pain**
- ▲ **Immune system**
- ▲ **Sleep**
- ▲ **Smooth muscle function**

Serotonin, one neurotransmitter, was found in low levels in some FMS patients by I. Jon Russell, M.D. Serotonin helps to control depression, anxiety, pain levels, immune system function, vascular (blood vessel) constriction and dilation, smooth muscle function, sleep, and many other functions. Researchers have found evidence of a problem in the conversion of tryptophan to serotonin. Tryptophan, an amino acid, is needed to produce serotonin.

↑ Substance P ↑

- ▲ **Switched on nerve endings**
- ▲ **! Pain !**

Substance P is another neurotransmitter that was found to be three times higher in FMS patients' spinal fluid by Dr. Russell and also by Dr. Henning Vaeroy. This neurotransmitter is responsible for pain transmission. It is theorized that when serotonin is low and substance P is high, we feel more pain.

When serotonin is low and substance P is high, pain is high.

In the past, many doctors did not believe in the diagnosis of FMS because there was not a blood test available to test for the illness. Although there is still not a blood test targeted specifically for FMS, researchers have found proof that levels of numerous biochemicals are abnormal in patients who are diagnosed with fibromyalgia. This knowledge will lead to better treatment and understanding of the disease in the future. We will explore some of these findings in this section on research.

Adrenal-pituitary-hypothalamus Axis

This is a complex network that interacts closely—seems to be dysregulated.

- ▲ **Hypothalamus**
- ▲ **Pituitary gland**
- ▲ **Adrenals**
- ▲ **Thyroid**
- ▲ **Central nervous system**

The hypothalamus, pituitary, adrenals, thyroid, and central nervous system are part of a complex network in which all work closely together. It seems that many chemicals involved with these systems are low or dysregulated in FMS patients. The hypothalamic-pituitary-adrenal axis (HPA) is the body's major stress response system and can be activated by psychological as well as physical stressors. This system may interfere with the body's pain-filtering system and with how the nervous system responds to stress and painful stimuli.

RESEARCH

The thyroid gland - Some FMS patients develop thyroid disorders such as hypothyroidism, which occurs when the thyroid gland does not produce enough thyroid hormone. When this happens, weight gain, muscle pain, dry or itchy skin, constipation, and cold sensitivity can occur. If you have too much thyroid hormone, you will experience hyperthyroidism with nervousness, rapid heart rate, irritability, weight loss, and difficulty sleeping. There are other problems that can occur with the thyroid as well. Your doctor can help you with these. Patients were found to have a low response to thyrotropin-releasing hormone (TRH), which is released by the hypothalamus and causes the pituitary to secrete thyroid stimulating hormone (TSH). This may cause problems for the FMS patient.

If you would like to consider natural methods to enhance thyroid function, some supplements may be of benefit. L-tyrosine is an amino acid that helps stimulate thyroid production. The recommended dosage is 250-500 mg per day. Iodine is needed for proper thyroid functioning as well. Make sure your daily intake is not too high or too low. Look at your supplements and the foods you eat to keep track of this.

Please refer to the Appendix for physician's information on thyroid supplementation. Thyroid hormone supplementation may not help all of your symptoms, but it may help some symptoms. Each individual responds differently. This may be another piece of the FMS puzzle. Please confer with your physician for appropriate evaluation and treatment.

There is a Dysregulation of Many Neurochemicals in this Network Including

▲ Catecholamines
▲ Norepinephrine
▲ Epinephrine
▲ Dopamine
▲ Nerve growth factor
▲ NMDA Receptors
▲ Neuropeptide Y

▲ Prolactin
▲ Cortisol
▲ DHEA
▲ Corticotropin-releasing hormone
▲ Nitric oxide
▲ Growth hormone

Catecholamines, norepinephrine, epinephrine, and dopamine - Other neurotransmitters, called catecholamines, were found in low concentrations in the spinal fluid by Dr. Russell. These are the substances produced during the metabolism of norepinephrine, epinephrine, and dopamine. These chemicals are needed for various processes in the body, but their main job is to prepare the body to react in times of stress. When the fight or flight stress response is activated, we experience increased blood pressure and faster heart rate and respiration.

Nerve growth factor, a protein necessary for the repair of certain neurons, helps to trigger the release of substance P, which causes an increase in pain. Nerve growth factor was found elevated in FMS patients. Remember that when substance P is high, pain is high. Serotonin blocks the release of nerve growth factor. The antidepressant medication your doctor prescribes for you helps increase serotonin in your body which, in turn, may reduce or block some of these substances that can cause painful sensations. Substance P also stimulates the NMDA receptors, which play an important role in painful sensations. We discuss NMDA receptors in the section on wind-up.

Neuropeptide Y was found in lower amounts in patients with FMS by Dr. Daniel Clauw of the University of Michigan. This is supposed to be the most abundant neuropeptide in the brain. It is a member of a family of proteins that help regulate circadian rhythms (body clock), sexual function, anxiety responses, food intake (obesity), and vascular resistance (constriction of blood vessels). It affects the autonomic nervous system and can cause low blood pressure, fast heart rate and anxiety.

Prolactin, produced by the hypothalamus, has been found in lower amounts in FMS patients. It is thought to play a role in immune function.

Cortisol - In another study, Glenn McCain, M.D., found low cortisol levels in FMS patients. Cortisol is a steroid hormone produced by the adrenal gland in response to stress. Too much stress can cause the adrenals to become fatigued and unable to produce enough cortisol, which can lead to increased susceptibility to infections, fatigue, and anxiety. You can be tested for an adrenal insufficiency, and if one is found, you can be treated with small doses of a prescriptive medication called cortef. Refer to Dr. Teitelbaum's book *From Fatigued to Fantastic* for more information on this subject. You can also look at his protocol in the back of this book for information on which medications and supplements he recommends for low adrenal function. If your adrenal glands are exhausted and not producing enough cortisol, you will feel exhausted, have "brainfog," and become easily overwhelmed. It is important that you and your physician determine if this is a problem for you.

DHEA is also secreted by the adrenal gland and is thought to play a role in immune function, as well as being involved in cellular growth and development. It naturally decreases with the aging process, but has been found to be even lower in some FMS patients. Low levels corresponded with high pain levels. Many physicians are testing for DHEA levels, and when they are low, supplementing with DHEA doses from 5-60 mg. You can purchase DHEA over the counter, without a prescription; however, potency is not guaranteed. It is important to be tested for your DHEA levels before you treat yourself with over-the-counter DHEA, as too much can cause acne, lowered voice, or excess facial hair growth, particularly in women.

The Stress Response System Is in Overload with a Reduced Capacity to Handle Stress

Corticotropin-releasing hormone (CRH), produced by the hypothalamus, stimulates the production of cortisol and has been an area of study for scientists, particularly Leslie Crofford, M.D., of the University of Kentucky. CRH levels are normal in FMS, but the CRH responses to stress are low. Stress responses can be increased by emotional and physical stress, serotonin, and estrogen. Substance P and nitric oxide—the pain-enhancing neurochemicals—can decrease the secretion of CRH. **It is as if the body is in a chronic stress state and cannot turn off the chemicals activated by the stress process.** FMS patients need a turn-off switch! Most patients will describe not being able to respond well to acute stress, and it seems they cannot tolerate the little everyday stressors of daily living as well. Everything is amplified; not only pain, but also the stressors which we all have on a daily basis.

Nitric oxide was found in increased amounts. It dilates blood vessels, is increased when serotonin levels are low, and increases muscle pain by decreasing the amount of ATP (energy) found in muscle cells. This can cause cell death. Substance P and the excitatory amino acids stimulate nitric oxide production. Refer to Dr. Jorge Flechas's protocol in the back of this book for more information on this topic.

Serotonin, norepinephrine, and dopamine stimulate growth hormone, which has been found in low amounts in some FMS patients. Growth hormone is needed for normal muscle metabolism and repair, and 80% of it is secreted by the pituitary gland during deep sleep. Since FMS patients experience disturbed sleep, they are not producing enough growth hormone to aid the body in its repair process. Robert Bennett, M.D. of Oregon, has been studying this problem for many years now, and has found that when patients are properly tested for growth hormone deficiencies and have growth hormone supplemented, some symptoms of FMS diminish, although pain levels are not reduced.

Growth Hormone Deficiency

Symptoms of a growth hormone deficiency are

▲ Low energy levels
▲ Feeling of poor overall health
▲ Reduced exercise capacity
▲ Muscle weakness

▲ Cold intolerance
▲ Impaired memory and concentration
▲ Depressed mood
▲ Decreased muscle mass

Growth hormone is available as an injection.
Drugs may be developed to improve growth hormone production.

Dr. Bennett and other physicians use specialized tests to test for deficiencies in growth hormone. Growth hormone can only be increased by injections, and the therapy is very expensive: $500-$1000 per month. Your insurance may pick up the cost of treatment if an endocrinologist performs the diagnostic test. It may take up to six months to respond to treatment. Although growth hormone therapy may not alleviate your pain, it could improve your exercise capacity, and your overall sense of well-being, as well as improving your energy levels.

Studies have shown that when FMS patients exercise they do not manufacture as much growth hormone as normal controls do. In fact, healthy people produce eight times more growth hormone than FMS patients while exercising. This may be one of the reasons some FMS patients feel so bad after exercising and experience muscle soreness for days rather than the 24-48 hour postexertional soreness experienced by healthy people. It may be due to a lack of growth hormone.

Dr. Robert Bennett has been testing the drug mestinon (pyridostigmine), which blocks the release of somatostatin. Somatostatin, produced by the hypothalamus, is found in high levels in FMS patients. It blocks the release of growth hormone, which we know is low in FMS.

Bennett and his staff gave FMS patients 30 mg of Mestinon one hour prior to exercising and found that after the patients completed their workout, they showed an eight-fold increase in growth hormone production! This medication had no effect on healthy controls. Russell and his staff believe the increase in growth hormone may be due to Mestinon's blocking effect on the release of somatostatin, which inhibits growth hormone. Mestinon may be a promising treatment for patients, but more study needs to be done to find the proper dose and appropriate time to take the drug. Mestinon is an inexpensive and rather benign medication currently used to treat myasthenia gravis. See Jacob Teitelbaum's protocol in the Appendix for information on taking this medication.

There are natural supplements that are heavily marketed in the media proclaiming to be the precursors to growth hormone. Manufacturers of these supplements say they will help increase growth hormone naturally. There have been no studies done on FMS patients to determine if these supplements work to increase growth hormone. You might wish to speak to your physician before you take any of these supplements.

Muscle Abnormalities

Is There Something Wrong with FMS Patients' Muscles?

- ▲ No inflammation
- ▲ Uneven distribution of oxygen
- ▲ Low levels of ATP, ADP, and phosphocreatine
- ▲ Low aerobic capability
- ▲ Erratic breathing pattern
- ▲ Low exercising blood flow
- ▲ Reduced grip strength
- ▲ Heightened response to muscle microtrauma
- ▲ Low levels of a substance which helps repair muscle tissue
- ▲ Phosphodiester peaks—normally appears in elderly

For many years, researchers thought the problem of FMS was in the muscles themselves. This would make sense, because that is where FMS sufferers feel their pain. Yet studies done on the muscles have not proven that the pain is coming from the muscles. For one thing, researchers have not found evidence of any inflammation in the muscles, but they have found other abnormalities. Biopsies of FMS patients' muscles studied by Bengtsson have shown low levels of ATP, ADP, and phosphocreatine. These are substances our bodies use for energy, and they come from the breakdown of food. Lund found the distribution of oxygen in our muscles to be uneven, Sharon Clark's group noted a low exercising blood flow. FMS sufferers will tell you they don't have much of an aerobic capacity while exercising, and this was found to be true when Bennett tested FMS patients' aerobic capacity. An erratic breathing pattern was found by Goldstein in one-fourth of FMS patients studied and may account for the shortness of breath some FMS sufferers experience.

Researchers have found a reduced grip strength in FMS patients, which is a reflection of the weakness many FMS patients report. Researchers do not feel the weakness is coming from the muscles themselves, but it could be coming from a dysfunction in the central nervous system. Kristin Thorson has stated in the *Fibromyalgia Network* that some researchers believe we have a heightened response to muscle microtrauma which normally occurs after unaccustomed exercise and causes pain and tenderness 24 to 48 hours after exercising.* Another study by Jacobsen found low levels of the chemical procollagen-type III aminoterminal peptide in the serum of FMS patients, which could suggest a decrease in the rate of muscle tissue repair. Researcher Robert Bennett, M.D., has found phosphodiester peaks in 100% of FMS patients' muscles, which is a phenomenon that usually occurs only in elderly patients.

Researchers are suggesting that the abnormalities of muscles in FMS patients are a result of having FMS, and not the cause of FMS.

This may be due to low levels of growth hormone or low DHEA levels.

Amino Acids

- ▲ They are the building blocks of protein.
- ▲ They are used in important processes in the body.
- ▲ They must be present in balanced amounts.
- ▲ Researchers found low levels of seven in FMS patients.
- ▲ Tryptophan is needed for serotonin production.

Amino acids are the building blocks of protein. We get them from the breakdown of food, and they are used in various important processes in our bodies. These compounds must be present in balanced amounts in our bodies, and if they are not, many malfunctions can occur. I. Jon Russell, M.D., found low levels of tryptophan, as well as six other amino acids, in the serum of FMS patients. Tryptophan is needed to produce serotonin, which we already know is low in FMS patients. In a study by Harvey Moldofsky, M.D., a sleep researcher, when tryptophan was given to FMS patients to see if it would help improve their symptoms, it helped them sleep better, but made their pain worse. Tryptophan is no longer available over the counter in the United States because of a contaminated batch that is believed to have caused many people to develop a serious condition called Eosinophilia Myalgia Syndrome. Dr. Russell has presented some studies that show that the conversion of tryptophan to serotonin might be dysregulated and could be the cause of some of our symptoms. Mohammed Yunus, M.D., found low levels of five amino acids in his study: histidine, methionine, tryptophan, leucine, and isoleucine. Supplementing with these amino acids has not yet been researched.

Magnesium

- ▲ **It is necessary for energy-producing activities in the cells.**
- ▲ **It helps the smooth muscles of the body relax.**
- ▲ **It increases blood circulation.**
- ▲ **FMS patients need a red blood cell magnesium test.**
- ▲ **Discuss supplementation with your doctor.**
- ▲ **Watch out for side effects.**

Magnesium is necessary for all energy-producing activities in cells. It helps the smooth muscles of the body relax and also increases blood circulation. A regular magnesium blood test will usually not show a deficiency in FMS patients' cells, but a red blood cell magnesium test will confirm if their level is low. Red blood cell magnesium levels were tested by Thomas Romano, M.D. He found low levels in some FMS patients and then supplemented these patients with oral magnesium–800 to 1200 mg a day or magnesium intramuscular injections. (The patient's dosage was based on his or her specific deficiency.) Some improvement was noted by patients, although it sometimes took weeks or months to feel a difference. The newer forms of magnesium, magnesium glycinate, magnesium aspartate, and magnesium chloride, seem to be better tolerated and better absorbed. Magnesium may be difficult to absorb orally and may take from two months to one year to increase levels. It is believed that injectables or intravenous magnesium will work faster. Magnesium in high doses can cause diarrhea, so it is important to discuss supplementing magnesium with your doctor. Another supplement to try is one that contains a combination of magnesium and malic acid. Some health food stores carry a supplement like this, or you can order it. One of these supplements is called fibro-care and can be ordered from To Your Health, a resource listed in the back of this book. A 1200-mg dose of malic acid has been suggested for daily use. If you would like more information on nutritional aspects of FMS, please refer to the chapter "Diet and Nutritional Supplements."

Symptoms of a magnesium deficiency are

- ▲ Cognitive deficiencies
- ▲ Fatigue
- ▲ Muscle pain
- ▲ Depression
- ▲ Weakness
- ▲ Insomnia
- ▲ Muscle cramps

Fibromyalgia - The Result of Abnormal Pain Processing by the Body?

▲ **Genetic factors may increase the likelihood of getting FMS**
▲ **Multiple causes can contribute to FMS symptoms**
▲ **Pain processing involves many body systems and chemicals**

"Wind-up" and "central sensitization" cause increased pain in FMS.
Medications and behavioral therapies may help reduce their effects on pain.

Researchers believe that many fibromyalgia symptoms are caused or worsened by abnormalities in how the body processes pain. While the central nervous system is the primary entity in pain processing and perception, a number of other body systems play a role in worsening the pain of FMS.

Research indicates that the primary problem causing fibromyalgia pain is that the pain processing centers in the central nervous system are hypersensitive—as if someone turned their amplifiers way up. This may be in part due to a genetic tendency, and it may be partly due to the fact that women tend to be more sensitive to chronic pain than men (85% of FMS patients are women). A number of factors may contribute to the increased pain processing, including:

▲ **Chemicals (cytokines) released by the immune system in response to chronic infection by bacteria, fungi, or viruses**
▲ **Psychological or physical stress (illness, surgery, injury, etc.)**
▲ **Sleep deprivation (in particular, a lack of deep non-dreaming sleep)**
▲ **Neck injuries**
▲ **Hormonal imbalances**
▲ **Toxin exposure**

A large number of chemicals affecting pain nerves have been identified. Some increase the response to pain, some decrease it, and some increase it in certain nerves while decreasing it in others. The large number of chemicals and their complex activity is a major reason why researchers have had to work so hard at understanding how the system works! Some of these chemicals are:

Nerve growth factor	Neurokinins
Substance P	N-methyl-D-aspartic acid (NMDA)
Serotonin	Glutamate
Dopamine	Aspartate (in the sweetener aspartame)
Norepinephrine	Nitric oxide
Epinephrine	Gamma-aminobutyric acid (GABA)
Neuropeptide Y	Acetylcholine
and others still being discovered…	

Wind-Up

▲ **If pain is intense or long-lasting, the nervous system "learns" to be in pain.**
▲ **Pain processing cells change how they behave and even make physical changes to increase pain perception.**
▲ **This results in many more pain signals being sent to the brain.**
▲ **Everything hurts!**

When a pain nerve (or neuron) is stimulated, pain passes from the body up the nerve to the spinal cord, where it is processed. Signals are then sent up the spinal cord to the brain, where they are felt. In a normal person a stimulation of the pain nerve causes a brief burst of signals from the spinal processing center up to the brain. After less than a second, the discharges stop. If a few seconds later another signal arrives, another brief burst gets sent to the brain. Each time, the center becomes quiet between signals. Each input from the peripheral nerve causes the same brief effect.

In a FMS patient, however, the processing center's discharges take much longer—say, 10 seconds—to stop. If another signal comes from the nerve, it adds to the stimulation of the processing center and even more signals get sent to the brain. As signals continue to arrive every few seconds, the processing center sends more and more signals—it never has a chance to become quiet between them. Eventually, the increasing stimulation of the processing center causes it to send a huge number of signals up to the brain, which perceives it as severe pain. This process where each incoming signal from the pain nerve results in more and more signals being sent by the processing center to the brain is called "wind-up." Microelectrode studies have shown that this amplified pain response is present in fibromyalgia patients.

Pain signals are sent from the spinal cord to an area at the base of the brain called the thalamus. Here they are processed further and then distributed out to a number of other brain areas, including:

- ▲ **Memory areas (prefrontal cortex)**
- ▲ **The body's regulatory center (hypothalamus)**
- ▲ **The area where we experience pain (somatosensory cortex)**
- ▲ **The center of emotions (limbic system)**

Brain scans have shown that all these areas are affected by FMS, resulting in both physiologic and psychologic changes. If we get caught up in fear, negativity, and hopelessness, the pain centers become even more sensitive. If, on the other hand, we make a conscious effort to reduce negative feelings or thoughts, we can decrease pain's effect on these centers. This shows how keeping healthy positive attitudes and managing our stress can reduce the effects of fibromyalgia on the brain and ultimately reduce pain.

Central Sensitization

As the central nervous system continues to be stimulated by pain sensations, a variety of changes occur. (This ability of the CNS to change is referred to as "neuroplasticity.") The pain-processing cells undergo internal changes that make them much more responsive to pain stimuli. Actual physical changes occur, with increased connections between pain cells causing them to have a much greater impact on each other. The cells surrounding and supporting the pain cells (called "glial cells") swell up and start releasing chemicals that further irritate the pain-processing cells. And the cells that are supposed to inhibit the pain cells wither up and sometimes even die. All of these changes cause the central nervous system to become more and more hypersensitive to pain. Sensations that would normally hurt (nociceptive stimuli) feel much worse and sensations that would normally feel good (nonnociceptive stimuli) feel painful instead. Painful stimuli can be heat, chemicals, electrical sources, pressure or an injury. Nonpainful stimuli include light touch, massage or emotional stress. When painful stimuli become much more painful than expected, they are referred to as being in a state of hyperalgesia. Allodynia describes what occurs when normally pleasant sensations become painful. These changes can spread to adjacent areas of the central nervous system, causing all the pain to be felt in areas around the original pain site, and eventually they may spread throughout the entire nervous system, causing pain all over the body. Pain may also last longer after the painful stimulus is removed. This exaggerated response of the central nervous system is called central sensitization. Many FMS patients have had this experience first hand.

Pain Response System

1. Pain is generated in the periphery (muscles, joints, and skin).

2. Pain signals are sent via peripheral neurons to the dorsal horn of the spinal cord where they are processed.

3. NMDA receptor activation dramatically increases the number of pain signals sent upward.

4. The signal travels to the thalamus after making connections in the brain stem.

5. The thalamus acts as a relay center, sending information/pain signals to many areas of the brain, including the prefrontal cortex (memory areas), hypothalamus (regulates hormonal or endocrine system), the somatosensory cortex (where we experience painful stimuli) and the limbic system, affecting emotions, fear, despair and vigilance.

6. After the thalamus has relayed signals to various areas of the brain, signals can travel from the brain back to the spinal cord to inhibit pain processing.

7. In FMS, this inhibitory system (DNIC-diffuse noxious inhibitory control) is not as effective as it should be at filtering or inhibiting the pain signals going to the brain.

8. The result is even more pain signals being sent up to the brain.

> ▲ **Researchers are finding medications to interfere in this process and decrease pain**
> ▲ **Some antidepressants improve the ability to calm down pain processing**
> ▲ **Anti-seizure medicines and some muscle relaxants make nerves less irritable**
> ▲ **Keeping healthy attitudes and stress levels can also reduce pain**

Virtually all medications that are used to help fibromyalgia patients were actually developed to treat other conditions. Norepinephrine is a chemical that allows nerves to communicate with each other (neurotransmitter) which acts to reduce the activity of the nerves processing pain in the spinal cord. Antidepressants that increase norepinephrine—particularly Cymbalta, Effexor, and tricyclics—can cause these centers to reduce the number of pain signals they send up the spinal cord to the brain.

Some anticonvulsants (Neurontin, Topamax, Gabatril), muscle relaxants (Zanaflex, Baclofen), and the cough medicine dextramethorphan can block receptors in the pain nerve membrane that are stimulated by pain-causing chemicals. This helps calm the nerves down and reduce their activity. (Unfortunately, since they tend to calm down nerves, many of them also can cause drowsiness. This isn't all bad, however; if you take them at night, they can help with sleep.) Many clinicians are experimenting with using low doses of several of these medicines together to try to get more benefit with fewer side effects. How the medicines work in a given person can vary widely, so the particular mix must be worked out for each individual patient.

Stress causes the release of chemicals that excite the pain processing centers and therefore increases pain. Normal people living modern lifestyles lead highly stressful lives, so getting a chronic, debilitating disease can send stress levels skyrocketing! Research has proven that a number of techniques can be very helpful in reducing stress, including progressive relaxation, meditation, the release of pent-up feelings, lifestyle management, and others. Most fibromyalgia patients will benefit from training in one or more of these techniques.

The benefit of keeping healthy attitudes has been proven in many studies. Giving in to a feeling of victimization, helplessness, and despair is a key step in changing the frustration of living with fibromyalgia into full-blown depression, and depression significantly worsens fibromyalgia. The field of counseling that works primarily with attitudes is called cognitive therapy, and many studies have shown that FMS patients who engage in cognitive therapy improve their overall symptom levels and quality of life.

Central Sensitization Syndromes

Dr. Mohammed Yunus is a prominent FMS researcher who has theorized that fibromyalgia is one of a number of illnesses that appear to share this presence of hypersensitive pain processing nerves. Since these nerves are located in the brain and spinal cord (the "central nervous system"), he calls the condition "central sensitization."

Other illnesses appearing to share this problem include:

▲ **Migraines**	▲ **Temporomandibular joint syndrome**
▲ **Irritable bowel syndrome**	▲ **Chronic fatigue syndrome**
▲ **Primary dysmenorrhea (painful periods)**	▲ **Tension headache**
▲ **Periodic limb movement disorder**	▲ **Irritable bladder (interstitial cystitis)**
▲ **Restless legs syndrome**	▲ **Myofascial pain syndrome**

(Multiple chemical sensitivity and Gulf War Syndrome may some day be added to this list.)

Since these conditions appear to share a common underlying cause, they may respond to many of the same medications used to treat fibromyalgia. Why central sensitization may be associated with FMS in one person and migraines in another remains uncertain but may be due to genetic, physiologic, or environmental differences between the two people.

Another important factor in central sensitization is that it's not limited to touch or pain sensations coming from the body. Every sense can become hypersensitive. An odor that a non-sensitized person perceives as mildly unpleasant may be nauseating to a sensitized person. Somewhat loud noises become painfully loud, mildly bright lights may become blindingly bright, and mildly poor-tasting foods become disgusting. Even the sense of balance can become hypersensitive, resulting in a tendency to develop motion sickness. It's very likely that the princess in *The Princess and the Pea* had central sensitization! *It is very important to understand that these experiences of the person with central sensitization are not due to weakness or a desire to wallow in self-pity. They are the result of changes in the central nervous system. People suffering from these problems deserve compassion and understanding, not suspicion and criticism!*

Michael McNett, M.D. is the author of the sections on abnormal pain processing through central sensitization syndromes, pp. 33-36.

The Autonomic Nervous System (ANS)

Researchers have found ANS dysfunctions in FMS and CFIDS patients

▲ **Sympathetic nervous system produces "fight or flight" response**
▲ **Parasympathetic system helps the body calm, digest, rebuild**

The ANS is made up of two opposing systems, the parasympathetic and the sympathetic nervous system, that are constantly in a dynamic balance. The ANS regulates muscles in the skin, around the blood vessels, the eyes, stomach, intestines, bladder and heart. It also regulates actions of the glands, as well as digestion, breathing, metabolism, blood pressure, heart rate, bowel and bladder tone. While the ANS tends to run without our conscious knowledge (who wants to think about whether their heart is beating or not?), meditation, relaxation techniques and biofeedback can help us control it to some degree.

The Sympathetic Nervous System

The sympathetic system was very helpful back when we lived in caves. When we were in danger (say, a saber-toothed tiger was outside the cave), we needed to prepare our body for physical activity, either to fight it or to run away. This is called the "fight or flight" syndrome. The sympathetic system does this by increasing our heart rate and blood pressure, increasing our rate of breathing, and diverting our blood flow from the internal organs and skin to our muscles. It reduces the activity of the bowels and bladder and increases metabolism. Finally, it acts on the brain to make us intensely aware of threat and dramatically increases our response speed. (A good example of this is the way people tend to impulsively say things in the heat of an argument that they later regret.)

The Parasympathetic Nervous System

When we don't need to be active, the parasympathetic system kicks in. It sends blood back to the digestive tissues and skin (helping it to heal from any cuts or infections), lowers the heart rate and blood pressure, and calms the mind. It reverses changes produced by the sympathetic nervous system during non stressful times, so we can "rest and digest."

Researchers theorize that a FMS patient's sympathetic nervous system is hyperactive and the parasympathetic system is underactive. The sympathetic nervous system is particularly overactive at night, which may interfere with sleep. A technique using a noninvasive heart monitor was used to determine the activity of these systems by measuring heart rate variability. Patients with FMS were shown to have three times the intensity of sympathetic nervous system activity at night compared to controls. This could mean that the sympathetic nervous system is overworked, exhausted, and not responding properly to normal stimuli. Fibromyalgia patients exhibit the results of this by feeling overworked and exhausted. They have a difficult time handling the everyday stressors of life!

Some FMS patients may have problems with the autonomic nervous system that can be diagnosed by specialized laboratory tests.

Autonomic Nervous System Dysfunction (Dysautonomia)
- ▲ **It is diagnosed by a tilt table test.**
- ▲ **Its symptoms are dizziness, lightheadedness or fainting upon standing.**
- ▲ **It is treated with medication or an increase in salt and water.**

If you experience dizziness on standing or fainting spells, you may have one of the autonomic nervous system dysfunctions such as neurally mediated hypotension or postural orthostatic hypotension. Patients with these conditions often have low blood pressure which fails to rise adequately when going from sitting or lying down to standing up. Standing for prolonged periods of time will also produce symptoms.

It is not necessary to have low blood pressure for this condition to exist. Cardiologists perform the test for dysautonomia in the laboratory, using a tilt table test. During the test, patients lie on a table which is tilted upward (with head upright), while blood pressure and heart rate are monitored. This test can determine if the autonomic system is working properly. If your system is not working properly, your heart will not pump enough blood to your brain, and you may feel dizzy, nauseous, foggy, or tired. Many patients with FMS and CFIDS have this condition.

This author had experienced dizziness when going from sitting to standing most of her life and thought that was normal! It is not normal and can be treated somewhat effectively with a variety of medications including Florinef, atenolol, ProAmatine, certain anti-depressants, and others that increase blood pressure. Increasing salt intake and water consumption may help improve symptoms. If you have a history of hypertension, your doctor may not want you to increase salt. Speak to your physician before making any changes in your diet. Mild exercise and relaxation sessions or biofeedback can also help this condition.

Although treating this condition may not take away all of your FMS symptoms, it may help some of them. This is another area of fairly new research, so researchers hope that new medications without significant side effects will be developed in the future. Patients who have the most severe autonomic nervous system dysfunction may be unable to stand up and are required to be in a wheel chair all of the time. In severe cases of dysautonomia, death can occur. This condition is not restricted to mature individuals, but occurs in young children and teenagers as well.

There is a national association which offers information on dysautonomia. It is listed in the resource section in the back of this book. They have a Web site, www.familialdysautonomia.org, with links to other information about this condition. If you experience any of these symptoms, tell your primary physician, who can refer you to the proper center for testing. Many hospitals perform the tilt table test. Dysautonomia is a real medical condition, and treatment should be covered by insurance.

Limbic System

Limbic System Dysregulation

Jay Goldstein, M.D.

HYPOTHALAMUS
AMYGDALA
HIPPOCAMPUS

Controls:

- ▲ Body temperature
- ▲ Metabolic rate
- ▲ Memory
- ▲ Fatigue
- ▲ Appetite

- ▲ Immune system
- ▲ Pain
- ▲ Sleep
- ▲ Concept formation
- ▲ Autonomic nervous system

Triggering Events:

- ▲ Physical trauma
- ▲ Virus
- ▲ Emotional stress

- ▲ Toxins
- ▲ Infection
- ▲ Childbirth

Treatments:

- ▲ Antiviral medications
- ▲ Neurological medications
- ▲ Immune system enhancers

- ▲ Cognitive behavioral therapy
- ▲ Stress management

Jay Goldstein, M.D. has been involved in research on both chronic fatigue syndrome and FMS, and he believes the two syndromes overlap. He believes a limbic system dysregulation could be the cause of FMS. The limbic system is a portion of our brain that includes the amygdala, hippocampus, and hypothalamus. It controls body temperature, metabolic rate, memory, learning, fatigue, appetite, autonomic nervous system, sex drive, endocrine system, immune system, pain, sleep, concept formation, blood formation, and other functions. He believed people are predisposed to developing FMS or chronic fatigue, and a triggering event such as a virus, infection, surgery, toxin, childbirth, or severe emotional stress could set off a series of events in the limbic system that could lead to FMS or chronic fatigue. If his theory is correct, it may explain the variety of symptoms found in FMS patients, because different structures could be affected in different people—producing one symptom such as depression in one person and severe allergies in another, yet both would have pain. On a positive note, he believes symptoms can be treated with antiviral medications, neurological medications, and immune system enhancers, depending on each person's symptoms. Since our mental attitudes affect limbic structures, he also believes FMS and chronic fatigue can be treated with cognitive behavioral therapy and stress management techniques. His book is listed in the resource section at the back of this book. Dr. Goldstein, who retired from practice recently, is credited for making observations that are now being validated by research.

Brain Scans

- ▲ **BEAM, SPECT, and PET scans**
- ▲ **Expensive tests**
- ▲ **Marked reduction in blood flow**

Doctors are using sophisticated, expensive brain scans like the SPECT scan to target areas of brain dysfunction in FMS patients.* Jay Goldstein, M.D., found a marked reduction in blood flow to the right hemisphere of the brain. Another researcher, James Mountz, M.D., found a decreased blood flow to the caudate nuclei, which has connections to the brain's limbic system and may be involved in memory and concentration problems and pain regulation. The higher the pain score, the more the blood flow was reduced. Patients with chronic headaches were tested by Thomas Romano, M.D., who found differences in the blood flow between the right and left hemispheres. It may be that the cause of FMS is indeed in our heads! If you are experiencing severe cognitive deficits, your doctor might order one of these scans for you. There are some medications designed to ameliorate cognitive problems; you and your doctor can determine if these would be helpful for you to try.

When we feel pain, certain portions of the brain are activated. By comparing FMS patient responses with healthy controls or other pain patients, scientists can detect changes that occur which may ultimately aid in understanding the illness.

- ▲ **Patients with FMS were compared to healthy controls, depressed patients, and pain patients.**
- ▲ **FMS patients responded differently to pain stimuli.**
- ▲ **Studies show FMS is not related to depression.**

Another study, using functional MRI after a painful stimulus, showed increased activity in the somatosensory area of the brain. This area of the brain processes painful stimuli. Researchers believe this study shows how our beliefs about our ability to control pain may influence pain levels.

Depressed patients, FMS patients, and CFIDS patients were compared in another study that looked at brain blood flow when a painful stimulus was applied. FMS patients displayed significant increases in bilateral regional cerebral blood flow in the somatosensory cortex and the anterior angulate cortex. Healthy controls and depressed patients without FMS showed increases in blood flow into the contralateral thalamus, somatosensory cortex, and anterior angulate cortex. Patients with CFIDS only did not show bilateral blood flow responses as the FMS patients did. This seems to indicate that FMS may not be related to depression and that CFIDS-only patients react differently than FMS-only patients. **This does not mean you should not be treated for depression if you have depressive symptoms! You could be experiencing depression as well as FMS.**

Other studies have looked at how FMS patients and other chronic pain patients process pain in their brains and have discovered similar areas stimulated from a painful touch.

In normal patients, when a painful stimulus is applied to one side of the body, the brain regions on the opposite side of the body usually show activity. FMS patients and CFIDS patients show activation in both sides of the brain (bilateral), which is an abnormal response when compared to healthy controls. This further supports the theory of a central pain processing problem.

Other researchers found a reduced blood flow to the brain stem section known as the pontine tegmentum, which had not been previously noted. They also corroborated the finding of earlier researchers who found a reduced flow to the thalamus. The reduced flow to the brain stem was an important finding, as this is the area that channels brain functions for the entire body. It had not been associated with the pain processing centers prior to this research.

Immune System

- ▲ **Low natural killer cell activity**
- ▲ **Abnormal secretion of interleukin-2**
- ▲ **Low secretion of interleukin-1**
- ▲ **High incidence of immune reactive protein in the skin**

The immune system may be compromised in FMS sufferers. Normally, natural killer cells seek out and destroy foreign invaders in our bodies. When FMS patients' natural killer cells were tested by I. Jon Russell, M.D., they were found to be in normal amounts, but their activity was low. Researchers do not know why this is so, but serotonin may influence the activity of natural killer cells. Wallace has also found an abnormal secretion of interleukin 2, a cytokine (chemical) produced by the immune system that fends off infectious agents. When these cytokines are produced by the immune system, they can produce symptoms of pain and fatigue. Dr. Russell found a decreased production of interleukin-1 at the hypothalamic level of control. This chemical increases the secretion of growth hormone, corticotropin-releasing hormone (adrenals), serotonin, norepinephrine and epinephrine, and the beta-endorphins. Beta-endorphins have pain-relieving properties. A high incidence of immune-reactive proteins has been found in the skin of FMS patients. These are not normally seen in a healthy person's skin. In other words, proteins are leaking through the blood vessel walls and accumulating in surrounding tissues, which often occurs in conditions that have an immunologic component.

Sleep Disorders and Stress

- ▲ **They affect the immune system adversely.**

Some researchers believe an alteration in sleep can contribute to a problem with the immune system, or a disorder with the immune system could be causing a problem with the sleep cycle. The sleep cycle irregularities are covered in the section on sleep.

Immune Connection in Pain Processing

- ▲ **Immune system is in overdrive.**

- ▲ **Astroglial cells produce cytokines, which cause pain, fatigue, and cognitive dysfunction.**

- ▲ **May be due to viruses, bacteria, parasites, inflammation, toxic exposure, or physical trauma.**

Immune Dysfunction

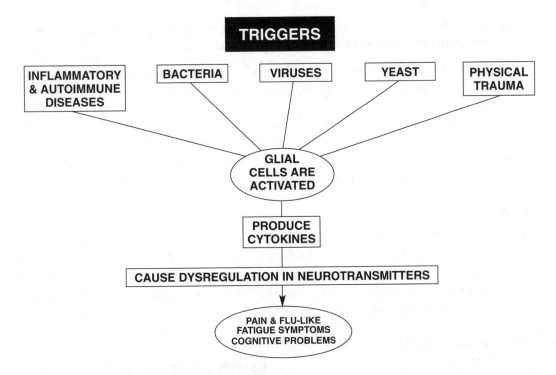

Recently, researchers have been looking at the immune system and how it may play a role in the development of FMS. They theorize that chronic immune activation may be one of the causes of FMS pain, fatigue, and cognitive problems. Researchers report that when immune system processes are activated, they can affect the peripheral nerves, portions of the spinal cord and brain, causing an increase in pain. Many people have a friend or relative who has experienced the painful condition known as shingles, which is a herpes virus that attacks nerves and causes horrendous pain!

It was not until the 1980's that scientists began looking at astroglial cells, which comprise 50% of the brain's cells and surround every neuron in the body. When they detect foreign invaders, they release proinflammatory cytokines, which can cause pain, fatigue, cognitive problems, sleep disorders, and a host of other symptoms, including anxiety and stress-related reactions. They can release a number of chemicals such as nerve growth factor, excitatory amino acids, nitric oxide, and substance P. This process may also affect hormone regulation. One of these chemicals, nitric oxide, can damage cell membranes, interrupt energy production, and reduce the ability of blood platelets to store serotonin. (Read more about nitric oxide in Dr. Jorge Flechas's protocol in the back of this book). The glial cells can be activated not only by infections or viruses, but also by inflammation caused by a physical trauma such as a whiplash, surgery, or sensory overload as in a toxic exposure. It appears the system becomes more compromised the longer it is left untreated.

Some of the cytokines produced by the glial cells are increased to twice that of normal people.

- ▲ Il-8 — produces pain through the body's sympathetic nervous system

- ▲ Il-6 — can increase pain and fatigue, alter mood, affect stress response, and cause brain fog

- ▲ Il-1 beta — can increase fatigue and muscle aches; blocks substance P

▲ **IL-IRA — blocks the action of IL-I (which causes pain) and aids in the body's stress reactions, as well as helping eliminate the production of IL-8**

▲ **Il-2 (TNF Alpha) — causes muscle aches, cognitive problems, fatigue, fever, brain fog, depression, and inflammation**

Because the glial cells surround every neuron it is easy to understand how the pain can spread throughout the body and produce so many symptoms, including feeling as if you have the flu.

It is interesting to note that the glial cells which researchers are describing are not well understood. More research needs to be performed to unlock their modes of action; scientists theorize that if you can block glial activation, you may be able to block some of the pain it produces. Some medications are currently being developed which may work for this purpose.

Infectious Agents

Since CFIDS is known to overlap with FMS symptoms, some of the research directed towards this illness has benefited FMS patients as well. Many patients feel as if they have the flu all the time. Although some studies have shown no evidence of a viral infection in the blood of CFIDS and FMS patients, others have found evidence in the central nervous system by analyzing the cerebrospinal fluid of patients with CFIDS and FMS.

Some of the infectious agents researchers found were

▲ **HHV-6**
▲ **HHV-8**
▲ **Chlamydia**
▲ **Mycoplasma**
▲ **Cytomegalovirus (CMV)**
▲ **Epstein-Barr virus (EBV)**
▲ **Coxsackie virus**

You may ask your physician to test you for different infections if your symptoms warrant testing. Treatment should be tailored to the results of the tests.

Although the Center for Disease Control has concluded that these viruses do not cause CFIDS, it is performing studies to search for undiscovered viruses in these patients. Many physicians providing a holistic approach for the treatment of these conditions are testing for viral, bacterial, and parasitic infections. They may use prescription drugs as well as nutritional and novel therapies to ameliorate these infections. Sometimes these treatments reduce symptoms. This author has had significant improvement in symptoms when treated with antibiotics, antivirals, and nutritional supplements for intestinal parasites, yeast infections, and EBV. The research being carried out on Gulf War Syndrome, which has some symptoms similar to FMS, may benefit all of us.

Another immune system modulator, the enzyme Rnasel, was found to be significantly increased in 72% of CFIDS patients when compared to normals. This enzyme interferes with protein synthesis and "gobbles up" ATP which is needed for energy production in cells. The greater the level of this enzyme, the more severe the symptoms. Because researchers believe CFIDS and FMS are overlapping conditions, this research may have some relationship to FMS patients who complain of severe fatigue and not just pain.

How does this information help you, the FMS or CFIDS patient? Most important, you can be tested for viruses or bacteria which may be affecting you. Your physician can test you for GI and urinary tract infections or many of the viruses thought to play a role in the activation of these cytokines. Chronic sinusitis and vaginitus should also be treated, as well as intestinal parasites. Autoimmune diseases like rheumatoid arthritis or lupus should be aggressively treated, as well as Lyme disease.

RESEARCH

Please refer to the "Pioneering Treatments" and "Diet and Nutritional Supplements" chapters to find out more about these treatments.

Pain Research and Gender

Women

▲ Process pain differently than men.
▲ Have lower pain thresholds.
▲ Have lower pain tolerances.
▲ Have less response to pain medications.
▲ Have a less effective DNIC system.

Men

▲ Have 7 times more serotonin.

Hormones may play a role.

Since nine out of ten people with FMS are women, it does not take a leap of faith to presume that there is a difference in the way women experience pain. Women also know how hormones can affect us and the men around us! Some researchers believe there are more men with FMS than we know about, because men do not go to doctors as often as women. Men may have a "grin-and-bear-it" reaction or may be using alcohol to dampen their pain. Please encourage any male you know with chronic widespread pain to see a physician, so he can receive proper treatment.

Pain researchers have been investigating how gender differences affect pain. They compare how men and women process painful stimuli. Researchers have found that women have lower pain thresholds and lower pain tolerance than men. Could hormones be creating pain for women? Estrogen and progesterone can influence serotonin production, and testosterone has been found in low levels in female FMS patients. Some recent animal studies have shown that testosterone may play a role in pain modulation. More physicians are prescribing low-dose testosterone for women in menopause or perimenopause, as it seems to improve energy levels, sense of well-being, sexual desire, and functioning. Many FMS patients complain of a flare-up of their symptoms premenstrually. Taking care of PMS symptoms may improve your overall sense of well-being. Speak to a knowledgeable physician if you experience premenstrual flare-ups.

There are many differences between men and women in how they process pain.

Studies show that women are more susceptible to prolonged painful stimulus than men, and women also experience pain sooner than men. Studies have also shown that there is not a discernable difference between the incidence of pain reported in female and male children prior to puberty (age 13 or thereabouts). The difference may be in hormonally related changes.

In studies, men showed a greater response to opioid system activation in a number of brain regions involved with pain control, whereas women responded with a reduction in opioid action. Endorphins, part of the body's opioid system, are natural pain relievers and as effective as morphine in controlling or reducing pain.

Researchers have also found that the DNIC (pain-filtering) system inhibits pain sensations in the spinal cord before they reach the NMDA receptors (which, when activated, can cause wind-up). This system works less effectively in women. Effectiveness in this system also declines with age. It works with the use of several pain-relieving chemicals including serotonin, norepinephrine, and the body's own opioids. Men have seven times more serotonin in their spinal fluid than women. We know that serotonin modulates pain and mood. Further research is needed, but scientists have made great strides in this area.

Unfortunately, the pain medications currently on the market do not work as well for woman as for men. Most research in the past has been carried out on males, due to concerns with pregnancy and the effects that hormones have on female systems. The government has mandated that future research include women, which may give us further clues to the pathogenesis of pain processing in females and how they respond to pain medications. This will provide new and more effective medications for females.

Ibuprofen, an NSAID used to treat pain and inflammation, does not work as well in women for relief of noninflammatory pain as it does in men. Opioids, such as morphine, work faster for men and produce less over all pain relief for women. Women need more time for these drugs to be effective, and they wear off faster than for men. Some pain-relieving patches such as lidocaine, which are used to treat specific areas of pain, work better for men. Researchers have just begun to delve into this area, and continued study may have a profound effect on how pain is treated, depending on your sex and age.

One study in Michigan showed that physicians actually gave less than optimal pain-relieving medications for women as compared to men. Why do you think this happens, and does it not make you wonder about the rational for this behavior?

Genetic Studies

- ▲ **Does FMS run in families?**
- ▲ **Some evidence indicates a predisposition to FMS.**
- ▲ **Studies are being done to evaluate the possibility.**

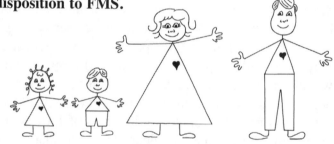

In one study by Mark Pellegrino, M.D., 50% of the children of FMS patients developed FMS. Another study by Waylonis and Heck reported that 12% of their FMS patients studied had symptomatic children and 25% had symptomatic parents. Many FMS patients report having relatives who had undiagnosed aches and pains. Or after receiving a diagnosis themselves, they alert other relatives, who then find out they have FMS, too. This is an area of research that is being further studied by M.B. Yunus, M.D., and others and will certainly be of help in putting the puzzle together.

Other studies have shown higher percentages of relatives with FMS, from as few as 23% to as many as 45%. Researchers believe that genetics may play a role in pain sensitivity, as well as in inheriting sleep disorders. Other studies have found a genetic relationship between FMS and the serotonin transporter gene 5-HTT. It seems that some people may process serotonin differently than others, which could contribute to symptoms.

The NIH (National Institutes of Health) is currently performing twin studies on FMS and CFIDS patients in Sweden where there is a large twin registry. FMS and CFIDS will be studied to identify genetic, gender, and environmental factors implicated in these illnesses. Other studies are being done to ascertain DNA abnormalities, genetic linkages, and familial inheritance.

Summary

Research = Cure

▲ **Get more physicians interested in research.**
▲ **Support NIH appropriated funds for research.**
▲ **Write letters to Congress.**

In the last 15 years, FMS has become the focus of research and interest for a handful of physicians. The physicians interested in FMS are to be applauded for their dedication and belief in a condition that frustrates both patients and doctors alike. In fact, there are still doctors who do not believe in the diagnosis of FMS. Fortunately for us, more doctors are becoming aware of the disorder and are diagnosing it. As more research is carried out and more doctors become interested in FMS, knowledge will grow and treatments will become more advanced. We will all feel better! The National Institute of Health's Web site www.nih.gov is a good resource for current information on FMS research.

$ $ $ = CURE

In the fall of 1999, the National Institutes of Health appropriated $3.6 million for FMS research. Never before had there been this much money allocated for FMS research. It is very important for all FMS sufferers to let their congressional representative know how this syndrome has adversely affected their lives. The research money was given because of the letters and calls that FMS patients made to their representatives. Your continued support will help ensure further funding for FMS, as progress cannot be made without funds for research. Please write! National FMS/CFIDS organizations are an appropriate place to donate funds for research. A list is found in the "Resources" section of this book.

Pain affects a large percentage of people around the world, with studies showing that 11% have chronic widespread pain and up to 20% have chronic regional pain. People searching for pain relief cost billions of dollars in medical expenditures—not to mention loss of work time and decreased job performance. Future research may develop new drugs that will aid those suffering from chronic and acute pain. Drugs tailored for treating pain in women are also on the horizon.

More effective treatments in physical therapy continue to be developed from the results of research on FMS patients. Occupational therapy treatments and recommendations will also be enhanced by further research. This will benefit all workers who will need modifications at work to continue to be productive.

We cannot predict what unusual treatments will be discovered to enhance the treatment of pain. Perhaps light or laser therapy, sound waves, or electrical stimulation in varying frequencies will work. Maybe we're not aware of a researcher who is currently working on a novel way to reduce pain. Humans are very creative, and we will some day discover hidden secrets to provide pain relief.

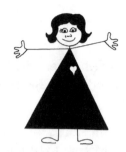

SLEEP DISTURBANCE IN FIBROMYALGIA

One of the most prominent features of fibromyalgia is sleep disturbance. When your head drops to the pillow each night, do you feel as though you spend the next eight hours just skimming on the surface of sleep, hovering in a state of semiconsciousness? Do you get to sleep, but then awaken frequently after the first three to four hours of sleep? It doesn't seem possible that a person could wake up in the morning feeling more tired than when he or she went to bed the night before, but this is recognized as one of the major symptoms of fibromyalgia.

Five Stages of Sleep

During the night, we normally pass through five stages of sleep in 60- to 90-minute cycles, four to five times per night. These cycles can be traced through the electrical brain waves that occur during sleep, via an EEG (electroencephalogram). The sleep cycles normally progress from very light sleep in stage 1 to progressively deeper sleep in stage 4. Stages 1-4 are referred to as nonREM sleep (nonrapid eye movement). During these stages, electrical brain waves become progressively slower, muscles further relax, and the body's metabolism slows. The well-rested, restored feeling we get from sleep comes from stages 3 and 4. It's during these stages that our bodies produce growth hormone for tissue repair and substances for recharging our immune system. The combination of stages 3 and 4 is often referred to as slow-wave or delta sleep. Stage 5 sleep follows stage 4 and is referred to as REM sleep (rapid eye movement). It is the sleep that occurs when the brain is experiencing increased electrical activity. Your breathing is faster in this stage, and your heart rate and blood pressure become irregular. REM sleep is the stage of sleep that is most associated with dreaming. After stage 5, sleep typically progresses through the five stages again, taking 60 to 90 minutes to complete a sleep cycle.

Sleep Disturbance

Many people with fibromyalgia do not progress through these five stages of sleep. They go to sleep easily, but wake up in the early morning (3 to 5 A.M.), unable to fall back to sleep. Others may have difficulty getting to sleep and then have interruptions during the night. Still others may sleep through the night unaware of any sleep difficulties, but may not be experiencing a deep, restorative sleep. Many people with fibromyalgia experience similar sleep disturbances.

Alpha-delta Sleep Anomaly

It's at stages 3 and 4 that disturbances in the brain's electrical activity occur, resulting in arousal, preventing the normal progression through the sleep cycle.

↓

Body is not restored.

The sleep disturbance in fibromyalgia occurs in stages 3 and 4 of the sleep cycle. A disturbance in the brain's electrical activity occurs, resulting in arousal, preventing the normal progression through the sleep cycle. The sleep disturbance is referred to by researchers as the alpha-delta sleep anomaly, a condition in which brief periods of awake-like brain waves (alpha waves) interfere with deep level (delta wave) sleep. This disturbance can be described as a state of partial wakefulness within sleep itself. When this disruption occurs, the body is not restored during sleep. Nonrestorative sleep is believed to be associated with the pain, fatigue, and other symptoms of fibromyalgia. Jon Russell, M.D., studied 44 fibromyalgia patients and discovered the following sleep disorders: alpha-delta sleep anomaly (43%), sleep apnea (25%), sleep myoclonus (16%) (involuntary arm and leg jerking during the night), and teeth grinding (14%).

Sleep Disorders

▲ Alpha-EEG sleep (Most common is phasic alpha-EEG.)
▲ Periodic limb movements during sleep
▲ Restless legs syndrome
▲ Sleep apnea
▲ Teeth grinding
▲ K-alpha sleep

Suely Roizenblatt, M.D., Ph.D., in collaboration with Harvey Moldofsky, M.D., identified three different patterns of alpha-EEG sleep: phasic, tonic, and low alpha. They analyzed symptoms in their study patients (FMS and healthy controls) before and after sleep to look for associations between alpha-EEG sleep characteristics and symptoms upon awakening. Phasic alpha was the most common alpha-EEG pattern identified in the fibromyalgia patients (50%) and concurrently was seen with the least frequency in healthy controls (7%). Phasic alpha-EEG sleep is defined as occurring episodically during slow-wave sleep in stages 3 and 4. In this study, it was also associated with the FMS patients who reported the most severe symptoms, especially a worsening of symptoms throughout the night and upon awakening. No association was identified between sleep apnea and any of the three alpha-EEG sleep patterns.

Periodic limb movements during sleep (PLMS) is another sleep disorder that occurs in some FMS patients. It is associated with alpha-wave arousals during sleep, which cause patient's limbs to move or jerk involuntarily during the night. Researchers believe that PLMS is caused by an episodic central nervous system processing abnormality. The different patterns of alpha-EEG sleep, K-alpha, and PLMS all are associated with periodic alpha intrusion arousals in sleep, but only PLMS causes the patient's limbs to move. It's important to note that while the patient may not be aware of any involuntary movements during the night, a bed partner will likely be able to report the jerking movements in detail!

When a patient finds it hard to sit still, especially in the evening, and experiences muscle cramps or twitching, he or she may have restless legs syndrome (RLS). It's interesting to note that if one fights the urge to move, muscle pain and tension usually build; as soon as one moves, the discomfort vanishes. RLS, like PLMS, also produces movement arousals with alpha-EEG during sleep and is linked to low levels of dopamine in the central nervous system.

Sleep apnea is a disorder that causes an interruption of breathing, often followed by a partial arousal or full awakening. It's described as obstructive if the airways are blocking the flow of oxygen during sleep. Apnea can be caused by the patient's tongue falling back into the throat or by fatty tissues in the throat that obstruct air passages. Snoring is also frequently associated with apnea. When apnea is caused by problems with the body's central nervous system control mechanisms, it's called central apnea. Some patients have components of both obstructive and central apnea, which is considered mixed apnea. An overnight sleep study is often ordered to identify the type of apnea that a patient is experiencing so that the appropriate treatment can be prescribed.

Teeth grinding or bruxism affects between 10-15% of FMS patients. It is often diagnosed by a dentist who may see wear and damage to various teeth from frequent grinding during sleep.

Another sleep disorder that Harvey Moldofsky, M.D., and colleagues have identified in some FMS patients is K-alpha sleep. This sleep pattern is noted on an EEG and is characterized by brief alpha arousal intrusions, occurring every 20 to 40 seconds, primarily in stage 2 sleep. Patients with a K-alpha sleep disturbance have a normal duration of all sleep stages and symptomatically have light, unrefreshing sleep and daytime fatigue.

Important Note

- ▲ **Sleep study may be ordered by your physician.**

- ▲ **Medications and treatment will be individualized depending on your sleep disorder(s).**

Another important component of the sleep disturbance in fibromyalgia involves serotonin, which is the major neurotransmitter essential for the induction of deep level, slow-wave sleep. (A neurotransmitter is a chemical that helps nerves transmit their messages.) People with fibromyalgia have been found to have low levels of serotonin in their blood and spinal fluid. At this time, doctors are prescribing medications that increase the availability of serotonin in the body with the ultimate goal of improving the patient's quality of sleep (more time in delta sleep) and reducing pain sensitivity. More research must be done on the relationship between these medications and the various sleep disturbances. While these medications do influence the availability of serotonin, the exact mechanism by which they operate is not understood. There are still many questions to be answered!

Options That May Improve Sleep Quality

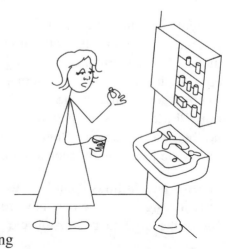

If you're waking frequently during the night, discuss with your doctor the option of taking a medication to help improve your sleep quality. (These medications are discussed in detail in the "Medications" chapter.) If your nighttime awakenings do not decrease after trying a medication for two to three weeks, discuss this observation with your doctor. An increase in dosage, the addition of another medication, or a change to a completely new medication may be prescribed. If you or your bed partner suspect that you might have periodic limb movements during sleep, restless legs syndrome, or sleep apnea, it's important to discuss these concerns with your physician. An overnight sleep study may be recommended to further assess your sleep and guide your physician in prescribing the appropriate medication and/or treatment. If your sleep does not improve after trying any newly prescribed treatment for several weeks, notify your physician. You may need to try different treatments in order to find one that works well.

The following medications and treatments are examples of some of the ways in which sleep disorders are treated. Your physician will individualize your treatment and prescribe what he or she feels is most appropriate for you. Sedating antidepressants (i.e. trazadone) or sleep-promoting hypnotics (e.g. Ambien) are often used to treat the alpha-EEG disorders, including phasic alpha. Ambien has been helpful in reducing K-alpha sleep in some patients. Treatments for PLMS often include dopamine agonists (e.g. Sinemet or Mirapex) or antiseizure medications (e.g. Klonopin or Neurontin). The medications used to treat RLS are similar to those used for PLMS with the extra precaution of ensuring that the dose of dopamine agonists isn't too high in the evening. A high dose of Sinemet or Mirapex may worsen evening restlessness. Treatment for sleep apnea may include continuous positive airway pressure or CPAP, a dental appliance to bring the lower jaw forward, or surgery to remove the fatty skin folds in the throat that could be obstructing the airway during sleep. The medications are discussed in detail in the "Medications" chapter. Bruxism is best treated by a dentist who may provide special mouth guards to be worn at night to protect the teeth from damage due to grinding. Some individuals who find it difficult to wear a traditional mouth guard may benefit from being fitted for an NTI mouth guard that is worn only on the front two teeth on the upper jaw. It is impossible for the biting surfaces of your teeth to make contact when wearing either of these mouth guards.

In addition to medication, listening to a relaxation tape before going to bed can be very helpful for many individuals. Often, patients report that they are able to get to sleep more quickly after listening to a relaxation tape. Some of these individuals will replay the tape during the night, often using headphones, if they're having difficulty getting back to sleep. (There is further discussion of relaxation tapes in the "Stress Management and Relaxation" chapter in this handbook.) Stress reduction, aerobic exercise, and other tips on improving sleep quality listed at the end of this chapter may further improve your sleep. We encourage you to try these tips and see what works for you!

Example of Bedtime Routine

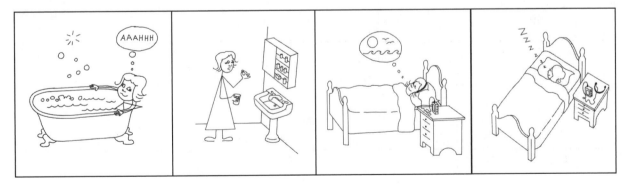

Sleep Log

A sleep log can provide a sample of what your sleep patterns are and how they may vary from night to night. It will be more accurate than your recall and will reflect a general sense of the quality of your sleep. It's helpful for both you and the health professionals working with you to see logs from three to four nights that are sampled over a two-to three-week period. It may also be beneficial for you to keep additional sleep logs when trying a new medication or implementing a new relaxation technique to document whether or not your sleep improves.

We encourage you to make copies of the "Sleep Log" below and put it in your fibromyalgia journal.

Sleep Resources

American Academy of Sleep Medicine *(includes list of sleep clinics)*	www.aasmnet.org	**708-492-0930**
Narcolepsy Network	www.narcolepsynetwork.org	**513-891-3522**
Restless Legs Syndrome Foundation	www.rls.org	**507-287-6465**
National Sleep Foundation	www.sleepfoundation.org	**202-347-3471**

Sleep Log

Date	Time to bed	Time of first awakening	Number of subsequent awakenings	Approximate range of time it took to get back to sleep	Time out of bed in A.M.	Medication taken before bed and/or during the night	Comments
Sample *2/15/97*	10:30 p.m.	3 A.M.	3	Few minutes to half hour	7 A.M.	Elavil - 9 p.m.	Sleep after 3 A.M. seemed light and disrupted. Sometimes I wasn't sure if I was sleeping or just resting with my eyes closed.

*Include things that disrupt your sleep and suggestions for improving your sleep.

Sleep Log

Date	Time to bed	Time of first awakening	Number of subsequent awakenings	Approximate range of time it took to get back to sleep	Time out of bed in A.M.	Medication taken before bed and/or during the night	Comments

*Include things that disrupt your sleep and suggestions for improving your sleep.

Sleep Disruption Journal

Check all of the following that are disrupting your sleep. Then write down possible problem-solving strategies for as many of them as you can. You may want to refer to *No More Sleepless Nights* by P. Hauri and S. Linde for some suggestions.

Sleep Disruptions

Δ Pain

Δ Need to urinate

Δ Pets

Δ Crying babies or children

Δ Snoring spouse

Δ Uncomfortable pillow or mattress

Δ PMS symptoms

Δ Menopausal symptoms

Δ Arguing with family member(s) before bed

Δ Irregular bedtime schedule

Δ Stimulant medications

Δ Jerking arms and legs

Δ Eating a large meal late

Δ Inside or outside noises

Δ Too much light

Δ Uncomfortable temperature in bedroom

Δ Worries

Δ Napping too late

Δ Caffeine

Δ Alcohol

Δ Nicotine

Δ Exercising too late

Δ Teeth grinding or clenching jaw

Problem-solving Strategies

TIPS *for Improving Sleep Quality*

▲ Consult your doctor about taking a medication to improve your sleep quality.

▲ If you are experiencing morning grogginess while taking a medication to improve your sleep quality, take the medication as early as 6 P.M.

▲ Take time to wind down before bed.

▲ Follow a bedtime ritual (e.g., warm bath, listening to relaxing music, reading, and other relaxing activities).

▲ Limit caffeine to one-two cups in A.M.

▲ Reduce or eliminate fluid intake after 6 P.M. if you need to urinate during the night. Medications such as diuretics and blood pressure medications that get rid of excess fluid should be taken earlier in the day whenever possible. (You will need to consult with your physician first.)

▲ Use relaxation tapes or exercises before bedtime.

▲ Develop a program of aerobic exercise, but avoid exercising in the evening.

▲ Actively deal with problems that interfere with sleep (e.g. pain and discomfort, crying baby, uncomfortable mattress or pillow, snoring spouse, concern about safety issues, etc.).

▲ Seek treatment for depression, anxiety, and/or stress if you are experiencing these.

▲ Avoid taking a nap late in the day. (It may be more difficult for you to go to sleep at your normal bedtime. Or you may sleep for a few hours, find yourself awake, and then be unable to get back to sleep.)

▲ Don't work in your bedroom.

▲ Drinking a glass of milk before bed may be helpful.

Caffeine, Alcohol, Smoking

When you have fibromyalgia, it's important to do all you can do to help ensure good quality sleep. You can begin by reducing caffeine, limiting alcohol, and eliminating smoking.

Caffeine

Caffeine causes people to take longer to get to sleep, to awaken more, and to lower their quality of sleep. Individuals vary in their sensitivity to caffeine. For those people who are exceptionally sensitive, sleep may be disturbed after only one cup of coffee or can of caffeinated softdrink in the afternoon. This sensitivity to caffeine often increases with age. Other symptoms that can be caused by too much caffeine include irritability, nervousness, heart palpitations, dizziness, diarrhea, stomach discomfort, and frequent urination.

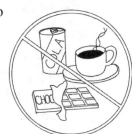

The following tables will help you determine how much caffeine you may be consuming on a daily basis. If you are sensitive to caffeine, try to eliminate it from your diet whenever possible.

Caffeine Content of Beverages and Foods

Coffee (5 oz. cup)
Brewed regular, drip method	106-164 mg
Brewed regular, percolator	93-134 mg
Instant, regular	47-68 mg
Decaffeinated	2-5 mg

Imported Loose-leaf Tea (5 oz. cup)
Black	25-110 mg
Oolong	12-55 mg
Green	8-36 mg

Tea - Major U.S. brands
1-minute brew	21-33 mg
3-minute brew	35-46 mg
5-minute brew	39-50 mg

Bottled Teas
Snapple Iced Tea, all varieties (16-oz.)	42 mg
Lipton Iced Tea, assorted varieties (16-oz.)	18-40 mg
Nestea Pure Sweetened Iced Tea (16-oz.)	34 mg
Green Tea (8-oz.)	30 mg
Arizona Iced Tea, assorted varieties (16-oz.)	15-30 mg
Celestial Seasonings Herbal Tea, all varieties (8-oz.)	0 mg

Cocoa and Chocolate
Cocoa Beverage (mix) (6-oz.)	2-8 mg
Chocolate milk (8-oz.)	2-7 mg
Milk Chocolate (1-oz.)	6-15 mg
Dark Chocolate (1-oz.)	5-35 mg
Baking Chocolate (1-oz.)	35 mg
Ovaltine	0 mg
Chocolate flavored syrup (1-oz.)	4 mg

Caffeine Content of Soft Drinks

BRAND	MG/12 OUNCES
Mountain Dew	54
Surge	52.5
Coke and Diet Coke	46
Tab	45
Sunkist Orange	42
Dr. Pepper	40
Pepsi	38
Diet Pepsi	36

Caffeine Content of Soft Drinks (continued)

BRAND	MG/12 OUNCES
Diet Rite Cola	36
Barq's Root Beer	22.5
Barq's Diet Root Beer	0
7-UP or Diet 7-UP	0
Sprite or Diet Sprite	0
Fresca	0
Caffeine-free Coke or Diet Coke	0
Caffeine-free Pepsi or Diet Pepsi	0
Minute Maid Orange	0
Mug Root Beer	0

Caffeine Content of Drugs

PRESCRIPTION DRUGS	CAFFEINE, MG/TAB
Cafergot (migraine headaches)	100
Fiorinal (tension headaches)	40
Darvon (pain relief)	32

NONPRESCRIPTION DRUGS	
Excedrin	130
NoDoz	100
Midol	64
Anacin	64
Triaminicin	30
Dristan	30
Neosynephrine	15
Sudafed	0
Actifed	0
Contact	0
Bufferin	0
Aspirin	0

Sources: FDA, Food Additive Chemistry Evaluation Branch, based on evaluations of existing literature on caffeine levels. Information from research conducted by The U. S. Department of Nutritional Services (all figures are approximate). National Coffee Association. National Soft Drink Association. Tea Council of the USA. Information provided by food, beverage, and pharmaceutical companies.

Smoking

Nicotine can keep you awake because it's a stimulant. Cigarettes cause a smoker's blood pressure and heart rate to increase and brain-wave activity to be stimulated. Smokers often have greater difficulty falling asleep, and they also tend to wake up more often during the night.

Smoking can be a difficult habit to quit, even if you know that your sleep would likely improve. The rate of success is often better with professional help. You may want to consult your physician or a psychologist or try a stop-smoking program recommended by a healthcare professional.

Alcohol

While many people find that alcohol at bedtime helps them to relax and fall asleep more easily, their sleep is often more disrupted and fragmented. By morning, they've often had less sleep than they would have had without any alcohol. A glass of wine or a cocktail before dinner will likely have less impact on one's quality of sleep, but as with caffeine, people vary in their sensitivity to alcohol.

Remember to use caution when consuming alcohol and taking medication. This combination may lead to serious side effects, especially with some of the medications used to treat fibromyalgia. For advice on the effect of specific medications and alcohol, it's best to consult your physician.

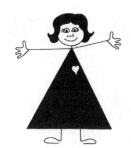

VICIOUS CYCLE OF FIBROMYALGIA

Researchers now feel that fibromyalgia can be caused by a variety of triggers which may include infections, physical trauma, hormonal problems, sleep disruption, emotional distress, or toxic exposure. They believe a person has an inherited tendency to develop FMS, but what we do not know is how many triggers it may take to develop FMS. It may take only one in some individuals, or a number of triggers may be needed for it to develop in other individuals. No matter how many triggers are needed to produce symptoms of FMS, once you have it, certain processes begin to take place which can lead to FMS getting worse over time. As this occurs, you may experience a

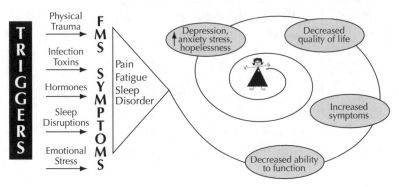

decreased ability to function in your daily life. Normal chores may become difficult to perform; cleaning your house, yard work, grocery shopping, or just picking up your baby may cause pain and increase your symptoms so much that you cannot perform these chores. You may even have to give up hobbies or activities you once enjoyed, such as exercise, hiking, golf, or even knitting if they are too painful to perform. Getting dressed in the morning can be impossible for some. Your pain may become so great that you may need to limit or give up your job as well. A decreased quality of life may result. Soon, you may find yourself spending less time with friends and begin to feel isolated and lonely. The unusual collection of symptoms you experience from your illness may cause you excessive worry. Is it any wonder that depression, anxiety, or irritability result from these changes in your lifestyle? Any normal person could become depressed over time if they lived in constant pain and had to give up their feelings of independence.

If you are not getting better from medical interventions, hopelessness can set in. You may feel that you will never experience improvements. Some people feel so hopeless that they give up trying. If you do not receive the appropriate help, this vicious cycle causes you to spiral further and further downward.

In the remainder of our book, we hope to educate you about treatments that will improve your symptoms. Some of these treatments should be done with the aid of your healthcare professionals, who may include a doctor, nurse, physical therapist, massage therapist, trigger point therapist, chiropractor, nutritionist, or psychological counselor. These professionals can help supply you with the treatments you may need such as medication, education, physical therapy, and supportive counseling. We have also included numerous self-care techniques and coping skills that you can use to take charge of your fibromyalgia. All of these together can lift your hopes and help to pull you out of the vicious cycle of fibromyalgia.

TREATMENT PYRAMID

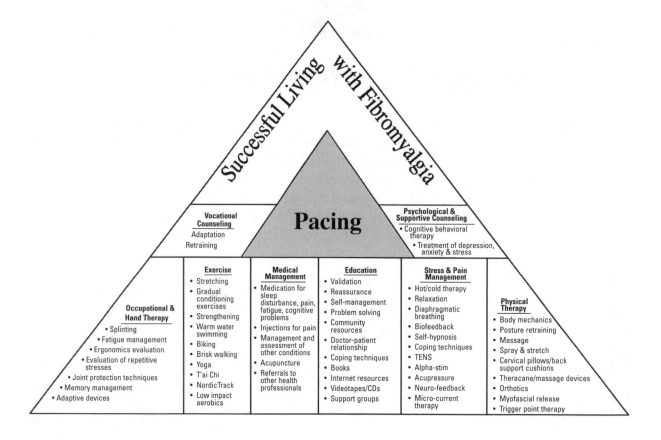

Successful living with fibromyalgia depends, for many, on the incorporation of a variety of treatments as illustrated in our treatment pyramid. Some of these treatment components may work better for some individuals than for others. Physical symptoms, environmental factors, and emotional states vary among patients, and all contribute to the varying individual success of each treatment. We encourage everyone to try treatment options in every category, and if they are helpful, begin to incorporate them in daily life. One of our aims is to help you improve your symptoms and your quality of life. If each part of the treatment plan helps you feel a small percentage better, when you add them all up, you can feel over 50% better. Pacing was deliberately made to stand out as a critical component in one's successful management of fibromyalgia. The way and degree in which one paces certainly vary among individuals, but we believe that pacing is necessary for everyone on some level. If they incorporate a variety of treatments in exercise, medical management, education, stress and pain management, etc., and are intentional about pacing their activities, many individuals will learn to successfully manage their fibromyalgia. We wish you courage to make the necessary changes in your life!

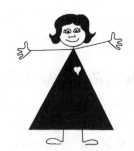

MEDICATIONS

Patient, Know Thy Medication!

It is important that you be knowledgeable about the medication you are taking. This includes knowing the dosage you are to take, the color of the pill, and it's shape. Please make sure the medication your pharmacist gives you is the one your physician has prescribed for you. Even pharmacists can make errors when dispensing pills. They may inadvertently put the wrong dosage in your pill bottle. How can you tell? If your pill suddenly changes color or shape, you may have a different dosage or a different medication.

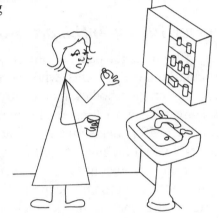

Many patients want to know if they can use the generic form of their medicine. Dr. Thomas Romano reports that it is up to you and your physician to determine if a generic equivalent can be substituted. He believes some generics are not as effective as the brand name drug, and if the generic drug is not as helpful as the brand name drug, you should insist on the name brand medication!

The severity of your FMS will determine which medicine, dosages, and in what combination medicine is to be taken. Other medical conditions you are experiencing will also determine the medication you will be prescribed.

Please note that dosages are variable, and it is up to you and your physician to determine effective dosages and timing schedules that are appropriate for you. Some medications cannot be taken with other medications you may be on or are not to be taken when other medical conditions are present. Your doctor may decide to use two or more medications in various combinations to treat your symptoms.

Several medications that are normally used for other purposes or other illnesses can decrease pain, improve sleep quality, improve cognition, and/or decrease fatigue in FMS. Although some medications have not been adequately researched for use specifically with FMS, numerous doctors are using them with good results. Other medications have been the subject of research. In this chapter, we have included as many medications found useful by physicians and patients for FMS as possible at this time.

For those who have tried many medications that have not worked, it is up to you to seek out a doctor who can help you sort out the problem, or to use other techniques such as acupuncture, relaxation, exercise, biofeedback, or hypnosis to control your pain. We hope that researchers will find a medication specifically for FMS and we will all feel better! Until that time, we have to experiment to see what works and what doesn't. It is also important to know that everyone reacts to medications differently, and what works for you might not work for another person.

Why Antidepressants? How Do They Work?

Antidepressants have been used for years to modulate pain, sleep disturbances, and fatigue—symptoms FMS patients can all relate to! Although these medications were not specifically developed for FMS, doctors have found that they seem to help some patients control their FMS symptoms. They may work by increasing the levels of the neurotransmitters norepinephrine, epinephrine, dopamine, and serotonin in the brain. They help us sleep, reduce pain, and elevate mood. At higher doses, they are used for treating depression.

You May Need to Try Several

Since each person reacts differently to medications, you may need to experiment with a few different drugs before you find one that works for you. Occasionally, medications can cause the behaviors or feelings they are designed to reduce, for example depression, nightmares, muscular pain, or insomnia. If these or unusual symptoms occur, notify your physician immediately.

Fear of Taking Antidepressants

Many fibromyalgia patients are concerned about taking a medication labeled antidepressant, particularly those patients who have been told their symptoms are all in their heads. The chemicals in our bodies that control pain and sleep also control mood, which is why the antidepressants work for some people. If you are depressed, these medications in the low dosages given for FMS patients may not treat your depression at all. They can, however, improve some patients' overall feelings of well-being and reduce pain somewhat, and for those reasons they are worth trying! You could use the example of a diabetic who needs to take insulin every day. We might need the serotonin-boosting effects of these medications just to keep our heads above water! Living with a chronic illness such as FMS increases your likelihood of becoming depressed. Remember, it is important to speak to your physician about treatment options if you do become depressed. Your physician might increase the dosage of your current medication, prescribe another medication, and/or suggest counseling. Studies show that from 20-50% of patients with FMS will experience depression during the course of the illness.

Safety

Many FMS patients are concerned about the safety of these medications. When taken under a doctor's supervision, they are safe in the majority of cases. Be sure to report any changes or adverse reactions to your doctor immediately. It is not always necessary to make an appointment with your doctor to discuss side effects or concerns you are having about your medication. A phone call is often all that is necessary. One of the doctor's nurses may also be able to answer your questions. If not, you may ask the nurse to discuss your situation with the doctor and call you back.

It is not advisable to drink alcohol while taking some of these medications, as it can magnify a number of the medication's unpleasant side effects.

These medications can interact with other medications, supplements, and herbal remedies (even some over-the-counter medications), so remember to tell your doctor about everything you currently use, including cough and cold remedies.

Use Your Pharmacist

Ask your pharmacist questions you have about your medication. He or she has a wealth of knowledge and is often delighted and willing to answer your questions. Request the paper insert from the medication box from your pharmacist. It is free and will list side effects, adverse reactions, and drug interactions, among other things.

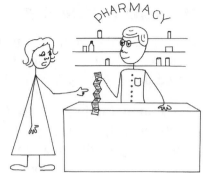

Important Note

You may want to show this section on medications to your physician; this information might help him or her decide what medication is best for you.

As research continues on FMS, we will find new medications being used in novel ways. Some of these are covered in the chapter "Pioneering Treatments."

Medications Most Commonly Used for FMS

TRICYCLIC ANTIDEPRESSANTS
Elavil-amitriptyline
Flexeril-cyclobenzaprine
Pamelor-nortriptyline
Sinequan-doxepin

OTHER ANTIDEPRESSANTS
Desyrel-trazodone
Effexor-venlafaxine
Wellbutrin-bupropion
Remeron-mirtazapine
Cymbalta-duloxetine

SSRIS
Prozac-fluoxetine
Zoloft-sertraline
Paxil-paroxetine
Luvox-fluvoxamine
Celexa-citalopram
Lexapro- escitaloparam

SLEEPING MEDICATIONS
Ambien-zolpidem tartrate
Sonata-zaleplon

ANTIANXIETY
Buspar-buspirone
Xanax-alprazolam
Klonopin-clonazepam
Ativan-lorazepam

MUSCLE RELAXANTS
Norflex-orphenadrine citrate
Skelaxin - metaxalone
Zanaflex-tizanidine
Soma-carisoprodol
Baclofen-lioresal
Flexeril-cyclobenzaprine

OTHERS FOR PAIN RELIEF
Neurontin-gabapentin
Gabatril-tiagabine
Tegretol-carbamazepine
Depakote-valproic acid

NSAIDS
Advil/Motrin-Ibuprofen
Feldene-piroxicam
Naprosyn-naproxen
Relafen-nabumetone

COX-2 INHIBITORS
Celebrex-celecoxib

PATCHES/TOPICALS
Capsaicin
Aurum
Lidoderm
Duragesic-fentanyl transdermal
Ketalar-Ketamine
Neurontin-gabapentin

SHORT-ACTING OPIOIDS
Lortab-hydrocodone+Tylenol
Vicodin-hydrocodone+Tylenol
Norco-hydrocodone bitartrate+Tylenol
Morphine-morphine sulfate
Percolone-oxycodone hydrochloride
Percocet-oxycodone+Tylenol
Tylox-oxycodone+Tylenol
Darvocet-propoxphene+Tylenol
Tylenol #3-Tylenol+codeine

LONG-ACTING OPIOIDS
Avinza-sustained release oral morphine
Kadian-sustained release morphine

MS-Contin-sustained release morphine
Oramorph SR-sustained release morphine
Oxycontin-sustained release oxycodone
Duragesic patch-Fentanyl

OPIOID-LIKE MEDICATIONS
Ultram-tramadol
Ultracet-tramadol+Tylenol

COGNITION/MEMORY/FIBRO-FOG/FATIGUE
Piracetam-nootropyl
Deprenyl-selegiline-hydrochloride
Hydergine-dihydroergotoxine
Ritalin-methylphenidate
Concerta-methylphenidate hydrochloride
Metadate CD, ER-methylphenidate
Dexedrine-dextroamphetamine sulfate
Adderall-amphetamine sulfate
Provigil-modafinil
Strattera-atomoxetineHCL

RESTLESS LEGS SYNDROME PERIODIC LIMB MOVEMENT OF SLEEP
Mirapex-pramipexole
Sinemet-carbidopa/levodopa
Klonopin-clonazepam

UPCOMING MEDICATIONS FOR PAIN
Pregabalin
Milnapracin

Tricyclic Antidepressants

Studies have shown that the tricyclics can improve symptoms in one-third of FMS patients and after taking them for at least six months, another one-third may feel improvement. When an SSRI is used in conjunction with a tricyclic, it may enhance the tricyclic's benefits.

Elavil (amitriptyline) - Dose is typically 2.5-50 mg at night. It is known for its pain-relieving effects and helps you sleep. To avoid morning hangover, you could take it earlier in the evening or take half your dose in the early evening and the other half at bedtime. You can purchase a pill-cutter at your local drugstore which is easier than trying to break the pills in half or cutting them with a knife. If you feel headed for a flare-up, you can try taking half your usual dosage in the daytime. Of course, you should discuss these or other options with your physician. Be careful when driving a car or operating any machinery, as this drug can be sedating. This medication has been around for decades and used to be the medication of choice for treating FMS. Elavil is sometimes used in combination with other antidepressants, which may increase its effectiveness. Elavil may not be as effective as some of the newer medications, although some people may benefit from its use.

Flexeril (cyclobenzaprine) - Dose is typically 2.5-30 mg at night. This is a tricyclic drug similar to Elavil, which has more muscle relaxant properties than Elavil. Flexeril can also be taken in combination with other medications. It may be sedating.

Sinequan (doxepin) - Dose is typically 25-75 mg. This is another tricyclic similar to Elavil that has helped some patients. As it has antihistamine properties, it may be beneficial to those who experience allergies. It comes in both liquid and tablet forms, which can be beneficial in dosing options.

Pamelor (nortriptyline) - Dose is typically 10-50 mg per night. It is another tricyclic that has helped some FMS patients. It has the same side effects as Elavil, although it may not be as sedating.

Side Effects of the Tricyclic Antidepressants

▲ **Morning hangover** ▲ **Heart rate abnormalities**
▲ **Constipation** ▲ **Dry mouth and eyes**
▲ **Weight gain** ▲ **Headache**
▲ **Drowsiness** ▲ **Increased sensitivity to sunlight**

Many of the tricyclics have side effects that may be intolerable for some patients, such as experiencing a morning hangover feeling, constipation, weight gain, drowsiness, heart rate abnormalities, dry mouth and/or dry eyes, and an increased sensitivity to sunlight. You can try taking these medications earlier in the evening to avoid feeling "hung over" in the morning. For constipation, eating high-fiber foods or taking a natural bulk laxative may work well. Drinking water or sucking on sugarless hard candy can help with the dry mouth feeling, as well as using some of the over-the-counter products, such as chewing gum specifically formulated to help with the symptoms of dry mouth. Weight gain is difficult to deal with, and many patients find they cannot lose weight no matter what they do while on these medications. As you may also become more sensitive to sunlight, wearing extra protection such as a high SPF sunscreen or extra clothes can help. Medicine drops are available for dry eyes.

Sometimes, side effects decrease after you have been on a drug for some time. If not, please do not be afraid to tell your physician your concerns, as he or she may want to have you try a different medication.

Other Antidepressants

Desyrel (trazodone) - Dosage is typically 25-75 mg before bedtime. It is a novel antidepressant that increases serotonin concentrations in the synapses, is moderately sedating, and is useful for sleeping difficulties. It is usually well tolerated.

Wellbutrin (buproprion hydrochloride) - Dosage is typically 75-150 mg per day. It is an antidepressant also used to improve attention and concentration and for smoking cessation. It can cause headaches in some people, especially those with a history of migraines.

Effexor (venlafaxine hydrochloride) - Dosage is typically 37.5-225 mg per day. It is not related chemically to any of the other antidepressants; it not only boosts serotonin, but also increases norepinephrine. Effexor may increase blood pressure and cause sexual difficulties.

Remeron (mirtazapine) - Dosage is typically 15-30 mg given once a day. It enhances serotonin and noradrenergic activity and is commonly used in the treatment of depression. Remeron can be used at bedtime to enhance sleep quality.

Cymbalta (duloxetine) - Newly approved, its suggested starting dose is 20 mg/day and may increase as high as 60 mg/day. Cymbalta is the first of a new line of antidepressants called NSRIs, because they are norepinephrine and serotonin reuptake inhibitors. Most common side effects include nausea, dry mouth, and constipation.

Serotonin Boosting Medications (SSRIs)

This is a class of medications which has experienced an explosion in research, as well as being written about and talked about extensively in the news media over the last decade. New ones are being developed faster than we can write about them. Because serotonin controls numerous functions in the body other than depression and anxiety, the serotonin-boosting drugs are sometimes used to treat a variety of other illnesses, too. When used in combination with a tricyclic, they increase the tricyclic's effects. Due to this, it is important that you have a physician who is knowledgeable about the usages of these medications—whether in combination or when used alone.

Prozac (fluoxetine) - Dose is 5-60 mg. This is a specific serotonin-boosting medication and was one of the first developed in this category of drugs. If it gives you insomnia, you might have to take it in combination with one of the more sedating drugs or take it in the morning. Prozac also comes in a liquid form, enabling you to take it in smaller amounts than normally supplied by capsule.

Zoloft (sertraline) - Dose is typically 25-200 mg. It has been shown to be effective for some patients, although you may need a sedating medication in the evening, as it can cause insomnia or nervousness.

Paxil (paroxetine hydrochloride) - Dose is typically 5-60 mg. This is similar to the other SSRIs and is often found to be useful in treating anxiety. Paxil is the most potent of these types of medications and might prove beneficial for you.

Luvox (fluvoxamine) - Dose is typically 25-50 mg. This drug has been approved for the treatment of obsessive compulsive disorder and is also used for the treatment of depression.

Celexa (citalopram hydrobromide) - Dose is 20-40 mg once a day. Used for the treatment of depression.

Lexapro (escitalopram) - Dose is 10-20 mg once daily. This is a newer SSRI used for the treatment of depression.

Side Effects of the Serotonin-Boosting Medications

- ▲ Stomach distress
- ▲ Anxiety or nervousness
- ▲ Insomnia
- ▲ Sweating
- ▲ Mood swings in a small percentage of people
- ▲ Headache
- ▲ Sexual difficulties
- ▲ Weight loss or weight gain

Upset stomach, headache, and feeling nervous are often experienced in the first few weeks of treatment, but they often resolve over time. If the side effects become bothersome or too intense, speak to your physician about them. He or she may change your prescription. Sexual side effects may take longer to become apparent, with an inability to experience orgasm and loss of sexual desire affecting many people. If this happens, your physician may offer to change you to another medication, or in some instances, may add a different medication to counteract the unwanted side effects.

These medications can sometimes cause unusual mood swings or behaviors in a small percentage of individuals. Be sure to report any unusual feelings, strange thoughts, or odd behaviors to your physician immediately. Some people report they have bizarre or very vivid dreams while on these medications. If you are concerned about your weight, note that while some of these medications can cause weight loss, they may cause weight gain in certain people. Give your medication at least a month to work or for side effects to resolve. Your physician may have to increase or decrease the dosage to provide the best results. You may need to try a number of different SSRIs before you find one that works well for you. Remember, only you can judge how you feel!

Sleeping Medications

More physicians are prescribing sleeping medications for FMS patients, as they know that without a good night's sleep, their patients will have a difficult time improving.

Ambien (zolpidem tartrate) - Typical dosage is 5-20 mg at night; some patients may need 20 mg. Ambien seems to be well tolerated by many patients. In a clinical trial of Ambien, patients reported fewer awakenings and a significant improvement in sleep quality. As its effects last for only four hours or so, if you wake up in the middle of the night and have difficulty falling back to sleep, you may need to repeat your dose.

Sonata (zaleplon) - Typical dosage is 5-20 mg at night. Sonata has been found to decrease the time it takes to get to sleep, but has not been shown to increase total time sleeping or decrease the number of awakenings.

Benedryl (diphenhydramine hydrochloride) - Dose is typically 25-50 mg taken before bedtime. This is an antihistamine with sedating properties and can be purchased over the counter. It is found in Tylenol PM.

Xyrem (GHB or Gamma-Hydroxybutyric Acid) is a promising sleep aid being researched for its use in FMS. Read about it in our "Pioneering Treatments" chapter.

Side Effects of Sleeping Medications

- ▲ Minimal side effects
- ▲ Grogginess
- ▲ Morning hangover
- ▲ Rebound insomnia when discontinued

Side effects seem minimal for these medications. When taking Ambien or GHB, it is possible to be so deep in sleep that if something happens around you, you may not hear it or wake up. This can be dangerous.

These medications may not work at all for you, or conversely, they could make a big difference in your sleep time or sleep quality.

Antianxiety Medications

Anxiety can make pain worse, and pain can make anxiety worse! Decreasing anxiety may help alleviate some of your pain and help you sleep better.

Xanax (alprazolam) - Dose is typically .25-1.5 mg at night. I. Jon Russell, M.D., has published a study that proves Xanax's effectiveness for fibromyalgia. It has been found to be more effective if taken with ibuprofen (2,400 mg per day). For best results you may also need a small dose in the morning. Please be careful if your stomach is sensitive to ibuprofen; consult with your physician.

Klonopin (clonazepam) - Dose is typically .5-1 mg at night. It is effective particularly if you have arm or leg jerking spasms as you attempt to fall asleep. If you have this problem and take a tricyclic, it might make you feel worse. It is also useful for those who have TMJ or those who grind their teeth at night. This medication works by calming the GABA and NMDA receptors.

Ativan (lorazepam) - Dose is typically .25-.5 mg two to three times a day and .5-1 mg at night. It's primary purpose is as an anti-anxiety medication.

Buspar (buspirone hydrochloride) - Dose is typically 5-10 mg three times per day with the maximum being a total of 60 mg per day. Buspar is formulated specifically to reduce anxiety and is chemically unrelated to other antianxiety medications. Buspar tends to have a gentler onset and longer acting mechanism than medications such as Valium or Xanax. Its side effects include nervousness, dizziness, headache, and fatigue. It could have the opposite effect by increasing your symptoms.

Antianxiety Side Effects

▲ Habit forming   ▲ Depression
▲ Sedation   ▲ Decreased memory
▲ Withdrawal symptoms

Some of these can be habit forming (addictive) and very sedating, so be cautious when taking them if you are driving or operating machinery. It is important to note that discontinuing these medications abruptly can produce severe withdrawal symptoms, such as tremors, heart palpitations, and seizures. Be sure to discuss this with your physician before you discontinue any of these medications. Side effects can also include depression and decreased memory.

Muscle Relaxants

These medications are designed to help relax muscles and have been found useful by many patients for reduction of pain.

Zanaflex (tizanidine) - Dose is 2 mg-36 mg and varies with individuals. This is a central alpha-2 adrenergic agonist used to treat muscle spasms in multiple sclerosis. It decreases substance P. FMS patients' pain was reduced in studies; morning stiffness decreased, and sleep improved. It may be sedating, and it can cause dizziness and liver function abnormalities. It can also lower blood pressure.

Skelaxin (metaxalone) - Dose is 200-400 mg three to four times a day. Its mechanism of action is not known. It can cause nausea, drowsiness, dizziness, headache, and nervousness or irritability.

Flexeril (cyclobenzaprine) - Dose is typically 2.5-10 mg at night. It also has antidepressant properties and is discussed in the tricyclic antidepressant section.

Norflex (orphenadrine citrate) - Dose is typically 50-100 mg twice a day. Many patients do not experience increased fatigue with this compound, as they might with the other muscle relaxants, so it may be useful for daytime. Side effects include dizziness, dry mouth, tachycardia, headache, and constipation.

Soma (carisoprodol) - Dose is 350 mg four times a day. Provides muscle relaxation. Side effects include drowsiness, dizziness, irritability, insomnia, and depressive reactions. Allergic reactions include rash.

Baclofen (lioresal) - Starting dose is 5mg. It is a centrally acting skeletal muscle relaxant that works on the GABA receptors. It is also used for multiple sclerosis and for muscle spasm. It can cause sedation, dizziness, headache, weakness, confusion, and low blood pressure.

Muscle Relaxant Side Effects

- ▲ Sedation
- ▲ Impaired coordination
- ▲ Impaired memory and concentration
- ▲ Muscular weakness
- ▲ Addiction
- ▲ Depression

Muscle relaxants can make you feel groggy, so it is important to take them when you do not need to be alert. If they make you too sleepy, try halving the dose to see if they work better for you. Specific side effects are noted for each drug separately, as they all have different side effects.

Pain Relief

This is a mixed category of medications found useful for pain control for FMS. Some of these were originally developed as antiseizure medications and seem to help when patients experience numbness, burning, tingling, and shooting pains.

Neurontin (gabapentin) - Dosages of up to 2,400 mg per day and higher have been used. Neurontin stimulates GABA receptors and was introduced as an antiseizure drug. It is used for chronic pain relief and may require higher doses than recommended by the pharmaceutical company. Reversible kidney problems have been reported.

Gabatril (tiagabine) - Starting dose is 1 mg. It is similar to neurontin in action. Side effects include dizziness, drowsiness, insomnia, weakness, and nervousness.

Tegretol (carbamazepine) - Dose is 100 mg and up. It is an anticonvulsant that is used also for trigeminal neuralgia pain and migraines. Side effects include dizziness, sedation, nausea, and vomiting.

Depakote (valproic acid) - Starting dose is 250 mg twice a day up to 1,000 mg per day. Depakote is an antiseizure medication; it prevents migraines and is used for the reduction of manic episodes. Side effects include abdominal pain, abnormal thinking, breathing difficulty, constipation, depression, dizziness, and emotional changeability.

Catapress (clonidine) - Dose is .01-.03 mg per day in divided doses. This medication blocks the sympathetic nervous system and is useful for sympathetically maintained pain. Sedation can be a problem.

Dolophine (methadone) - Begin low at 2.5-5 mg for three days, then increase to 10 mg every three to four hours as indicated. Methadone is a narcotic analgesic that does not interfere with most antidepressant medications. It is low in cost and may work as an NMDA receptor antagonist. It is used for severe pain, for detoxification treatment of narcotics addiction, and for temporary maintenance treatment of narcotic addiction.

NSAIDs

▲ Motrin   ▲ Relafen
▲ Advil   ▲ Naproxen

These are the nonsteroidal anti-inflammatory medicines which can cause stomach distress, and some patients can develop bleeding ulcers from the use of the NSAIDs. There are some NSAIDs that claim not to produce as much stomach distress. Ask your doctor about them.

Cox-2 Inhibitors

▲ Celebrex

This is a newer medication that is similar to NSAIDs but which causes gastrointestinal distress or bleeding in only a small percentage of individuals. It can be less effective in treating FMS pain, but if you have arthritis pain as well, it may prove useful.

Topical Patches, Gels, and Creams: Used for Local Pain Relief

These are used for topical pain control, so they deliver medication only to the tissues beneath the skin. Their topical use may alleviate side effects and complications when the same medication is delivered orally or by injection. Some compounding pharmacists make patches or creams using a variety of ingredients. Your physician may wish to work with a compounding pharmacist in determining which one might fit your needs for specific pain relief. Side effects can include irritation of the skin at the site of application. Some can be purchased over the counter.

The following are the most commonly used topicals:

Topical Lidoderm patches and gels containing 5% lidocaine may be effective for regional myofascial pain problems: they are used currently for postherpetic neuralgia. The patches come in large sizes and can be cut to your needs. Prilocaine can be added to lidocaine to improve relief.

Duragesic patches contain fentanyl. Fentanyl is a potent narcotic (opioid) and should be monitored closely, as it can cause significant side effects, particularly in the elderly. It is effective for widespread pain and can be placed anywhere on the body.

Ketamine patches or gels. This medication reduces wind-up due to its action as an NMDA receptor antagonist. It is not useful for FMS patients as an intravenous therapy because of its dangerous side effects, but may be useful in a patch applied to the skin in painful areas. Orally, it is abused on the street and called Special K. Applied as a patch or a gel, the side effects are low and local pain relief may occur after one week's use. It is applied three times per day. Dextromethorphan may be added to improve its efficacy.

Neurontin can be added to the ketamine gel to improve its effectiveness.

Capsaicin. This is a cream made from hot peppers that can be purchased over the counter under a variety of names and in different strengths. Ask the pharmacist. The cream is absorbed into the skin and helps reduce substance P (the pain chemical). It is applied directly to the painful area three-four times a day, and it may take some time to notice any pain-relieving effects. It may produce a burning sensation if you take a hot shower or exercise after applying it. Do not place a heating pad over the area where you have applied the cream, and wash your hands after the application, so you do not inadvertently touch your eyes. Capsaicin can produce a burning and stinging sensation, especially on mucous membranes.

Nasal Sprays

Some of these medications can be compounded into nasal sprays. One such medication is ketamine 5% solution sprayed three times a day.

Opioids and Narcotics

- ▲ **Not the first choice for pain relief**
- ▲ **Best to use a physician who is knowledgeable in their use**
- ▲ **Addiction possibilities, physical dependence, tolerance**
- ▲ **Pain contract often used**

Opioids are not the first choice for pain relief for FMS, but physicians are feeling more comfortable with prescribing them for FMS pain, particularly when other treatment options do not provide sufficient relief. Some patients are concerned with addiction, but recent research has shown that addiction seldom occurs when these medications are used in chronic pain states. Addiction is different from physical dependence or tolerance. A person who has become addicted to a drug will spend a lot of time and money seeking the drug and often experience behavior changes that may become evident at work and home. Some may even resort to criminal activities as their need for more medication surpasses what is prescribed. **If patients have a history of addiction, these medications should be used with extreme caution.** When one is physically dependent on a drug, they will experience withdrawal if the medication is abruptly stopped and will need guidance on slowly tapering their dose. Tolerance occurs when one needs more medication to achieve the same pain relief. Of course, your physician may need to increase your dosage until they find the dosage that is correct for you. It is well noted in recent research that pain is often undermedicated by physicians, particularly for women. These medications can provide significant relief of pain when used appropriately. Your physician may wish you to enter into a pain contract if you are to be on an opioid for any length of time. This contract is required by law in some states. If you violate it, you will not be prescribed any further medication. This is for your protection. We offer an example used by Dr. Romano at the end of this chapter.

The goal of prescribing pain medications is to improve your quality of life by reducing pain without adding significant side effects. Although each person's response to pain is different, when you are on a dose that alleviates your pain, you should be able to perform more activities of daily living due to a decrease in pain.

Following is a list of some of the opioids used for pain relief. (This is a partial list; there are others and new ones coming out all the time.) You will need to speak with a specialist before acquiring a prescription for any of these medications.

Short-acting opioids, four-six hours

Lortab - hydrocodone + Tylenol
Vicodin - hydrocodone + Tylenol
Norco - similar to vicodin, but with less Tylenol
Morphine - morphine sulfate
Percolone - oxycodone hydrochloride
Roxicodone - oxycodone hydrochloride
Percodan - oxycodone + aspirin
Percocet - oxycodone + Tylenol
Tylox - oxycodone + Tylenol
Darvocet - propoxphene + Tylenol
Tylenol #3 or #4 - codeine + Tylenol

Long-acting opioids, 12 hours

Avinza - sustained-release oral morphine
Kadian - sustained-release morphine
MS-Contin - sustained-release morphine
Oramorph SR - sustained-release morphine
OxyContin - sustained-release oxycodone hydrochloride
Duragesic patch - contains fentanyl

Dr. Thomas Romano states: "As a rule, the opioids are safe medications when used as directed. Their side effects tend to be more annoying than dangerous when taken in appropriate doses. The reason they are so highly controlled is due to their street value and misuse by addicts, drug dealers, and criminals. However, when used appropriately, they can be very useful for symptoms of FMS."

Opioids' Side Effects

▲ Nausea   ▲ Sweating   ▲ Urinary retention
▲ Dizziness   ▲ Itching   ▲ Irritability
▲ Sedation   ▲ Depression   ▲ Constipation
▲ Confusion   ▲ Sexual complaints   ▲ Decline in hormone levels

Ask your physician about possible side effects and how to handle them.
Usually start with low dosages and increase slowly until optimum effects are achieved.

All of the opioids have side effects that may include nausea, dizziness, sedation, confusion, sweating, itching, depression, sexual complaints, urinary retention, respiratory depression, irritability, a decline in hormone production, and constipation.

Tolerance develops early in treatment (it may not take long for the side effects to go away), and it may take a few weeks to find the appropriate dosage for you. Constipation rarely goes away, so taking a fiber supplement may help. Ask your physician how to handle side effects before you begin therapy with these medications.

It is important to note that when Tylenol is taken in excessive amounts, liver damage or

death can occur. Many of the narcotics have Tylenol added, so if you are already taking Tylenol on your own, your doctor needs to know how much you take and how often.

Continue with current treatments while taking opioids.

While taking opioids, it is not advisable to discontinue other treatments your physician or healthcare professional has recommended, such as exercise, eating well, stress management, pacing, and utilizing good sleep habits. These are all good basic interventions that have proven beneficial for decreasing symptoms of fibromyalgia. They are important for overall health and well-being.

Treating fibromyalgia pain can be complicated; therefore, it may be wise to utilize a physician who is a specialist in managing pain. See our chapter on pain management for information on pain specialists. The American Pain Society has a list of pain specialists practicing in your area; their number is 847-375-4715 and their Web site is www.ampainsoc.org. The American Pain Society has published guidelines for rheumatologists and other physicians to aid them in prescribing opioids. These guidelines are available on their Web site. The American Academy of Pain Management is another good resource to contact; their number is 209-533-9744, and their Web site is www.aapainmanage.org.

Opioid-like Medications

Ultram (tramadol hydrochloride) - Dose is 50-100 mg every four-six hours. It works differently from the opioid-specific medications in that it inhibits the reuptake of norepinephrine and serotonin and also has opioid-like actions. Seizures in a few susceptible individuals have been reported, as well as dizziness, nausea, and sedation.

Ultracet (37.5 mg tramadol hydrochloride/325 mg acetaminophen) - Dose is usually two tablets every four-six hours. It is another version of Ultram with added acetaminophen to improve its effectiveness. It is important to increase your dose slowly on Ultracet and to consult with your physician before combining Ultracet with any product containing acetaminophen.

Dextromethorphan (DM) - Dose is up to 75 mg per day. DM may calm down NMDA pain. It may work by blocking the action of nitric oxide on the NMDA receptors to minimize wind-up. It is found in many cough medicine preparations and is also available by prescription. DM can be added to Ultram to increase Ultram's benefits or if tolerance has been built up. Ask your physician about the use of this medication for your symptoms.

Cognitive-memory-fibro-fog-fatigue

Piracetam (nootropyl) - Begin dosage for two days with 3,000-4,000 mg/day, then taper to 1,500-2,500 mg per day. It is only available from compounding specialists. Piracetam benefits alertness, attention span and short-term memory. Side effects are nominal.

Deprenyl (selegiline hydrochloride) - dose is 1-5 mg per day. It is a monoamine oxidase type B inhibitor useful for depression. It increases alertness and inhibits the ability of toxic substances to destroy astroglial cells. It is a standard treatment for Parkinson's disease. Side effects include nausea, heartburn, irritability, and insomnia.

Hydergine - Dose is 2 mg per day. Hydergine is an ergot alkaloid. It improves alertness, short-term memory, and is an antioxidant for the brain. Side effects include headaches and nausea.

Ritalin, Concerta (long-acting Ritalin), Metadate, Dexedrine or Adderall - Dosages depend on your need. These medications are commonly used for Attention Deficit Disorder and may help your brain fog or improve your concentration difficulties. Dexedrine and Adderall are also used for the treatment of narcolepsy.

Provigil (modafinil) - Dose is 50-400 mg in the morning, depending on you and your physician's determination. Provigil was originally formulated for the fatigue of narcolepsy and Parkinson's disease. It may be useful if you experience excessive daytime sleepiness. Provigil studies for FMS show it is effective in improving daytime alertness. Side effects are headache and insomnia.

Strattera (atomoxetine-HCL) - Dose is typically 10-60 mg per day. It is a selective norepinephrine reuptake inhibitor and is the only nonstimulant medication FDA approved for ADHD. In Europe it is used to treat depression and anxiety.

Restless Legs Syndrome/Periodic Limb Movements of Sleep

Mirapex (pramipexole) - Dose is .125 mg to start; work up to .25 mg before bedtime. This is a new dopamine-3 receptor antagonist-like drug used for the treatment of Parkinson's disease. Lowered pain levels and an overall sense of well-being have been reported. Main side effects are nausea, insomnia, and dizziness.

Sinemet (carbidopa-levodopa) - Dose is usually started with 10 mg carbidopa/100 mg levodopa three-four times per day. Dosage must be individualized. This is another drug that is used to treat the muscle stiffness, tremor, and weakness of Parkinson's disease. Side effects can include lowered blood pressure, arrhythmias, depression, hallucinations, nausea, constipation, and fatigue.

Klonopin (clonazepam) - Dose is typically .5-1 milligram at night. This medication was described earlier under the antianxiety section. It is also used to treat restless legs syndrome.

Injection Therapies

Injection therapies are used for patients who have comorbid painful conditions such as myofascial pain syndrome, nerve entrapment and slipped discs. These may include

- ▲ **Botox injections**
- ▲ **Nerve blocks**
- ▲ **Facet blocks**
- ▲ **Epidural steroid injections**
- ▲ **Trigger point injections**

Botox injections - Botox can be injected into a trigger point to block the pain in that area. It works by preventing muscles from contracting. Botox, a purified form of the botulism toxin, is also used to reduce wrinkles. Its effects may last for three-four months or longer. Botox may reduce regional pain and is worth a try if you can find a physician who is knowledgeable in the technique.

Nerve block - This is a procedure in which an anesthetic agent is injected directly near a nerve to block pain. It is a form of regional anesthesia.

Facet joint blocks - This is actually a test and a type of treatment. A local anesthetic such as lidocaine or novacaine (sometimes with cortisone added) is injected into the facet joint. If the pain goes away, then the doctor can assume that the facet joint is a problem. Relief is usually temporary. This is an invasive test that doctors do not like to perform unless they feel it is absolutely necessary. Risks include infection of the joint and an allergic reaction to the medication being injected.

Epidural steroid injections - This is very similar to a cortisone injection, except that the cortisone is injected into a space near the spinal cord. A physician will utilize an X-ray to help guide the procedure. Often, a series of injections spaced a week apart is given before relief is noticed. Relief can be temporary or long lasting. Side effects may be infection, bleeding, nerve damage, or dural puncture. Another side effect of the steroid medication is an increase in blood sugar levels, so diabetics must be careful with any cortisone injection.

Trigger point injections - These are injections of a short-acting, local anesthetic into areas of the body which cause referred pain. Temporary pain relief and inactivation of the trigger points injected are possible if done properly. It is important to stretch the muscles surrounding the injection site immediately afterwards for full benefits.

Medications for Other Syndromes Associated with FMS

- ▲ Irritable bowel syndrome
- ▲ Mitral valve prolapse
- ▲ Autonomic nervous system dysfunction
- ▲ Infections
- ▲ Nutritional deficiencies

- ▲ Migraine headaches
- ▲ Allergies
- ▲ Sinusitis
- ▲ Hormonal problems
- ▲ Arthritis

Other conditions need to be treated with the appropriate medications.

There are number of symptoms that many FMS patients seem to have besides pain, a sleep problem, fatigue, and cognitive dysfunction. We cover these briefly here and review some of the available medications commonly used for them. You will need to talk to your physician about **all your symptoms, so you can receive the most effective treatment available.** Some patients forget to tell physicians about all their symptoms. This may not be a full list of medications used for these problems. Consult with your physician.

Irritable Bowel Syndrome

- ▲ Prilosec
- ▲ Metamucil
- ▲ Histamine H-2 blockers such as Tagamet (which may also improve slow-wave sleep)
- ▲ Reglan
- ▲ Levsin/Levbid
- ▲ Antacids
- ▲ Librax

Mitral Valve Prolapse

- ▲ Beta-blockers (Inderal)
- ▲ Calcium channel blockers

Autonomic Nervous System Dysfunction

- ▲ SSRIs
- ▲ Tricyclic antidepressants
- ▲ Appropriate salt and water intake
- ▲ Beta-blockers
- ▲ Florinef
- ▲ Midodine (ProAmatine)

Bacteria and Viruses

- ▲ Antivirals
- ▲ Antibiotics (may be long-term therapy)
- ▲ Diflucan, Sporanox, nystatin for yeast infections

Migraine Headaches:

- ▲ Excedrin Migraine
- ▲ Amerge
- ▲ Duradrin
- ▲ Bellergal
- ▲ SSRIs
- ▲ Tricyclyic antidepressants

- ▲ **Zomig**
- ▲ **Beta-blockers**
- ▲ **Calcium channel blockers**
- ▲ **Imitrex**
- ▲ **Midrin**
- ▲ **Botox injections**
- ▲ **D.H.E. 45 (dihydroergotamine mesylate) in a nasal spray form**

Some of these medications are given to prevent migraines and others to stop migraine attacks. There are certain foods that can trigger migraines. Speak to your physician about ones to avoid. Low magnesium levels may play a role in premenstrual migraine attacks.

Allergies and Chronic Sinusitis

- ▲ **Decongestants**
- ▲ **Antihistamines**
- ▲ **Steroid nasal sprays**

Hormonal Problems

- ▲ **Cortef**
- ▲ **Progesterone**
- ▲ **Growth hormone**
- ▲ **Thyroid**
- ▲ **Testosterone**
- ▲ **Estrogen**
- ▲ **DHEA**

Arthritis

- ▲ **NSAIDs**
- ▲ **Cox-2 inhibitors**

Nutritional Deficiencies - Need to be evaluated with your health professional.

Upcoming Medications

These are not yet available for FMS patients at this writing, but may be by the time you read this book. Talk to your physician about new medications as they become available and remember to keep up to date on new research.

Pregabalin - Dose is 150-450 mg per day. Pregabalin is a cousin of neurontin in that it acts on the GABA receptors and is effective in reducing neuropathic pain and anxiety. It has been tested on FMS patients, and it reduced their pain, sleep problems, and fatigue. Dizziness and tiredness were the only side effects noted, and they were mild.

Milnapracin - This norepinephrine and serotonin reuptake inhibitor with weak NMDA receptor antagonist activity has shown promise in the treatment of FMS, and it has a good safety profile.

Medication Dosage, Timing, and Treatment during Flare-ups

- ▲ **FMS changes from day to day.**
- ▲ **So can your medications.**
- ▲ **Consult your physician.**

Because FMS does have flare-ups and remissions and tends to change from day to day, it is very important to talk to your doctor about increasing your medication during a flare-up. It is also very important to make sure your increased pain or new pain is actually related to your FMS and not to some other medical problem that requires different medical attention. It might help you feel better if you know in advance that it is okay, with your physician's approval, to add an extra dose of a muscle relaxant, increase your regular

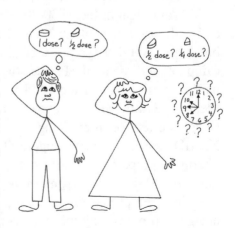

medication, take more NSAIDs, or add a sleeping pill for a few days, depending on your circumstances. Many women need to add more medication premenstrually because they tend to have a flare-up every month at that time. Some people feel worse in the winter when it is colder and the sun is not out as much, and they could benefit from added medication or light therapy. When physical or emotional stress aggravates your symptoms, this may be another time to add more medication. Talk to your doctor about proper dosages and times of the day when you could benefit from more medication. It will take some time for you and your physician to determine proper dosages and appropriate times to take them, so please be patient.

Options During a Flare-up

▲ **Increase medication.**
▲ **Add muscle relaxants.**
▲ **Add a sleeping pill.**
▲ **Add anti-inflammatory.**
▲ **Try a topical cream.**

Dosages vary from person to person.

Get physician's approval before a flare-up occurs.

Topical Creams or Gels

Zostrix cream (capsaicin 0.025%) - This is a topical analgesic you can buy over the counter that is effective for relieving the pain of arthritis in specific areas and has recently been shown to help FMS patients. It is recommended that you use this cream three to four times a day for days or weeks for maximum effectiveness. The actual ingredient in Zostrix or its generic form is capsaicin, which is made from hot peppers. It is absorbed into the skin and actually reduces substance P, which is the neurotransmitter responsible for sensations of pain. It might be useful to try rubbing it in a specific area such as the neck, shoulder, or hip to see if it helps alleviate some of your pain. Rubbing it all over your body for fibromyalgia is not recommended. Be careful and follow the warnings on the label. Remember to wash your hands well after applying, because it can be extremely irritating if you accidentally touch your eye with even a tiny bit of this cream. It can also create a burning sensation (which usually diminishes with time) and can actually burn your skin if you place a heating pad over it. It also may produce a burning sensation if you exercise or sweat, so you might want to wash it off of your skin before exercising or sitting in a hot tub. Other companies have begun to manufacture creams containing capsaicin, and the preparations go by many different names. Ask your pharmacist for the brands, as some of these are less expensive than Zostrix. One, called Capsin, is packaged with a unique applicator so that your hands do not even come in contact with the cream. Another new brand is called Pain-Free, which is distributed by To Your Health, Inc. (800-801-1406). This company also supplies some other natural vitamin and herbal supplements that have been useful for some FMS patients. They can send you a free brochure. Another type of topical cream is called Aurum and is composed of methylsalicylate, camphor, and menthol. In one study done by Dr. Romano and Dr. Stiller, Aurum helped reduce pain in almost half of the FMS patients. These creams are certainly worth trying! Dr. Phillip Mease of Seattle believes a new cream called Myo Rx, which contains omega-3 and omega-6 fatty acids, is effective in reducing pain levels. Sanford Roth, of Phoenix, Arizona, studied a topical NSAID cream called Hyanalgese-D, which was also effective in reducing pain levels. Ron Partain, Pharm D, prepares a customized topical pain reliever called Arizona Pain Gel. You may contact him at 800-400-7406; ronscompoundrx@aol.com. ArthoFlex Max (TDS) is a topical pain-relieving gel produced by Medical Merchandising, Inc. ArthoFlex Max-Cap is an external analgesic produced by the same company. If you have questions or wish to order either of these two topical creams, you may call 800-277-9167, fax 501-221-9946, or visit www.docholt.com. Biofreeze is a cooling gel that is helpful for some patients. You may order this product by calling 800-246-3733 or on their Web site: www.biofreeze.com.

Important Notes

▲ **Medications can lose their effectiveness over time.**
▲ **Try a new one.**
▲ **Practice creative prescribing between you and your physician.**
▲ **Stay in touch for news in drug treatments.**
▲ **Use a medication diary.**

Some patients do not need to take these medications every day or in the dosages suggested. Sometimes one half or one quarter the suggested dosage is all that is required every other day or every two days during those times when you are not experiencing a flare-up. To make it easy to cut your pill in half or quarters, you can purchase an inexpensive pill cutter at the drugstore. Remember, many FMS patients are very sensitive to these medications and sometimes the less, the better. Only you and your doctor can determine what works best for you. It may take some creative prescribing on your doctor's part, but it can be worked out.

If you begin to awaken more frequently at night, discuss with your doctor the option of making a change in your medication. An increase in dosage, the addition of another medication, or a change to a completely new medication may be suggested. Postponing this decision for weeks or months may contribute to a flare-up of symptoms if your sleep continues to be disrupted.

Some of these medications seem to lose their effectiveness after a period of time, so it may be necessary to change to another antidepressant for a period of time to give your body time to adjust. You might then be able to go back to your original medication after a few months and find that it works again.

Summary

▲ **Take an active role.**
▲ **New medications will be discovered.**

As more people are diagnosed with FMS and demand effective treatment, new medications to alleviate symptoms will appear. Researchers are experimenting at this very moment. Since it takes a long time for this information to filter down to you and your doctor, it is very important for you to take an active role in following advances in medication. It would be good if you stayed in touch with a support group, subscribed to an FMS newsletter, attended conferences, and kept in touch with a physician interested in your case.

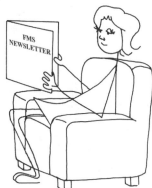

We have added a medication diary for you to include in your FMS journal. Keeping a written record of your medication, its side effects, dosages, and timing will be helpful to see how your medication is working for you. It will also enable your physician to make better judgments when prescribing your medications.

Questions to ask your physician about your medications

1. What dosage? _____

2. When? Morning or night? _____

3. Possible side effects? _____

4. How long should I try it? _____

5. Do I take it with food? _____

6. Does it interact with any other medications I take? _____

7. Does it interact with any vitamins? _____

8. Can I call the office with questions, or do I need to make an appointment? _____

9. What time can I call and with whom do I speak? _____

10. What does the medication look like? What shape is it? What color? Are there different

    dosages? _____

11. Can a generic be substituted? _____

12. What medications can I take and in what dosages when I am experiencing a

    flare-up of symptoms? _____

Comments _____

_____

_____

_____

_____

_____

_____

_____

_____

_____

_____

_____

_____

Medication Diary

MEDICATION	DOSAGE	DATE STARTED	TIME TAKEN	COMMENTS*	DATE DISCONTINUED

*Side effects, impact on sleep quality, etc.

Sample Contract for the Management of Opioid Maintenance Therapy for Nonmalignant Pain

1. Should be considered only after all other reasonable attempts at analgesia have failed.

2. A history of substance abuse should be viewed as a relative contraindication.

3. A single practitioner should take primary responsibility for treatment.

4. Patients should give informed consent before the start of therapy; points to be covered include recognition of the low risk of psychologic dependence as an outcome potential for cognitive impairment with the drug alone and in combination with sedative/hypnotics, and understanding by female patients that children born when the mother is on opioid maintenance therapy will be likely to be physically dependent at birth.

5. After drug selection, doses should be given on an around-the-clock basis; several weeks should be agreed upon as the period of initial dose titration, and although improvement in function should be continually stressed, all should agree to at least partial analgesia as the appropriate goal of therapy.

6. Failure to achieve at least partial analgesia at relatively low initial doses in the nontolerant patient raises questions about the potential treatability of the pain syndrome with opioids.

7. Emphasis should be given to attempts to capitalize on improved analgesia by gains in physical and social function.

8. In addition to the daily dose determined initially, patients should be permitted to escalate dose transiently on days of increased pain; two methods are acceptable:

   a) Prescription of an additional four-six "rescue doses" to be taken as needed during the month.

   b) Instruction that one or two extra doses may be taken on any day, but must be followed by an equal reduction of dose on subsequent days.

9. Patients must be seen and drugs prescribed at least monthly.

10. Exacerbations of pain not effectively treated by transient small increases in dose are best managed in the hospital, where dose escalation, if appropriate, can be observed closely and a return to baseline doses can be accomplished in a controlled environment.

11. Evidence of drug hoarding, acquisition of drugs from other physicians, uncontrolled dose escalation, or other aberrant behaviors should be followed by tapering and discontinuation of opioid maintenance therapy.

_____   _____
Patient Signature   Physician Signature

_____   _____
Date   Date

This sample contract has been reproduced with permission by Thomas Romano, M.D.

MEDICATIONS

TIPS Medication

▲ Never take your medications without fluids. Take a sip of water first an[...]

▲ One of the possible side effects of the tricyclics could be a dry mouth. A dr[...] long periods of time can increase the chance of tooth decay, particularly in peo[...] Sjogren's Syndrome, so do not forget to mention this to your doctor or dentist.

▲ Tricyclics can cause increased sensitivity to sunlight, so take precautions by using a su[...] block of at least SPF 15.

▲ Do not put your medications in a medicine cabinet that will be exposed to hot, humid weather. It is not wise to leave them in your car or purse where they might be exposed to heat build-up.

▲ Give up caffeine! It alters and interferes with your sleep pattern. Do not forget that there is caffeine in tea, iced tea, chocolate, and cola drinks. Also, many over-the-counter pain and cold medications contain caffeine.

▲ Alcohol interferes with your sleep quality and does not mix with these medications.

▲ Nicotine can affect medications.

▲ If you are just trying a new medication, ask for samples. Many fibromyalgia patients complain that their drawers are filled with unused medications.

▲ If you cannot tolerate these medications and want to try an alternative, there is a homeopathic remedy called Rhus Toxicodendron 6C that has been studied in England and found effective in treating fibromyalgia. There are homeopathic stores in larger cities, as well as homeopathic doctors. You can call 1-800-264-7661 (a consumer line of Boiron Labs) and they will give you the name of a pharmacy where this can be ordered.

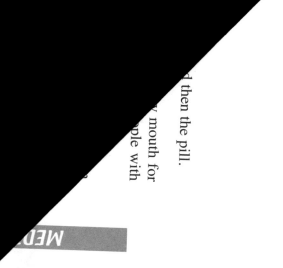

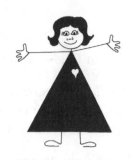

AIN MANAGEMENT

ndividuals vary in the way they describe their pain, express its
Their experience of pain often has both physical and emotional
n whether their pain is chronic or acute, on their past experiences
with pain, and on the degree of support that they have in their daily life. When pain begins to impact one's ability to function, the decision is often made to seek assistance from health professionals. For many, the goal is to decrease or eliminate pain, if possible, or at the very least to find ways of coping with it. Whatever one's goal, everyone experiencing pain deserves to have pain evaluated by a health professional and to receive guidance in its management.

Physical Medicine, Including Physical Therapy and Hands-on Modalities

There are a variety of physicians and other health professionals who treat the pain and dysfunction of fibromyalgia. Fibromyalgia was initially treated by rheumatologists, who are specialists in treating arthritis-related diseases. As treatment for fibromyalgia has evolved over time, other specialists have come to the forefront in treating the pain of fibromyalgia. They include

- ▲ **Physical medicine and rehabilitation physicians and clinics**
- ▲ **Pain specialists and pain clinics**
- ▲ **Fibromyalgia treatment centers**
- ▲ **Osteopathic doctors**
- ▲ **Chiropractors**
- ▲ **Physical therapists and physical therapy clinics**

Doctors of Physical Medicine and Rehabilitation

Doctors of physical medicine and rehabilitation, also known as physiatrists, are M.D. physicians specially trained in treating musculoskeletal and neurological problems. They are proficient in treating a wide range of problems, from sore shoulders and brain injuries to spinal cord injuries. They treat acute and chronic pain, and they see people who have been in car accidents or who have suffered strokes. They also treat paraplegics and those suffering from multiple sclerosis. They have become very important in the treatment of fibromyalgia patients, particularly for those who have other conditions along with fibromyalgia, such as arthritis and back or neck injuries. Their philosophy is one of treating the whole patient by addressing not only physical problems and injuries, but also the person's emotional, vocational, and social needs. The focus is on restoring function and improving quality of life for patients. Physiatrists may work in rehabilitation centers, hospitals, or private practice and may specialize in treating certain conditions such as brain injury or sports medicine. They have the ability to diagnose problems, prescribe medications, and direct physical therapy treatment programs.

Pain Specialists and Pain Clinics

Pain specialists and pain clinics include physicians and other health professionals who have expertise in pain management. Pain specialists may be found in hospital pain management clinics or may direct freestanding clinics. Large clinics located in hospitals are often multidisciplinary and include a team of doctors, nurses, psychologists, social workers, physical therapists, vocational counselors, and other health professionals who can contribute to treatment. Pain clinics in large hospitals are often closely linked to a variety of departments in the hospital such as physical medicine and rehabilitation, orthopedic surgery, neurosurgery, nutrition, psychiatry, and psychology. Physicians should be board certified in pain management. In large clinics, both inpatient and outpatient treatment may be offered. Large clinics may also have a pain management program that patients attend every day, a few times a week, or sometimes all day for weeks at a time. A referral is often needed from a primary physician to attend one of these programs. Different modalities for treating pain may be prescribed including medications and injection therapies to relieve specific pain, such as nerve blocks, bioelectric treatments, acupuncture, and others. These clinics may specialize in treating specific problems such as headaches, back pain, or sports injuries. When you are searching for a clinic, please be certain that the health professionals there are knowledgeable in treating fibromyalgia.

Fibromyalgia Treatment Centers

Some clinics are opening that specifically treat fibromyalgia. They may be directed by many types of physicians, including family practice doctors, internists, chiropractors, osteopathic doctors, physiatrists, rheumatologists, or neurologists. These clinics may or may not have pain specialists on staff and may or may not provide all of the forms of physical medicine described in this chapter.

Doctors of Osteopathic Medicine

Doctors of osteopathic medicine are physicians who are trained in a "whole person" philosophy to healthcare. A routine part of the osteopathic patient examination is a careful evaluation of the musculoskeletal system. Physical manipulations are often used to treat patients. These physicians can also prescribe medications and perform surgery.

Chiropractors

Chiropractors were once thought of as alternative physicians, but increasingly they work with M.D.s or as part of clinics that offer a broad spectrum of services. These specialists may provide treatment in physical medicine and rehabilitation centers, pain clinics, or solo practice.

Physical Therapists and Physical Therapy Clinics

Physical therapists are specially trained, licensed individuals who may work in hospitals, rehabilitation clinics, medical offices, nursing homes, athletic facilities, and private practice. Their goal is to restore physical function, improve mobility, relieve pain, and prevent or limit permanent physical disabilities in patients suffering from injuries or disease. Some physical therapists specialize in treating specific conditions such as low back pain, arthritis, heart disease, fractures, head injuries, and cerebral palsy. They strive to reduce pain, increase flexibility and range of motion, build strength, and correct posture. Physical therapy is often prescribed following spine or joint surgery to treat soft tissue trauma, nerve inflammation and injury, muscle spasms, arthritis, and fibromyalgia. Physical therapists may help set up a stretching, exercise, and strengthening program for patients. A physical therapy clinic may be a freestanding clinic or part of a larger hospital program, such as a pain clinic or rehabilitation clinic. A physician's referral is needed for treatment by a physical therapist.

If your doctor refers you to a physical therapist, make sure the therapist understands fibromyalgia and its treatment.

Physical Medicine Program

A physical medicine program can be an important component of your fibromyalgia treatment. Of course, the physician directing your treatment and the health professionals carrying out the modalities need to be knowledgeable about fibromyalgia. They need to know what is effective and what is not for helping with fibromyalgia's pain and dysfunction. Treatment that is too aggressive can cause a flare-up or increase your pain. Physicians will determine which modalities will be beneficial for your individual situation. Health professionals will work with you and your physician in mapping out a plan for you that may include

- ▲ Physical therapists
- ▲ Massage therapists
- ▲ Myofascial trigger point therapists
- ▲ Exercise physiologists
- ▲ Chiropractors

- ▲ Nurses
- ▲ Psychologists
- ▲ Social workers
- ▲ Hypnotherapists
- ▲ Biofeedback practitioners

- ▲ Occupational therapists
- ▲ Hand therapists
- ▲ Rehabilitation counselors

Components of a Physical Medicine Program May Include

- ▲ Myofascial trigger point therapy
- ▲ Therapeutic massage
- ▲ Myofascial release
- ▲ Spray and stretch

- ▲ Stretching with heat
- ▲ Heat, ice, or acupressure
- ▲ Ultrasound or TENS
- ▲ Craniosacral therapy

These Treatment Programs Offer Education on

- ▲ Adaptive equipment
- ▲ Footwear and clothing
- ▲ Pacing principles

Myofascial Trigger Point Therapy

Myofascial Pain Syndrome (MPS)

Myofascial pain syndrome is often confused with fibromyalgia. Some physicians, including Mark Pelligrino, M.D., believe that myofascial pain syndrome and fibromyalgia are similar conditions and can be related. Others feel that the two conditions are very different. You may have both conditions at the same time. If you have both, each condition can amplify and exacerbate the other. Myofascial pain syndrome is characterized by painful muscles and the presence of trigger points and taut bands of muscle fibers which are ropey and painful when palpated. Fibromyalgia is diagnosed by the presence of tender points, which do not refer pain and are not hard or knotted.

Some people who experience myofascial pain may be misdiagnosed as having fibromyalgia. A physical trauma may set up conditions for a localized myofascial pain syndrome to develop such as in the neck, shoulders, or back. If trigger points and tight ropey muscle bands are not present, then localized pain may be called regional fibromyalgia. If myofascial pain is not treated properly, or if one is predisposed to developing fibromyalgia, some doctors theorize that myofascial pain may spread to become widespread fibromyalgia pain. **It is important to have a thorough**

assessment by a qualified professional to determine if you have myofascial pain syndrome, fibromyalgia, or both and which treatment options will be most beneficial for you.

Myofascial pain syndrome is found equally in men and women, while 90% of patients who are diagnosed with FMS are women. MPS is usually more localized than fibromyalgia. People who have myofascial pain syndrome may feel fatigued and have problems with sleep. Fibromyalgia patients generally experience more widespread pain and an achy, flulike feeling all over. They also have sleep difficulties and more cognitive problems. You may have both MPS and FMS at the same time.

MPS can be treated by myofascial trigger point therapy, trigger point injections, anti-inflammatory medications, muscle relaxants, pain medications, and other treatments. If you have fibromyalgia and do not have trigger points, then some of these treatments may not benefit you.

Trigger Points vs Tender Points

▲ **Trigger points refer pain; tender points do not.**
▲ **Trigger points cause numerous symptoms.**
▲ **Trigger points can be caused by a variety of problems.**
▲ **Trigger points can be treated.**
▲ **Tender points are unique to fibromyalgia.**

Many FMS patients are confused about the difference between tender points and trigger points. Trigger points are small, contracted knots in the muscles that can be felt with your fingers and may feel like a small lump or stone under your skin. They emit their own electrical signals, which can be measured by specialized electronic equipment. They are different from tender points.

Tender points are the specific points on the body that, when touched, feel tender to the person being touched. Tender points are the areas physicians touch or feel to determine the diagnosis of FMS and are not areas in which the muscles are knotted or have a lumpy feel. (Tender point areas used in diagnosis are noted on a diagram in the "Symptoms and Diagnosis" chapter.)

Trigger points have been well studied by two physicians, Dr. Janet Travell and Dr. David Simons. Their classic textbook *Myofascial Pain and Dysfunction: The Trigger Point Manual* describes trigger points in detail. Many massage therapists, physical therapists, and myofascial trigger point therapists have training in defusing trigger points.

Trigger points can cause patients a lot of pain and discomfort. A confusing aspect about them is that they can cause pain in an area far away from the actual site of the trigger point. This is called referred pain. Tender points do not refer pain. For instance, trigger points in your scalene muscles located on the side of your neck can cause pain in your chest, upper arm, lower arm, thumb, and forefinger, as well as in an area near your shoulder blade. Many FMS patients suffer with Temporal-Mandibular-joint pain which could be set off by trigger points located in the masseter muscles in the jaw. Trigger points in this area can cause pain in the front of the face near the sinuses, in the teeth, and in the ear, along with ringing in the ears. Trigger points are common, can be found in any muscle of the body, and can last indefinitely if they are not deactivated by proper treatment. Muscles affected by trigger points feel hard; they may limit your range of motion and cause stiffness in your joints.

Trigger points may arise after surgery or after a joint is forced to remain immobile by the use of splints or braces. They can begin after a physical trauma such as whiplash, sprain, fracture, or dislocation. Repetitive movements can cause them, as can poor body mechanics or asymmetry of a body part. Trigger points can cause numerous symptoms besides pain, which may include weakness, dizziness, blurred vision, goose bumps, headaches, pain during intercourse, nausea, diarrhea, numbness, and cold extremities—depending on the location of the trigger point. Dr. Travell believed that fibromyalgia could begin with the appearance of trigger points in various places of the body.

Treatment of Trigger Points and Myofascial Pain

The good news about trigger points is that they can be treated by a technique called myofascial trigger point therapy. Specially trained massage therapists, and myofascial trigger point therapists can treat them, or you can treat them yourself once you have some education in this area. Biofeedback or relaxation therapy can help patients learn to relax tense, tight muscles. Trigger point injections may be helpful as well.

Relieving the referred pain of trigger points requires pressing and compression on the knot for 30-60 seconds, slowly releasing the pressure, and then massaging it. Massage is better done with tools, rather than your fingers, as your fingers will tire quickly. Deep, stroking massage is best done in one direction only. Massaging the muscle can be done for as long as you like and you can perform this technique up to 12 times per day for better relief. Although this process may be painful, when done in the right "spot," it should eventually lead to less pain. If the trigger point returns in the future, you can treat it again with the same technique. Tender points cannot be treated in this manner.

Acupressure is a compression technique. Many fibromyalgia patients constantly rub their shoulders or may ask their family members to rub their sore knots. Tools are available to help facilitate breaking up the knots or tight bands, allowing your fingers to rest! Two that you can try are the Thera Cane and the Backnobber. These tools are made of fiberglass and designed to allow you to put pressure on the knots or tight bands easily. The Thera Cane is available from the Thera Cane company at www.theracane.net or by calling 800-587-1203. The Backnobber can be ordered from the Pressure Positive company at www.backtools.com or by calling 800-603-5107.

Other useful tools are available from these companies. There are larger balls to roll on and long cylindrical foam rollers which can be useful in performing compression. Your therapist can help you decide which tools are best for you to try. A smaller device called the jacknobber can be ordered from Orthopedic Physical Therapy Products at 888-819-0121 or at their website www.optp.com. Videos and instructions on the product's use can be ordered from the respective companies.

You can also place tennis balls into a stocking or sock and roll on them on the floor or up against a wall to put pressure on the trigger point areas. Body rolling as a form of myofascial release involves the use of five-, six-, or seven-inch therapy balls to provide blood flow and circulation to tight, constricted areas. Cheryl Soleway has an excellent instructional video and ball to use. Contact FitBALL,USA at 800-752-2255 for ordering information or go to www.balldynamics.com.

Self-care

Treating Trigger Points and Myofascial Pain Yourself

By Mary Biancalana B.S., M.S., C.M.T.P.T.

Mary Biancalana, B.S., M.S., C.M.T.P.T., is a Nationally Board Certified Myofascial Trigger Point Therapist, Director of Self-Care at the Fibromyalgia Treatment Centers of America based in Chicago, Illinois. She has graciously provided this information on treating trigger points that includes her self-care protocol. Mary is also a certified personal trainer with the American Council on Exercise and holds a master's degree in education. She has many years of experience working exclusively with fibromyalgia patients and patients experiencing myofascial pain. She has conducted seminars and exercise classes, and she trains other professionals in the techniques outlined here. She can be reached at The Fibromyalgia Treatment Centers of America by calling 773-604-5321 or faxing 773-604-5231.

A good self-care routine consists of

- ▲ **Warm-up or heat**
- ▲ **Use of compression tools**
- ▲ **Stretching and relaxation of the muscles**
- ▲ **Full range of motion of the joint close to the compression**

These steps are extremely important in coping with and decreasing the pain from trigger points or fibromyalgia pain symptoms if trigger points are present. By using simple, self-care protocols, you will gain power over your pain, feel less helpless, and begin to live a fuller, more pain-free life.

Compression helps you become aware of areas held in chronic tightness. By becoming aware of tightness or tension in the muscles, you will be able to begin to notice when the muscles are contracting for no reason, and you can breathe and concentrate on relaxing held tension.

This self-care technique helps to break up the pain-tightness-pain cycle present in myofascial pain and fibromyalgia patients. Self-care activities allow you to feel empowered and proactive in your journey to achieve reduced pain and fuller function in your life.

Because a large percentage of fibromyalgia patients may have developed trigger points in their muscles (myofascial pain syndrome), it is important that you evaluate your pain on a muscle-by-muscle basis to determine if trigger points are a source of pain for you.

Many muscle pains are actually referred from a distant trigger point location. In realizing that muscle pain from trigger points is referred to a distant area, it is important to know that pressing where it hurts probably will not help much with reducing your pain. A far distant muscle may actually be causing the deep ache, sharp pain, or weakness you are feeling. *To effectively reduce the pain, it is important to locate the exact trigger point area that is causing the referred pain.*

Recommended Self-care Protocol

- ▲ **Warm-up or heat** - Try to apply some form of heat to the area that you will be compressing. A warm shower, bath, hot tub soak, Fomentek water bag, or another type of moist heat wrap will provide heat to areas that have hard, tight muscles or dysfunctional tissue. This heat helps to provide local circulation and will help you break up the pain-tightness-pain cycle. A warm-up can also be five to ten minutes of light exercise or local movement. Fomentek bags are filled with water and placed on the area to be treated. They are available at 800-562-4328 or at www.fomentek.com.

on - Using a good referred pain index or chart such as those provided in the
in our resource section at the end of this chapter, locate muscles and trigger
end to treat. This can help you determine exactly where to apply
Press on the area of hard, tight tissue, gently but firmly, breathe, and
ng for 30 to 60 seconds. Try to relax any tightness in the area that you are
ng. It is important to keep the muscle in a position of good neutral posture or
a slight stretch. Breathe from the diaphragm, not from the chest, and hold for a cycle
of three relaxed breaths. Slowly remove the pressure and relocate your tool (or finger) to
another spot. As you become experienced with this technique and learn what feels best,
you may hold for a shorter or longer time depending on your ability to relax the area.
Follow immediately with the next step in the protocol, which is stretching.

▲ **Stretch or actively contract and relax** - After you have compressed a particular group of
muscles or area, you are ready for a gentle and relaxed stretch of those muscles. Breathe
in as you begin the stretch. Stay relaxed and do not pull to the point of pain, just a feeling
of stretch. Hold and try to relax into the stretch as far as you can. Take a final breath and
exhale as you complete your stretch. Actively contracting the muscle, holding, then
exhaling and releasing into a further stretch is another technique to use. Go on to the next
and final stage.

▲. **Range of motion movement** - This component is extremely important when you have
fibromyalgia or myofascial pain syndrome, because having pain usually causes us to hold
and guard a joint or area. When muscles are inhibited, they develop more trigger point
areas and worsen the pain-dysfunction-pain cycle. Remember, we are trying to break up
these muscle-holding patterns. Movement should be done in all different planes: forward,
back, rotation, twist, flex and extension are all important. Put on your favorite music and
breathe while aiming for a smooth, gentle range of motion and movement.

This self-care protocol can help you improve your function and experience less pain. Follow this
sequence as many times a day as possible.

Enjoy and feel empowerment over some of your fibromyalgia symptoms!

Examples of trigger point therapy or self-care:

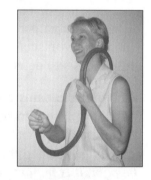

▲ The Backnobber and Thera Cane are tools that are specifically
designed to apply trigger point pressure with the best ergonomics in
mind. In this example, you can see the Backnobber on the upper
trapezius muscle (upper shoulder area). This muscle area can be a
cause of headache pain, ear pain, and pain at the spot.

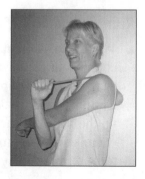

▲ A tennis ball in a stocking or sock can be a useful tool for myofascial
compression in many areas. The key is to be relaxed and not to use
any muscular effort in the area that you are compressing.

The Trigger Point Therapy Workbook: Your Self Treatment Guide For Pain Relief, by Davies, is an excellent resource to help guide you in treating your trigger points. This book show where trigger points are located in every muscle of the body and how to treat them. Devin Starlanyl, M.D., also has written two excellent books that explain myofascial trigger point treatment. If you intend to try this yourself, get a book to guide you or seek professional guidance.

Perpetuating Factors

You must eliminate or correct perpetuating factors before eradicating trigger points indefinitely. If you have abnormal bone structure or postural problems due to poorly designed chairs or work stations, perform repetitive movements that aggravate muscles, or are sedentary, you may have to change those factors before feeling better. Sometimes, your sleeping position can aggravate symptoms, particularly if you sleep on your stomach or in a fetal position. Using a pillow between your knees while sleeping can help relieve knee, leg, or back pain, and a pillow at your chest to rest your arm on while sleeping can help reduce arm, neck, or shoulder pain. Some people have one leg that is shorter than the other, differences in their hips, short arms, foot or toe abnormalities, or spinal rotation that can contribute to pain. Specially trained myofascial trigger point therapists, hands-on therapists, physicians, or chiropractors can evaluate these problems and help correct them.

Dr. Travell believed that, vitamin deficiencies must be cleared up before trigger points can be defeated. Vitamins that she felt are important and may be deficient are B1, B6 and B12, C, folic acid, calcium, iron, magnesium, and potassium. She also theorized that metabolic disorders such as thyroid insufficiency, estrogen insufficiency, hypoglycemia, and high levels of uric acid present in the blood must be corrected before trigger points can be erased. Dr. Travell believed that nicotine, caffeine, and alcohol should be avoided because of their negative effects on metabolism.

Many physicians and patients are finding that in order to help reduce FMS symptoms, patients must improve their nutrition, balance their hormones and watch their diet. They may also try guaifenesin, which removes uric acid from the blood. Check the chapter "Diet and Nutritional Supplements" for more information.

Some other modalities which help relieve trigger points include spray and stretch, trigger point injections, botox injections, myofascial release, acupressure, and compression and stretch.

Taking care of your trigger points, if you have them, may help reduce your pain levels.

Myofascial trigger point therapists are specially trained in treating this problem. To find a trained therapist in your area, contact the National Association of Myofascial Trigger Point Therapists at www.myofascialtherapy.org.

Massage

▲ **Promotes deep muscle relaxation**　　▲ **Loosens tight muscles**
▲ **Increases circulation**　　▲ **Relieves pain and spasms**
▲ **Reduces stress**

Heat is often used before massage to help relax painful and tight muscles. While many people with fibromyalgia initially receive massage as a part of their physical therapy, many continue massage with a massage therapist after physical therapy has been completed. Massage therapists often practice in health clubs, local YMCA or YWCA facilities, or private offices. Check your yellow pages for certified massage therapists and ask to be scheduled with a therapist who has worked with clients who have FMS. Full or partial-body massages are usually available, with prices ranging from $50 to $125 for a full hour. Although massage therapy is often not covered by insurance, it may be well worth the cost if it helps you to feel better and remain active and productive. Many massage products are available at www.massagewarehouse.com; 800-507-3416.

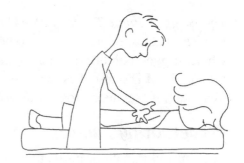

Myofascial Release

▲ **Frees up constricted areas**
▲ **Releases pressure**
▲ **Relieves pain**
▲ **Promotes the flow of blood and lymph**
▲ **Improves range of motion**

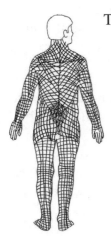

The fascia is a tough connective tissue that surrounds every muscle, bone, nerve, blood vessel, and organ of the body. When it surrounds muscle, it's called myofascial tissue. (This drawing illustrates myofascial tissue.) It can be described as a three-dimensional stocking that runs from head to toe. Fascial restrictions often occur in people with fibromyalgia and feel like "knots" or "bands" of tight and painful muscle. The fascial restrictions may be altered by myofascial release. When the therapist has determined where the contracted "bands" or "knots" are in the muscle, he or she applies gentle pressure in the direction of the restrictions. This gentle, hands-on technique can free up constricted areas, release pressure, relieve pain, promote the flow of blood and lymph, and improve range of motion.

Spray and Stretch

▲ **Use to manage myofascial pain**
▲ **Spray skin over tight muscle group**
▲ **Stretch muscle gently**

This technique uses a vapo-coolant spray on a particularly tight muscle group or to manage myofascial pain. The spray deadens the pain while the contracted muscle is stretched by the therapist. This technique can help stretch tight muscles and deactivate trigger points. After receiving instructions on how to perform spray and stretch from your therapist, you may use the technique at home. It is helpful to request that a family member or friend also be instructed in this technique by your therapist because it is difficult to do by yourself. Ice can be used instead of the spray to elicit a similar response. A product called Spray and Stretch is available by prescription only. Another product, Instant Ice, is available at some drugstores without a prescription. You will need to ask the pharmacist for Instant Ice as it is not on the shelf. For additional information on vapo-coolant sprays, contact the Gebauer company at 800-321-9348, or on their Web site at www.gebauerco.com.

PAIN MANAGEMENT

Stretching with Heat

▲ **Apply moist heat.**
▲ **Stretch muscle gently.**

It can also be helpful to use heat before stretching a muscle group. In order to facilitate stretching, the muscle must be as relaxed as possible. This can be accomplished through moist heat in the form of hot packs, a hot tub, or by directing a hot shower on the muscle. Apply the moist heat for 10 to 20 minutes. Then gently stretch the muscle until an easy stretch is felt; hold for 10 to 20 seconds or a bit longer and then relax. This technique can gradually stretch out the contracted muscle and surrounding myofascial tissue. Adding Epsom Salts or essential oils to the bathwater may be helpful.

Stretching without the use of ice or heat throughout the day can also be helpful, but remember to stretch gently.

Important Note

If you have had recent surgery or have a muscle or joint problem, including hypermobility, consult your healthcare professional before stretching.

Heat, Ice, and Acupressure

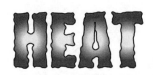

Heat may be helpful before a massage and before your stretching exercises; heat may also be used to aid relaxation, pain relief, and muscle stiffness. Microwavable gel packs, heating pads, warm baths and showers, whirlpools, down quilts, long underwear, and paraffin baths are examples of heat sources. Paraffin baths are designed to be used especially on hands and fingers. Liquid paraffin has the advantage of applying even heat to all joints of your hands and fingers, decreasing pain and stiffness and increasing blood flow. One source for a paraffin wax heat therapy bath is www.vitalityweb.com; 800-796-9656. If you choose to use a hot pack, place a light towel between your skin and the hot pack and leave it on the area for approximately 20 minutes.

Important Note

Avoid prolonged exposure to heat sources that could cause burns. Check your skin periodically! Do not go to sleep with a heating pad on.

The local application of ice can decrease pain, muscle spasms and swelling. Frozen gel packs, ice packs, and packages of frozen vegetables are examples of ice sources. Place a light towel between your skin and the ice pack and leave the pack on the area for approximately 10 to 20 minutes.

Important Note

Check your skin periodically. If the area being treated turns white or blue, discontinue treatment immediately.

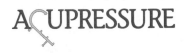

Some people with fibromyalgia experience some pain relief when they put gentle pressure on tight palpable bands or knots. This technique is called acupressure. For additional information on acupressure, see page 84.

Ultrasound and TENS

Some health professionals recommend ultrasound and/or TENS in the initial treatment phase to reduce pain and muscle spasms. Ultrasound is often administered by a physical therapist. It uses high frequency sound waves to direct heat deep into soft tissues, promoting circulation, relaxing muscles, and reducing pain. TENS (transcutaneous electrical nerve stimulation) practitioners tape electrode patches on the skin in painful areas and connect the patches by a wire to a battery-operated stimulator. Stimulation to the nerves by TENS may cause some tingling as it works to block pain impulses. A portable TENS unit may be prescribed for daily use if found to be helpful in therapy. The amount of pain relief from ultrasound or TENS varies from person to person. Talk with your health professional about whether either or both might benefit you.

Craniosacral Therapy

Developed by Dr. John Upledger, this manual technique is applied to the spinal cord. It enhances the flow of cerebrospinal fluid. It is a relaxing and gentle treatment that is noninvasive.

These Treatment Programs May Also Offer Education on

▲ **Adaptive equipment**
▲ **Footwear and clothing**
▲ **Pacing principles**

Adaptive Equipment

Many therapy devices are recommended by physical therapists. They include cervical pillows, lumbar supports, portable massage wands, hot and cold gel packs, portable shiatsu massagers, pen and pencil grips, and Thera Canes. The following catalogs include many of these helpful products and more that can make working, playing, and simply living a bit easier. The 800 phone numbers for each catalog are included, so you may call and order a catalog to be sent to your home. Many of these products may also be purchased in drug, department, or specialty stores. Brookstone, a specialty store found in many local shopping centers, carries a nice assortment of adaptive equipment. Talk with your physical therapist about what items might be best for you.

Adaptability	**800-243-9232**	www.ssww.com
BackSaver products	**888-867-2225**	www.sitincomfort.com
Many different brands	**800-303-7574**	www.comfortchannel.com
Enrichments	**800-323-5547**	www.sammonspreston.com
Gebauer Co.	**800-321-9348**	www.gebauerco.com
Functional Solutions	**800-235-7054**	www.beabletodo.com
Ortho. Physical Therapy Products	**888-819-0121**	www.optp.com
Pressure Positive	**800-603-5107**	www.backtools.com
Saunders Group Inc.	**800-778-1864**	www.thesaundersgroup.com
Solutions	**877-718-7901**	www.solutionscatalog.com

Footwear

Comfortable shoes with good support and extra cushioning are an important investment. Both Easy Spirit and Rockport make excellent walking shoes with extra cushioning to help absorb the shock of walking. Nike, New Balance, and other athletic shoe companies make similar shoes. Socks with extra cushioning may also be a good investment.

If you have a lot of pain when walking on the front part of your foot, or the metatarsus, you may benefit from having a metatarsal orthotic fitted for your shoes. The orthotic will redistribute the weight on your foot when walking and help to decrease your discomfort. If this is a concern for you, discuss this with your physician. (You will need a prescription.)

If you are experiencing a lot of pain in your feet, you will want to consider having your physician or podiatrist further assess them. It's important to find out if a condition other than fibromyalgia is causing your discomfort. Various orthodics or other treatments may be helpful and make walking less painful.

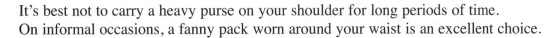

Clothing

Dress comfortably whenever you can! Loose knit clothing that is easy to put on and to take off works especially well when you're experiencing a flare-up of fibromyalgia symptoms.

It's best not to carry a heavy purse on your shoulder for long periods of time. On informal occasions, a fanny pack worn around your waist is an excellent choice.

Pacing Principles

The importance of pacing is often discussed by physical therapists and other health professionals as they guide individuals with fibromyalgia in developing an exercise and stretching program. Pacing needs to be incorporated throughout the day in order for fibromyalgia to be successfully managed. Although pacing can be a challenge for many of us, we encourage you to embrace the following pacing principles as you strive for a better balance of work, rest, and leisure.

▲ Take frequent breaks throughout your day to rest, stretch, and relax your muscles.

▲ If you need to sit or stand for long periods of time or are working on a lengthy demanding task, take frequent short breaks to change positions and to move around.

▲ When you're engaged in activities that include a lot of repetitive movements (e.g. computer work, household cleaning tasks, etc.), you may need to take breaks even more often than usual. A general guideline is to break from a repetitive activity every 20 to 30 minutes.

▲ Alternate activities in order to use different muscles and give other muscles a rest.

▲ If you're in a car for an hour or more, stop and get out for a short walk and stretch.

▲ When you're having a "good" day, resist the temptation to overdo and to work or play with no breaks. Many people with fibromyalgia will pay later with increased fatigue, muscle stiffness, aching, and/or pain.

▲ Take breaks before you get tired and before you're experiencing increased muscle strain. You may need to set a timer to remind yourself to stop.

PAIN MANAGEMENT

Therapy Resources and Techniques

Pain Erasure by Bonnie Prudden gives some helpful tips on how and why massage and myotherapy can ease painful muscles. This may be a helpful resource for you and assist you in understanding why these techniques can be an important component of your overall treatment program.

Demonstration of Trigger Point Injections Video by Robert Bennett, MD. Order at www.myalgia.com

Fibromyalgia and Chronic Myofascial Pain: A Survival Manual, by D. Starlanyl and M.E. Copeland. New Harbinger Publications, 2001.

The Trigger Point Therapy Workbook: Your Self-Treatment Guide for Pain Relief by C. Davies. Harbinger Publications, 2001.

The Painmaster MCT patch is a topical patch that uses microcurrent technology to reduce pain. You can learn more about it at the Web site, www.paincontrolrx.net or call for information at 800-426-3179.

TIPS *Physical Medicine and Hands-on Treatments*

▲ Physical therapy and other hands-on modalities may help many people with fibromyalgia feel better. A health professional who is knowledgeable about fibromyalgia can help you find the treatment that is best for you.

▲ Remember that many times it takes three to four treatments before you begin to feel any benefit. Don't give up too soon!

▲ If you experience massage that is too deep for too long or stretching that is too much, you may have a "rebound effect" and feel increased pain and soreness the following day or two. Heat, particularly moist heat, can be very helpful.

▲ Remember to ask your therapist if you can bring a willing family member or friend to be instructed in massage, stretching, and/or spray and stretch. This family member or friend can be invaluable during times of a flare-up of symptoms and for those times that you cannot see a physical therapist.

▲ You need a doctor's prescription for physical therapy or myofascial trigger point treatments if insurance is to pay for it.

▲ Most insurance companies do not include massage therapists in their coverage. If you find that massage helps you remain active and feel better, you may want to have an occasional massage anyway. Your health and well-being are well worth the cost!

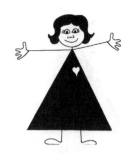

ACUPUNCTURE

Acupuncture is a traditional method of treating illness in Asia. It has been gaining acceptance in our Western World. It has been used for centuries by Asian physicians for all types of illness and has been noted to be especially helpful in alleviating musculoskeletal pain. A treatment consists of inserting very fine needles in specific points of the body. After the needles are inserted, the acupuncturist might use electrical stimulation, burn herbs, or manually stimulate the needles. There should be little or no pain upon insertion of the needles. Once they are in, the patient should not feel them at all and may even lapse into a state of drowsy relaxation. A treatment lasts for 30 minutes to one hour and prices can vary from $60 to over $100. Some of our Western physicians are trained in the technique; many Asian physicians have been using the technique for years. Make sure that the doctor you choose to do acupuncture is licensed and uses disposable needles for your safety.

It is not known how acupuncture works. Many believe it helps unblock chi, which is believed to be the life force that drives physical processes and motivates emotions. If chi becomes blocked, imbalances can result in our bodies, causing physical or emotional illness. Western physicians believe it works to relieve pain by blocking the pathways that send painful signals throughout our bodies. There have been a few studies done on acupuncture and FMS, and one in particular, using electroacupuncture, showed improvement in over half the patients participating in the study. A few patients felt worse after treatment, however. Acupuncture might be a modality for you to consider as part of your overall treatment plan, particularly if you have not benefited from medication and other methods of pain relief.

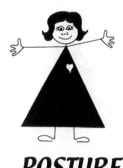

POSTURE

Good posture and correct body alignment are important in helping to alleviate undue strain on your muscles, joints, ligaments, and tendons. Take a moment to look in a mirror and examine your posture, both standing and sitting. It's important to stand or sit up straight with your shoulders back and your chin tucked in. If you become aware of what your posture and body alignment should be and try to maintain them, you will reduce the stress on your muscles and thereby relieve the pain and discomfort that occurs from holding muscles in a poor position for extended periods.

Many people with fibromyalgia have muscle aching and pain in their neck and trapezius muscle (a large muscle in the neck, shoulder and upper back). If they assume a forward lean posture (as shown in the illustration), for long periods of time, additional strain is added to these muscles and their pain and aching increases. A forward lean posture is easy to assume when working at a desk or computer, especially when you are not at the correct working height. Please refer to the diagram below, which shows an example of good posture and correct body alignment when sitting at a computer.

Learning to stretch muscles that may have become constricted over time because of poor posture can be important in helping you to maintain good posture and correct body alignment. Bob Anderson's book *Stretching*, is an excellent resource for stretching exercises. *Self-Help Manual for Your Back*, by H.D. Saunders, is also an excellent resource for posture, stretching exercises and good back care. A physical therapist can be very helpful in teaching you the correct stretching exercises and can instruct you in good posture and correct body alignment. An occupational therapist is trained to help people restructure their work and home environments to maintain good posture and decrease the energy required to do a specific task. Yoga can be a helpful adjunct to improving overall flexibility and strength. It also has the additional benefit of improving your posture! If you have concerns or questions regarding posture, don't hesitate to ask a physical or occupational therapist for an evaluation.

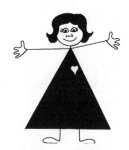

PRACTICAL COPING TIPS

The following tips are additional ways of coping that we've found to be helpful. Try some and see if they're helpful for you, too. The tips are organized in the following categories: fatigue, family and friends' support, memory problems, morning stiffness, and miscellaneous coping tips. You may want to write down other practical coping methods that you've discovered on your own at the end of this section. There are additional tips at the end of most sections in this book.

Fatigue

Fatigue can be one of the most debilitating and frustrating symptoms for FMS patients. The fatigue you are experiencing is most likely different from any fatigue you have experienced before and may be overwhelming. Some people describe this fatigue as being similar to experiencing constant jet lag. The levels of fatigue patients experience can range from mild to severe. Some people have enough energy to lead a fairly normal life, and others have a great deal of difficulty getting out of bed. Some find they are energetic for a few hours during the day and then a few hours later can barely move because fatigue has overcome them. FMS sufferers often say they feel they have "hit the wall" with their fatigue and can go no further. It definitely can be frustrating. Not knowing when the fatigue will strike is stressful and makes it difficult to plan your daily activities. It is reassuring to know that as your symptoms improve, your fatigue levels should improve as well.

Tips for Coping with Fatigue

▲ **Plan**
▲ **Pace**
▲ **Prioritize**

Helps to reduce fatigue and pain.

Plan

▲ Speak to your physician about medication to get a good night's rest. Lack of sleep is the major contributor to feeling fatigued. Waking up and going to sleep at the same time each day is important.

▲ Use schedules, lists, and calendars. These are also useful for coping with memory problems. You can purchase planners and calendars that will fit in a purse or can be left by a desk. Please do not try to fit too many activities into one day. A "to do" list is great for keeping you reminded of what you need to do each day, but be realistic about the number of items on your list. Cross off each "done" item and see how much you've accomplished!

▲ Plan for a rest period each day. Schedule a longer period of time during the week, an afternoon or even a day if possible, when you can relax and take care of yourself. This is particularly important to have planned into your schedule after you have a busy series of events.

▲ Plan to do an activity that you enjoy each day. We all feel less fatigued when participating in an activity we like doing.

▲ Organize your home so things are within easy reach for you. You shouldn't have to do any unnecessary reaching for items stacked in high cabinets or spend extra time sorting through cluttered closets and drawers. It may take some time to get organized, but it will be worth the effort.

▲ Drink plenty of water. Dehydration can result in fatigue.

▲ Are you eating well-balanced meals? Lack of proper nutrition robs us of energy. Eating smaller meals, evenly spaced throughout the day, will help keep blood-sugar levels controlled. See our "Diet and Nutritional Supplements" chapter for additional information.

▲ Exercise. If you do not overdo, exercise can increase your endurance and boost your energy level. Please refer to the "Exercise" chapter for help with planning an exercise program.

▲ Plan activities so you alternate a restful or an uplifting activity with a strenuous one. For example, do not plan to vacuum and scrub floors in the same day. Vacuum, then write letters or pay the bills. Scrub floors another day.

▲ Avoid errands or shopping during busy traffic hours. You will feel less stressed. Shopping during off hours will allow you to spend less time standing in long lines and will save your energy.

Pace

▲ Pacing is a challenge. It seems we all want to do everything during those times when we feel better, but then feel exhausted from overdoing and send ourselves into a flare-up! Be realistic about the goals and activities you set for yourself.

▲ Take frequent short rest breaks during the day. Stretch, take deep breaths, or just close your eyes and listen to soothing music.

▲ Use a relaxation tape when you feel most fatigued. You may be amazed at how refreshed you will feel afterwards. You might even feel better than if you had taken a nap!

▲ Try to do your heavy or difficult tasks when you know you will have more energy.

▲ Listen to your body. Rest before you get overtired. Sometimes this is difficult for FMS patients; we are tired all the time and do not realize when we have overdone it, until it's too late.

Prioritize

▲ Take care of the important things first. Your stress load might be reduced if you do the tasks you really dislike doing first. This will save you worry time, which will alleviate some fatigue caused by worry!

▲ Decide which activities you do not need to do. Which ones can you postpone? Sometimes we do things that might be better left undone.

▲ Ask other people to help you with tasks you find difficult.

- Learn to say no. Many of us are overcommitted. Weigh what you have to do against what you want to do.

- Make yourself and your health priorities.

Family and Friends' Support

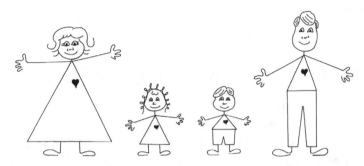

It's often difficult for family members and friends to understand the degree of pain and fatigue that you're experiencing, because fibromyalgia is an invisible condition. You may feel isolated and lonely and believe that "nobody understands." As you struggle with chronic pain and fatigue, you may have a tendency to conserve energy by further isolating yourself. By doing so, you may be cutting off the very support that you need in order to live successfully with fibromyalgia.

Take time to inventory your support system. Identify those individuals who are helpful and those who are not. Well-meaning family members and friends can't always give you the kind of support that's really helpful. During this inventory process, identify those family members and friends who are more supportive and helpful in certain situations. Clarify the strengths and weaknesses of your support network and begin to elicit support from those best able to help you. When you're able, nurture those individuals closest to you; your support network is a valuable asset.

Things to Say to Your Family and Friends:

- Although I look well and don't complain, please understand that much of the time I do not feel well. I am in pain and have overwhelming fatigue.

- Please understand when I tell you that I can't go on an outing or engagement. I wish that I could do all the things that I'd like to do.

- You are experiencing the loss of a healthy me. Share your feelings about this loss, but please don't be angry with me. I didn't choose to have fibromyalgia. It is not my fault, and I grieve too.

- Let's do things together on days when I feel good or schedule them earlier in the day when I have the most energy. Can we go out to brunch rather than dinner? Can we celebrate at home?

- When we go to the zoo, please understand I need frequent rest breaks. We can have fun and enjoy our times together, but we may have to adapt and do things a bit differently.

- When I'm having a flare-up, please ask me how you can help. Offer me a back rub. Remind me that even though the pain is bad now, it won't last forever.

- Believe me when I say I have pain. So much of the time, I suffer in silence! Tell me you believe me.

- Support me in all I must do to take care of myself—rest, sleep, relaxation, medication, medical care, support, and exercise.

▲ Keep telling me you care about me. Affirm my courage and my efforts to get better.

▲ Recognize that I often feel irritable when I am fatigued and in pain. I don't mean to hurt you.

▲ Hug me, give me warm touches and loving words of acceptance.

▲ I appreciate all you do to help support me, even when I forget to tell you so.

▲ Always remember how important your love and support are to my well-being and my success in meeting the challenges of living with fibromyalgia.

Memory Problems: CRS—Can't Remember Stuff!

Many individuals with fibromyalgia experience cognitive problems. Trying to remember a name, putting the wrong word in a sentence, forgetting what your supervisor just told you to do five minutes ago, misplacing things, an inability to concentrate on reading or studying are common complaints of many FMS patients. Sometimes these problems in cognitive functioning are referred to as "fibro-fog." When fibromyalgia symptoms flare-up, often memory and concentration problems will also be more severe. It is not fully understood why this occurs, because the brain's processing system is very complex. It is known, however, that poor sleep quality exacerbates cognitive problems. As you get better, your difficulties with memory and concentration should lessen. If your cognitive problems are extreme, discuss your symptoms with your physician. Further evaluation may be necessary.

Tips for Coping with Memory Problems:

▲ Use a desk calendar large enough to write in the activities you need to do each day. Check it every day.

▲ Make a list of important phone numbers for each phone in your house. Tape it next to the phone, to the wall, or inside a cabinet so it does not "walk away."

▲ Keep a pad of paper next to your favorite chair with a pen to jot down notes to yourself.

▲ Buy a pocket recording message tape player that you can speak into and leave audio messages to yourself. Don't forget where you keep it!

▲ Talk to your doctor about your memory problems. He or she can determine if you need medication and/or if depression is contributing to your memory problems.

▲ Consider seeing an occupational therapist. These health professionals will often suggest excellent memory compensation techniques to use until your memory and concentration improve.

▲ Exercise your mind. The more you use your mind, the more your memory may improve. Do crossword puzzles; read interesting articles or books.

▲ Try to avoid taking oral directions when traveling by car. Keep a notepad handy on which to write directions and any other important information you need to remember.

▲ Speak to your family about your memory problems. It will save you some worry!

▲ Don't feel bad when you ask people to repeat something they just said. Tell them you have CRS (Can't Remember Stuff)!

▲ If your memory is interfering significantly with work, you may need to talk to your supervisor or someone in your company's department of human resources. Explain the specific difficulties that you're having with your memory and ability to concentrate. Often it's better to get things out in the open. Allow yourself more time for projects at work or make the decision to do some extra work at home.

▲ Avoid stressful situations when you can. They often make memory problems worse.

▲ Leave tasks that require concentrated effort for those times of the day or week when you feel better.

▲ Divide tasks into smaller portions. Do a little at a time and the job will seem more manageable.

▲ Keep lists! Try to keep your lists in a planner or at a specific spot in your house, for example, on a desk or table in the kitchen or another room you frequently inhabit, such as the family room or den. Some individuals find Post-It notes helpful.

Morning Stiffness

Many individuals with fibromyalgia report experiencing stiffness in the morning when they get out of bed. Muscle stiffness can also reoccur throughout the day, especially after being in one position for an extended period of time.

Tips on Coping with Morning Stiffness:

Jenny Fransen, R.N.

▲ Prepare your clothes, lunch, transportation, etc., the night before.

▲ Choose easy-care clothing and hairstyles. Dress for comfort.

▲ Simplify your morning routine as much as possible.

▲ Always allow extra time to get ready in the morning. Avoid rushing when you are stiff and in pain.

▲ When you get out of bed, take a hot bath or shower to relieve pain and help loosen up muscles and joints, then stretch and do range of motion exercises.

▲ Hot paraffin may help relieve stiffness in your hands and fingers.

▲ Take medication upon awakening to reduce pain. You may even want to set an alarm early to take medication and then go back to sleep.

▲ Whenever possible, adjust your routine to accommodate morning stiffness. You may need to schedule certain activities later in your day.

▲ Isotoner gloves (turned inside out) have been found to reduce swelling in the hands when worn at night.

▲ Cushioned resting splints worn at night help to reduce swelling, pain, and stiffness in the morning.

▲ Upon awakening, slip on shoes with cushioning, like aerobic or walking shoes. They provide support and cushioning to stiff and painful feet.

▲ Use adaptive equipment with easy grip handles, building them up with adhesive back foam, foam curlers, or pipe insulation. Consider building up tooth brushes, hairbrushes, automobile steering wheels, and others.

▲ Report how long you are stiff in the morning to your physician. This information is important in planning your care.

▲ Ask for help from family members. Let them zip back zippers, assist with breakfast, and help with other early morning tasks.

Miscellaneous Coping Tips

▲ Take frequent breaks throughout the day to change positions. If you're sitting for a long time at your job, in a movie theatre, or in a plane or car, get up, move around, and gently stretch.

▲ A very hot bath once or twice a day can provide temporary pain relief and relax your mind.

▲ Take your favorite pillow along on trips. It will save your neck!

▲ Check muscle tension throughout the day–are you tensing your shoulders, holding your breath, or clenching your teeth?

▲ When you have to carry heavy items, use a fold-up luggage cart to make your load lighter.

▲ When you go on a trip, instead of taking one large, fully packed suitcase, take two smaller ones. Suitcases with wheels will make your travel easier, too.

▲ Invest in one of the electrical massagers that you can lean up against–it can help loosen tight muscles and take your mind off of the pain. It also will not get tired!

▲ Instead of carrying a heavy purse, try wearing a fanny pack to reduce muscle pain in the shoulder area. Carry your wallet and other necessities in your pockets.

▲ Keep a back pillow (lumbar support) in your car to relieve tension when driving. You can buy specially designed ones or place a rolled-up towel between the small of your back and the car seat.

▲ When reading, put your book or magazine on a pillow in front of you to reduce stress in your arms and to improve your posture.

▲ Shoulder pads can actually cause pain in your shoulders if they are too large. Remove them from your clothing, if necessary.

▲ Make sure bra straps are loose and comfortable. Tight ones can constrict circulation and be painful.

▲ Let family members help you whenever possible. It is hard to give up activities you have always done, but when you are feeling better, you can gradually do more.

▲ Make sure your work station is at a good height for you. It should not cause stress on your arms or your neck.

▲ Don't apologize for having fibromyalgia. Don't be put on the defensive by "well-meaning" friends or relatives. Learn to say no if you cannot or do not want to perform certain tasks. For your real friends, no explanation is necessary; for others, no explanation will ever suffice.

Coping Journal

Date	Planning Things to do	Pacing When to do them	Prioritizing In order of necessity

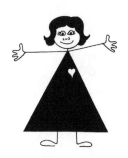

MY BATTLE WITH FIBROMYALGIA

Pain and fatigue
have come again
like an enemy
seeking to destroy life.

Like a storm at sea
the waves sweep over me
and threaten to dash me
to the rocks below.

But I have a lifeline.
I know my enemy well
and I know I will win.

I will ride out the storm
knowing that it will subside
and the sun will shine again.

Once more I have won.

Peggy J. Donahue

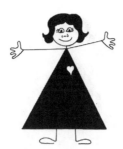

VICIOUS CYCLE OF PAIN IN FIBROMYALGIA

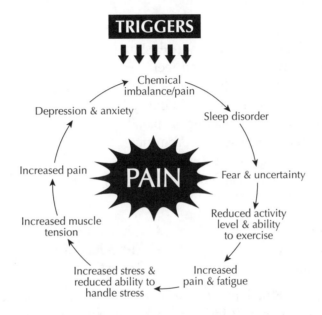

Breaking the vicious cycle of pain is an important step in taking charge of your fibromyalgia. Researchers recognize that a variety of triggers, including physical injury, emotional trauma, infection, hormonal changes, or an extended disruption in sleep, may create chemical imbalances, pain, and changes in the central nervous system. Individuals begin to experience disrupted sleep. Some may begin to feel uncertainty and fear about their health and its impact on their lives. Many begin to limit their daily activities, avoid exercise, and then, unfortunately, begin to experience increased pain, fatigue, and other FMS symptoms. Living with fibromyalgia and seeing its impact on relationships, work, and home life can be very stressful. Individuals often feel that life is passing them by and that they're unable to keep up with their daily tasks, which increases their stress even further. Poor sleep, chronic pain, and fatigue can diminish one's ability to cope with stress, causing the perception of life stressors to increase. Muscle tension increases as stress builds, and it leads to increased pain. Many individuals begin to experience symptoms of depression and/or anxiety due to this cascade of events, which creates further chemical changes in the central nervous system and an increase in pain. The sleep disorder often worsens, and the vicious cycle of pain continues.

Many of the treatments discussed in this book will help break the vicious cycle of pain. These include: medication, sleeping tips, relaxation and diaphragmatic breathing, psychological and supportive counseling, guidance in a conditioning program, heat, ice, gentle stretching, massage, acupressure, support from family and friends, education, guidance in self-management, coping tips, good posture and body mechanics, pacing, cognitive behavioral therapy, and stress management. As you are able to incorporate a number of treatment strategies, you may gradually feel your pain decrease and become more manageable.

▲▲▲

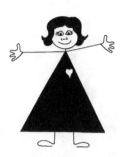

EXERCISE

Do you remember when you could lift your grocery bags without pain or run up a flight of steps and not get short of breath? Did you attend exercise classes and feel great afterwards? Now do you wonder when you will be able to walk around the block again without feeling as if every muscle in your body is screaming in pain? Yes, your body is not what it used to be! You must accept this reality or you will become frustrated and will not improve! Improving your physical fitness and the way you feel takes

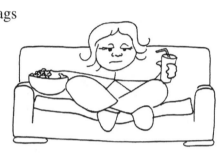

- ▲ Guidance
- ▲ Patience
- ▲ Perseverance
- ▲ Determination
- ▲ Time–lots of it
- ▲ Realistic goals

Some researchers feel FMS patients might have an inherited tendency toward exercise intolerance. Research has shown that FMS patients also experience muscle weakness.

Remember

- ▲ **Do not dwell on the past.**
- ▲ **Start with where you are now — not where you used to be!**
- ▲ **Don't compare yourself to others.**

Try not to dwell on the past; it doesn't serve any purpose except to make you feel bad about the things you can't do anymore. You can learn to substitute activities you can't do with activities you can do. You will need to start with activities you are able to do right now—even if that's only walking to the front door—and increasing your activity level as you are able. It is also very important not to compare yourself to others; you might not be able to do the same amount and types of activities others can do, but thinking about the difference will only frustrate you and make you feel bad about yourself. You don't need that! What you need is to feel good about yourself by honoring your body and treating it with the utmost care and respect. It will repay you with increased vitality and less pain.

Why Aerobic Exercise?

Several studies have confirmed the effectiveness of aerobic conditioning exercises for fibromyalgia patients. It

- ▲ **Reduces tender point pain.**
- ▲ **Floods muscles with oxygen.**

- ▲ Improves sense of well-being by releasing endorphins into the bloodstream.
- ▲ Helps sleep by making the body physically tired.

- ▲ May activate the immune system.
- ▲ Increases serotonin levels.
- ▲ Improves self-esteem.
- ▲ Reduces depression.

Getting Started

Those patients who can participate in some form of aerobic exercise seem to feel better over time, although not everyone benefits. Studies may determine why some feel better when they exercise than others. Problems with growth hormone production while exercising may contribute to exercise intolerance.

Some of you might be thinking that you hurt so much that just walking around the block is next to impossible! There are some obstacles you may have to overcome to work up to an exercise program.

- ▲ **Check with your doctor before you begin to make sure you don't have any joint, muscle, or disc problems that could be worsened by exercising too vigorously or inappropriately.**

- ▲ **Get your fibromyalgia under control with medications that might help alleviate some of the associated pain and stiffness.**

- ▲ **If possible, work with a physical therapist knowledgeable about fibromyalgia problems who can guide you in an exercise program.**

- ▲ **Make your approach gradual and progressive. Avoid overexercising. It will only make your fibromyalgia symptoms worse.**

The type of doctor who could guide you in an exercise program could be

- ▲ **Rheumatologist**
- ▲ **Internist**
- ▲ **Physiatrist**

Because fibromyalgia affects each person differently, you may find yourself having to start at the beginning of this exercise program if you have a severe case of fibromyalgia. If your fibromyalgia is not severe, you could begin at a higher level. If you are already in an exercise program, great! Keep it up!

The key is to start slowly. Fibromyalgia patients need to start slowly and increase their workouts much more slowly than the average person. If you have chronic fatigue syndrome as well, you might find that exercise makes you feel worse. Listen to your body! If you feel really terrible after exercising, cut back. Go slower. Spend more time stretching. If you feel any unusual pain, **STOP** and contact your physician. You may experience some muscle soreness at first. This is normal for fibromyalgia patients. If you keep exercising, you will gradually increase your ability to exercise with less muscle soreness. In his book *The Fibromyalgia Survivor,* Mark Pellegrino, M.D., reports that you are not hurting yourself by exercising and that the muscle soreness should decrease, so don't be afraid of the soreness.

EXERCISE

Aerobic Exercises Beneficial in FMS

- ▲ Walking
- ▲ Bicycling
- ▲ Warm water swimming
- ▲ Nordic Track or Elliptical trainer
- ▲ Treadmill
- ▲ Stationary bicycle
- ▲ Water aerobics
- ▲ Dancing

Pick an exercise you like.

It is important to pick an exercise that you enjoy. If you hate to swim and your physical therapist encourages swimming, you might not keep it up. Alternating aerobic activities helps keep some people motivated. Bouncing or jarring exercises are not good for people with joint, disc, or spinal problems, and may cause additional discomfort and injury. Many people prefer to exercise with a friend or in a class. If you do choose to exercise with others, make sure their level of physical fitness is similar to yours. If they can exercise longer or more vigorously than you, you will have a difficult time keeping up and will only become discouraged.

Before Beginning Your Exercise Program

Remember that you are not training for a sports event. You are training for your health and well-being, so training at 70% of your aerobic capacity may be too difficult. We feel it is more important to keep moving than to worry about training intensity.

One important reminder is to keep your arms close to your body when you exercise. This position will help reduce fatigue and pain during exercise, and during other physical activities as well, such as gardening, sweeping, vacuuming, folding laundry, painting, and computer work. Also try to keep any repetitive movement to 20 minutes or less. FMS patients' muscles seem to respond poorly to repetitive movements.

Stretching Is Important for Many But Should Be Avoided by Some

For many individuals with fibromyalgia, stretching before any workout is important. You may need to spend more time stretching those areas where your muscles are the tightest. Remember to stretch only to the point of resistance, then hold for 10-30 seconds, never forcing any stretch. We have some stretches pictured for you at the end of this section. A knowledgeable physical therapist or sports trainer can guide you in the proper method of stretching and may suggest a gentle yoga or t'ai chi class to help you gain flexibility and strength and reduce stress. For those of you who have very tight muscles, it is helpful to get in the habit of stretching throughout the day. The book *Stretching,* by Bob Anderson, is a great resource on this subject and is available at major bookstores.

Some individuals with fibromyalgia have hypermobile joints. Hypermobility is characterized by laxity of ligaments that allow the muscles to stretch beyond their normal range of motion. It is very important to avoid stretching techniques if you have been diagnosed with joint hypermobility or feel that you are "double-jointed."

We encourage you to discuss any symptoms of hypermobility with your health professional and consult a physical therapist who can guide you in a variety of exercises designed to stabilize the problematic joints.

Exercise Program

▲ Stretch before.
▲ Begin with amount you can do without pain.
▲ Choose low-impact aerobics.

▲ Increase slowly.
▲ Stretch after.
▲ Know your target heart rate.
▲ Set a goal: 20-30 minutes, three to four times a week.

▲ Stretch before every workout.

▲ For beginners: Start with the amount of time you can exercise without fatigue or pain. Try increasing that by two minutes every three workouts. If that produces a lot of pain, back off and increase more slowly. Try one minute every week.

▲ One method that works well is to break your exercise time into two times a day. Divide the amount of time you can comfortably exercise by two. Do one half in the morning and the other half in the afternoon or evening. Gradually increase this time until you reach ten or fifteen minutes without pain, and then drop back to one time per day. This method helps to avoid flare-ups.

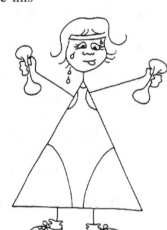

▲ Stretch after every workout. This is very important.

▲ If you wish to aim for a target heart rate, subtract your age from the number 220, then find 60-70% of that number: for example, 220 - 40 = 180 x 60-70% = 108-126 beats per minute for a 40-year-old.

▲ Goal: 20 to 30 minutes three to four times per week. (This time does not include time spent stretching before and after exercising.) If you feel fine after exercising for 20 or 30 minutes, of course you can exercise longer if you like. Just remember, if you overdo it, you will hurt!

▲ Keep up your exercise routine indefinitely.

Remember

▲ Improvement time varies from one individual to another.

▲ Adjust the intensity of your program according to how your body feels.

▲ Modify your workout to protect problem areas that need to be treated gently.

▲ There will be setbacks. FMS has a course of flare-ups and remissions. Don't overdo when you're feeling better; go easy when you are in a flare-up.

▲ Don't give up!

▲ Stretch throughout the day.

Exercise Diary

It is wise to keep an exercise diary. We have included a sample page for you to photocopy and use. It will enable you to keep a good record of how much progress you make and how you feel. If you do not keep a record of your progress, it is often hard to see the gains you have made, particularly if they happen very slowly as so often seems the case for FMS patients.

TIPS Exercise

▲ It may take as long as three to six months to see improvement. Remember that fibromyalgia people are not as predictable as others in their responses to exercise, so it is important not to measure yourself against others.

▲ Find a friend to exercise with. You will have more fun and feel encouraged to keep it up.

▲ Keep an exercise diary so you do not forget how much you exercised the day before.

▲ Exercise tapes are great to use. Pick a low-intensity one. The Arthritis Foundation offers exercise tapes that are great to try. PACE I and II (People with Arthritis Can Exercise) programs are excellent for senior citizens and wheelchair-bound patients. Some support groups offer tapes; a list is offered at the end of the book. Some tapes also include stretching and gentle yoga exercises. Some libraries and video stores offer these tapes as rentals so you can try before you buy!

▲ Try to incorporate the use of all your muscle groups into your exercise workout.

▲ Remember that many people who keep up an exercise routine feel better because of it.

▲ Nautilus weight-lifting machines tend to be too difficult for fibromyalgia patients and may aggravate fibromyalgia symptoms. You might be able to handle them as your strength increases, but don't be upset if you can't. You can add strength training after you are well-established in an exercise routine. Start out with very low weights (1 lb. or less) or try using elastic bands.

▲ Try an exercise ball for a fun alternative.

▲ Warm water swimming is an excellent aerobics program for fibromyalgia, because it is gentle on the joints and the warm water relaxes the muscles. Water temperature must be at least 86° F. Many communities and hospitals have therapeutic pools and classes. You might need a prescription from your doctor to use certain pools. Many FMS patients have found the AquaJogger belt to be a fun aerobic alternative. The Arthritis Foundation has a list of warm water pools in your area. Contact your local chapter for this information.

▲ Two good books for stretching exercises are *Stretching* and *Stretching in the Office* by Bob Anderson. They can be purchased in bookstores, and on www.amazon.com; or your local library might carry a copy you can check out. Bob Anderson has also developed *Stretchware,* the ergonomic software that reminds you to stretch. It's available both as a direct download and on a CD-ROM. Additional information is on the Web site: www.stretchware.com.

▲ The Arthritis Foundation offers exercise classes in many communities. You can call them for specifics. They offer a warm water exercise program designed for people with arthritis that might be good to try.

▲ Remember to be flexible in your exercise program. Adjust your level to avoid over-exertion. Do not exercise if you have the flu or are feeling bad. Skip a day and then start again the next.

▲ In some health clubs, people knowledgeable of FMS can guide you in an exercise program. However, some health club personnel do not understand that "no pain, no gain" does not work with the FMS patient. If you find your health club personnel or physical therapist are pushing you too hard, you will need to reassess your program. Only you know how you feel!

▲ Fibromyalgia exercise videos - A good one to try is by Patty Bourne, a kinesiologist who developed a 30-minute, upbeat, exercise videotape for FMS patients. Sharon Clark, Ph.D., has developed three exercise videos: *Stretching and Relaxation, Toning and Strengthening* and *Aerobic Exercise*. Ordering information for the videos is included in the "Resources" chapter of this book.

▲ Some FMS patients like using an elliptical trainer or ski machine at low levels. Many patients find they are most successful with them by starting only with their legs and gradually adding their arms.

▲ Two good sources for health and fitness products are

www.bodytrends.com   800-549-1667
www.optp.com   888-819-0121

▲ Do not give up!

"If you constantly think and talk about your pain, then you are living with it. You are never apart from it. Just as your thoughts can influence your feelings and behavior, so can your behavior influence your thoughts and feelings. If you try to act normal in everyday living as much as you can, then you will find yourself gradually less involved with your pain and less aware of it." Richard Sternbach, M.D., from *Mastering Pain: A Twelve-Step Program for Coping with Chronic Pain.*

Exercise Diary

Date	Stretching	Exercise time	How did you feel after?

EXERCISE

Samples of Stretches

The following are a sample of stretches that are often recommended for those with fibromyalgia. It may be helpful to take a hot shower or bath before stretching. Remember to stretch gently and to hold each stretch for ten seconds or longer, then relax. Never force a stretch; you will only experience more pain. Daily stretching can be a very beneficial component of treatment, but when it's done incorrectly, it can actually do more harm than good. Bob Anderson's book *Stretching* provides excellent stretching guidelines and has numerous illustrations that are helpful when learning specific stretches. A physical therapist can individualize a stretching program for you and help ensure that you are stretching both correctly and safely. Remember that accurate information and individual guidance form the foundation for a good stretching program.

Important Note

Please consult your physician before you begin a stretching program. Some individuals with FMS have complicating physical problems that can be aggravated by stretching—a situation which you certainly want to avoid!

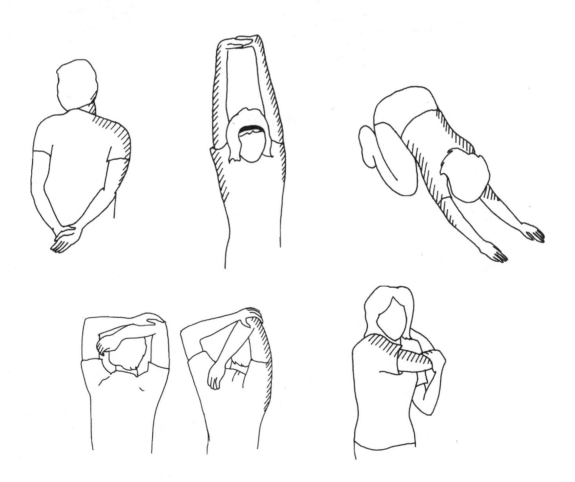

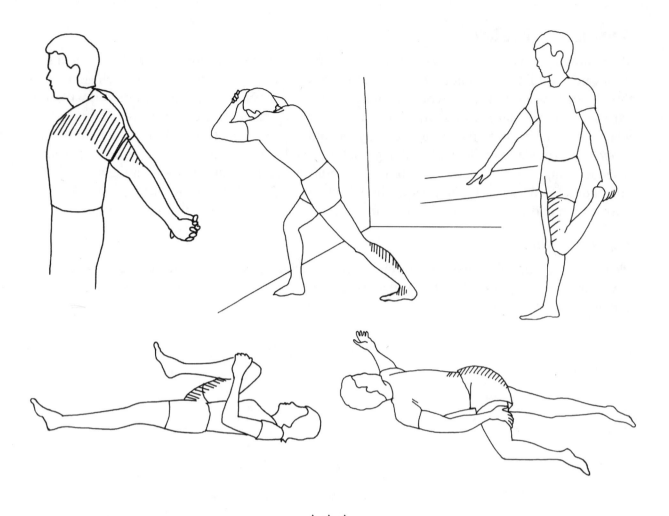

▲▲▲

112

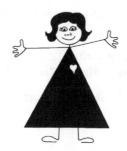

DOCTOR AND PATIENT RELATIONSHIP

The relationship you have with your doctor influences the success you have in learning to manage your symptoms. A positive relationship embraces good communication and listening skills and relies on accurate, timely information provided by both parties. Important components of good communication within the doctor-patient relationship are the following:

▲ **Have reasonable expectations.**

▲ **Exchange concise, accurate information.**

▲ **Exercise good listening skills.**

▲ **Ask questions of each other.**

▲ **Be willing to express feelings and concerns.**

The rewards and benefits of good communication between you and your doctor can be mutual respect and trust of one another. These attributes will empower you to take charge of your fibromyalgia.

Within this relationship, you have rights and responsibilities that you should recognize and commit to so you can receive well-coordinated health care that meets your individual needs.

Patient Rights

▲ **To have your needs and concerns listened to**
▲ **To be recognized and respected as an individual**
▲ **To receive quality medical care**
▲ **To be involved in the medical decisions that affect your life**
▲ **To ask for help and support**
▲ **To be informed and educated**

Patient Responsibilities

▲ **Provide concise, accurate information (e.g., medical history, current symptoms, sleep quality, current and past medications).**

▲ **Accurately report adverse fibromyalgia symptoms and side effects of medications.**

▲ **Become educated. (This will help enable you to ask the appropriate questions, form**

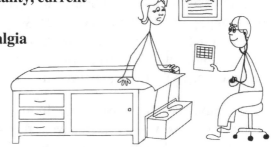

reasonable expectations, and recognize what information is important to record and report.)

▲ Be an active participant in your treatment. (Listen, ask questions, give feedback, follow through with treatment to the best of your ability.)

▲ Be honest in expressing feelings and concerns.

Office Visit

▲ Be concise and well organized.

▲ Ask your most important questions at the beginning of the visit.

▲ Summarize information that may help your doctor better assess your situation.

▲ Discuss types of treatment that you feel may be helpful.

▲ Develop a flare-up plan.

▲ If you are unclear about any part of your treatment or medical care, ask for clarification.

When preparing for your office visit, remember that you will need to be concise and well organized in order to discuss your needs and concerns with your doctor in a short period of time. Our changing health care environment with its myriad of insurance restrictions is putting increased demands on our physicians and limitations on the standard office visit. As a patient, you must strive to make good use of your allotted time and focus on those issues or questions that must be addressed by your physician.

Identify your three most important questions and/or concerns and be sure to ask them at the beginning of your visit. When choosing the questions to ask your doctor, review your list and consider who is the most appropriate health professional to answer each question. You may have questions on your list that would be best answered by your physical therapist, dietician, pharmacist, or nurse clinician. Weeding those questions out leaves more time in the office visit for those concerns most appropriate for your physician. If your doctor doesn't attempt to answer your questions, let him or her know how important it is that you discuss your concerns. If your situation is unusually complex and you have a number of concerns that cannot be addressed in a standard office visit, ask the individual who schedules the appointments how to handle this situation.

To help your doctor better assess your situation, it's often helpful to bring a summary of concise, accurate information to your office visit. For example, if you've been having difficulty sleeping in recent weeks, summarize your sleep patterns over the past several weeks and list the medications that you've been taking during that time with their specific dosages. If your symptoms have increased, be prepared to describe them.

If there are various types of treatment that you feel may be helpful to you in better managing your fibromyalgia, discuss them briefly with your doctor. Examples might be biofeedback training, counseling, physical therapy, or warm water pool exercise. If your doctor feels that you would benefit from a particular treatment, remember to obtain a prescription if necessary before leaving your appointment. It's also helpful to know what types of treatment are covered by your insurance and how many visits you are allowed.

Some individuals have benefited from developing a plan with their physician that can be implemented easily when they have a flare-up of their symptoms. This plan will certainly vary from doctor to doctor and patient to patient, but it may include several sessions of physical therapy, a small increase in medication or addition of another medication, or massage. Some physicians prefer to be notified of a flare-up that is difficult to manage and to individually assess the situation and make specific recommendations. Do not make any adjustments in your medication(s) without first discussing dosage options with your physician.

As you are coming to the end of your office visit, ask for clarification if you are unclear about any part of your treatment or medical care. You may benefit from taking brief notes during your visit or repeating back to your doctor, in your own words, what you understand your instructions to be.

The following questions may help you narrow the focus of your office visit and assist you in getting the most out of a short period of time. We encourage you to read through the questions and use them to organize your thoughts before your next appointment.

The patient can provide invaluable information to the doctor to use in diagnosis and treatment. Before your visit, ask yourself

- ▲ What is the main reason that I'm going to the doctor today?

- ▲ What are the three most important questions that I want to ask my doctor?
  (Write them down and take your list to appointment.)

- ▲ What else worries me about my health?

- ▲ What do I expect the doctor to do for me today?

During the office visit, ask your doctor any or all of the following (as appropriate):

- ▲ What tests need to be done?

- ▲ What is your diagnosis? (Ask doctor to write it down if necessary.)

- ▲ Medications? What? When? For how long? Possible concerns or side effects?

- ▲ Is there any treatment that could be helpful? What? Activity? Precautions?

- ▲ Are there any helpful patient education materials available for the condition?

- ▲ Any other recommendations?

At the end of the visit, ask your doctor any or all of the following (as appropriate):

- ▲ Am I to return for another visit? Yes or no? If yes, when?

- ▲ Should I report back to you by telephone for any reason? Yes or no? If yes, when?

- ▲ What symptoms and/or side effects from treatment or medications do you want to be informed of?

- ▲ Am I to call in for test results? Yes or no? If yes, when?

- ▲ If a problem arises with medication or treatment, may I call for an answer rather than make another appointment?

Phone Calls

If you're experiencing side effects from a medication and/or problems with a specific treatment, call your physician for advice. Adjustments in medication and/or treatments can usually be briefly discussed on the phone to help you avoid undue suffering.

- ▲ Don't expect your doctor to remember the details of your situation.

- ▲ Describe the problem or ask the question that concerns you most at the beginning of the conversation. It is often helpful to write down the specifics you wish to cover and put them by your phone.

- ▲ Be specific and concise. For example, if your question concerns your sleep and medication, know approximately how many times you've been waking at night and the range of total hours that you've been sleeping. Also have a list of your current medication(s) with specific dosage(s) by the phone.

- ▲ Have the phone number of your pharmacy handy in case your doctor wants to phone in a prescription for you.

- ▲ Be prepared to jot down any medical advice that you're given. For example, how long should you expect to take a new medication before noticing some improvement in your sleep quality?

- ▲ Ask your doctor when you should call again or come in for an office visit.

The memory and concentration problems that are common in many individuals with fibromyalgia often contribute to poorly organized and incomplete phone conversations. The work that you do in preparing for a phone call and the notes that you take during the call will help you obtain the information you need and ensure that you remember the important details.

Nurture a healthy, positive relationship with your doctor; the benefits are many. As a patient, educate yourself so that you will know what questions to ask and how to be proactive in your medical care. Take the responsibility of reporting to your physician undue side effects of medications, increased sleep disruptions, a flare-up of symptoms that doesn't respond to your efforts, and other issues that concern you. A physician who is sensitive to your needs can empower you to manage your symptoms from day to day and can use creative problem solving and management skills in coordinating an individual plan of care for you. Conversely, a physician who is not willing to work with you and provide guidance in the management of your fibromyalgia can actually contribute to the frustrations and challenges that you may already be experiencing. If you decide that you need to see a different physician, ask a leader of a local FMS support group for recommendations of physicians who are knowledgeable about FMS and who work well with FMS patients. A local arthritis care center may also be a resource for physicians.

"The quality of the doctor/patient relationship can mean the difference between a well-managed illness and needless wasted time and aggravation. Being assertive, believing in yourself, having confidence and possessing knowledge about your condition will help you enlist your doctor's cooperation and enhance your likelihood of successful treatment." Rebekah Milaro, FMS patient and contributing writer to *Fibromyalgia Network*, October 1991.

Doctor and Patient Resource

An excellent resource on evaluating the quality of your medical care is *Examining Your Doctor* by Timothy McCall, M.D. The book is available from www.amazon.com and at major booksellers. You may also want to check McCall's Web site for additional information: www.drmccall.com.

Disrespectful Medical Treatment

by Jenny Fransen, R.N., Co-author of *The Fibromyalgia Help Book.*

Only recently has medical science begun to understand the underlying mechanism of fibromyalgia. For many years it was not well understood; consequently, many people with this disorder spent years searching for a diagnosis and effective treatment to relieve their pain. Unfortunately, during this prediagnosis period, many people have met countless healthcare professionals who were insensitive, disrespectful, uneducated, and who blamed the patient for their pain. Patients were told they were crazy, "It's all in your head," and other damaging comments.

If you have had this experience, it is important to know you are not to blame for your symptoms. You are not crazy. You have a real medical condition, and you deserve respectful medical treatment. The damaging comments that were directed toward you were completely inappropriate. You have a right to be angry about this mistreatment.

Receiving this type of treatment over a prolonged period of time may cause you to distrust and feel angry toward all medical professionals. This anger and distrust, if left unchecked, can interfere in new relationships with healthcare professionals and refuel the cycle.

Guilt and shame are painful emotions felt by many people with fibromyalgia as a response to disrespect and blame from medical professionals. They are the feelings *I must be bad because I have this*, or *I must somehow be at fault for having this*. These feelings can lead to depression if they are prolonged and left unchecked. They can negatively impact one's adjustment to living with this medical condition.

Isolation is another painful experience people with fibromyalgia can experience as a result of not receiving the understanding needed to live with chronic muscle pain and fatigue. It is the result of feeling as if no one believes and understands what you are living with day after day. Feelings of isolation and loneliness are also extremely common, because fibromyalgia is invisible to the naked eye. No one around you can see or feel your pain.

Take some time to evaluate who has given you disrespectful care in the past and to assess what responses you have developed as a result of mistreatment. It might be helpful to make a list.

How can you express your anger toward those who have hurt you? You can write a letter and express how their treatment hurt you, how you now have received a correct diagnosis, and what they could have done to be more helpful. Some people choose to send the letter, and others do not. Simply writing it can help to put some closure on the relationship and help diffuse some of the anger toward the ones who have caused you pain. You may want to send information to educate them on fibromyalgia, so they don't continue to hurt others with this condition. However you choose to deal with your anger, it's important to focus it constructively toward those who hurt you, not toward anyone else. Continuing to feel anger for prolonged periods of time hurts you. Find constructive outlets to vent your anger. Try writing in a journal. Find people with whom you can talk to. Anger is an energy that can be used constructively to motivate you to help yourself feel better, to help other people, and to be proactive as a healthcare consumer and in your program of self-care.

Finally, you must not remain under disrespectful medical care. It will only continue to harm your sense of well-being, fuel depression and anger, and continue the cycle of distrust toward medical professionals. You must find respectful, caring medical professionals who believe you and do not blame you for your pain. You deserve respectful care, and you must have it.

Seek out an understanding person or counselor to help you resolve any painful experiences or emotions. By getting support, you can work through your experience so it doesn't continue to hurt you as deeply. Getting support can also help to reduce the isolation and depression that you may be experiencing. Remember to elicit support from those people who believe you and who are understanding.

TIPS *Working with Your Physician*

Jenny Fransen, R.N.

- ▲ Consider other resources for information, such as your pharmacist for medication questions.

- ▲ As there is no magic bullet for fibromyalgia, great patience is required to find a combination of therapies and medication to bring about improvement.

- ▲ Recognize that there will be inherent frustrations for patients and physicians when treating a condition that continues to hold many mysteries for the researchers.

- ▲ Realize much of your treatment is up to you: exercise, relaxation, stress management, pain management, and pursuing additional therapies and treatments such as biofeedback, spray and stretch, and massage.

- ▲ Learn as much as you can about your own disease, because you are the one who will manage the day-to-day problems that occur.

- ▲ Actively manage fibromyalgia-related problems such as pain and sleep problems.

- ▲ If you are having symptoms of depression, inform your physician. Depression can further disrupt sleep cycles. It needs to be treated.

- ▲ Reinforce and thank the doctor for specific behaviors and techniques you find helpful. "I appreciate that you really listen to me, Dr. Olson."

- ▲ Learn to ask for what you need from your physician. "Would you explain to me what can be done to help me sleep better?"

- ▲ Develop a good relationship with the doctor's nurse and receptionist. Identify rules of the office such as the doctor's day off and the best time to call and leave a message. Know the nurse's name and ask for him or her when you call. Be patient if healthcare providers cannot return your call immediately.

- ▲ Should you and your physician have difficulties, try to identify problems and work to resolve them. You can write your feelings in a letter if you can't express them in person.

- ▲ Avoid angry or defensive communication.

▲ If your physician has told you to return in three months, you can make an appointment sooner to discuss your questions or concerns if necessary.

▲ If a problem arises with medication or treatment, ask if you can call for an answer rather than make another appointment.

▲ Be assertive and take responsibility for your own treatment.

▲ Remember **you** are in charge of your treatment program.

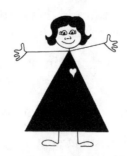

WORK-RELATED ISSUES

Fibromyalgia may affect a person's ability to perform on the job. The symptoms of chronic pain and fatigue and difficulties with memory and concentration can be especially challenging for some people. It's also recognized that certain work tasks or types of employment can aggravate fibromyalgia symptoms. In a study by G.W. Waylonis, M.D., and his colleagues, 321 individuals from across the United States completed a questionnaire regarding the effects of their current and past occupations on their fibromyalgia. The activities in this study that were reported to aggravate fibromyalgia symptoms were computer work or typing, prolonged sitting, prolonged standing and walking, stress, heavy lifting and bending, and repeated moving and lifting. Conversely, activities that did not appear to exacerbate the symptoms of fibromyalgia included walking, variable light sedentary work, teaching, light desk work, and phone work. In conclusion, light sedentary occupations that allow for varied tasks and changing positions appeared to be tolerated the best.

For many, it is worthwhile to spend time identifying potential problem areas in your job and then to begin identifying possible solutions. For example

▲ **Are you engaged in prolonged repetitive activities?**
   Can you take frequent short breaks to stretch, relax and/or do some biofeedback?

▲ **Are you in one position for sustained periods of time?**
   Changing positions frequently, if only for a few minutes, may be helpful.

▲ **Is your neck, shoulder, or back pain aggravated by postural strain?**
   Check the position of your work surface, chair, and computer to determine if you are at the proper height to maintain good posture.

▲ **Are you in a job with high stress?**
   Would it be possible to take short breaks to relax, do some abdominal breathing, practice biofeedback, or stretch? Can you delegate some tasks? Can you take a stress management class to learn ways to better manage stress?

Be creative in identifying potential solutions, try several, and then adapt them to your situation. An occupational therapist may assist you in assessing your specific needs and make various recommendations to you and to your employer. You might also ask yourself the following questions:

▲ **How can I do my job differently?**

▲ **How can I rearrange or modify the way various tasks are done?**

▲ **How can I pace myself and my work tasks better throughout the day?**

▲ **Can I adjust my work schedule or discuss the option of flexible working hours with my employer?**

▲ **Can I decrease my hours and work part-time?**

Continue to explore all of the options and make the necessary changes or adjustments that will help you better manage your FMS within your work environment. Your employer may be more willing to work with you in making these accommodations if you ask your physician to write a letter describing your fibromyalgia symptoms and explaining your specific limitations. Any suggestions that your doctor can include regarding changes or accommodations that might help you will help underscore your requests.

The Americans with Disabilities Act (ADA) requires employers to make reasonable adjustments and accommodations for people with disabilities and chronic illnesses. The ADA was amended in 1994 to exempt companies with fewer than 15 employees, while requiring those companies with 15 or more employees to follow the guidelines. You might consider asking your employer what resources and support services are available to help evaluate your specific needs and make recommendations for you. For more information on the Americans with Disabilities Act contact U.S. Equal Employment Opportunity Commission, Publication Information Center, P.O. Box 12549, Cincinnati, Ohio 45212-0549 or call 800-669-3362.

Some individuals with fibromyalgia may continue to experience difficulty in their jobs even after making a variety of changes and accommodations. Some may feel that they're unable to work in their current position, at least for a time. If you find that you are unable to perform your job, discuss this situation with your physician. Also, find out what other options are available to you at work. You may need to take a leave of absence from your current position and use that time to become more involved in a variety of treatments for your fibromyalgia, with a goal of better managing your symptoms and returning to work. You may also choose to explore other job options during this time or programs for retraining or vocational counseling. Check into whether you have short-term or long-term disability insurance benefits available through your job or through an independent insurance policy. Those individuals who were injured on the job may be able to receive worker's compensation benefits for medical expenses, retraining, or lost income.

If you have left work or been working part-time due to your fibromyalgia symptoms, you may benefit from gradually returning to work. Start with a minimum number of hours that you feel you can work and then slowly increase your work hours over the following weeks and months. Try to avoid overtime and shift work; the latter may be particularly troublesome. If you have the option, work a variety of days and times and vary the number of hours worked per day. See what works best for you! Continue to increase your hours while assessing your ability to function in your job and manage your fibromyalgia. If you experience increased symptoms that aren't tolerable as you work more hours, you may need to reduce your work schedule again for a time. Charting your progress in a journal can help you make wise employment decisions. Remember to work closely with both your physician and your employer during these times of transition.

Although many people with fibromyalgia continue to be employed, some individuals with this condition find that they are unable to do any kind of work despite a variety of attempts to do so. An option for these people is to apply for Social Security disability. This can be a difficult process for many, because claim administrators often don't have a good understanding of fibromyalgia, and sometimes patients find that their own physician is less than willing to write a letter in support of disability.

Attorneys experienced in fibromyalgia disability claims may provide invaluable assistance with the necessary paperwork, and hearings. They are also familiar with the steps that can increase the likelihood of a successful claim. If you need help in locating an attorney familiar with fibromyalgia, contact your state or local bar association for assistance. Members of a local support group may also be familiar with attorneys who are knowledgeable and experienced in fibromyalgia disability claims. Some national organizations may also supply you with a list of attorneys that specialize in this area.

The work status and prevalence of disability in people with fibromyalgia have been studied by Frederick Wolfe, M.D., and colleagues. In a survey of 1,668 FMS patients from seven centers with diverse socio-economic characteristics, they found that 65.4% reported being able to work most or all days, while 18.9% stated they could work few or no days. When assessing all disability sources, these investigators found that 25.3% of the patients had received a disability payment, while 74.7% reported that they had never received a disability award. In this same study, almost 15% of patients had received Social Security disability (SSD) payments, compared to 2.2% of the total U.S. population (U.S. Social Security Administration data). In an attempt to understand the reason for the SSD awards, a subgroup of 52 patients who had received Social Security disability was surveyed. Twenty-three percent reported an award specifically for fibromyalgia, 19.2% for arthritis, 23.1% for back problems or miscellaneous musculoskeletal problems, 1.9% for systemic lupus erythematosus, 9.7% for psychiatric reasons, 17.3% for nonrheumatic medical reasons, and 3.9% for unknown reasons.

While we know that fibromyalgia may affect your ability to perform on the job, we encourage you to explore a variety of options that potentially may help you better manage your FMS within your work environment. Be creative in identifying the possible changes, solutions, or adaptations that may benefit you. You may find that, as you implement some of these changes and adjust them specifically to your work situation, managing fibromyalgia and work can be a successful venture.

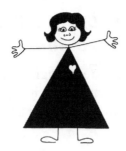

STRESS MANAGEMENT AND RELAXATION

Stress is not an external event that produces anxiety or frustration in our bodies; it is our own physical and emotional reaction to external events taking place around us and within us. Studies have shown that there are actual physical changes occurring in our bodies when we are stressed.

Changes That Can Occur Are

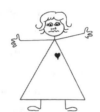

- ▲ Muscle tension and pain
- ▲ Stomach distress
- ▲ Headaches
- ▲ Heart irregularities
- ▲ Anxiety
- ▲ Depression

- ▲ Teeth grinding and/or TMJ
- ▲ High blood pressure
- ▲ Cold hands and feet
- ▲ Insomnia
- ▲ Ulcers
- ▲ Diarrhea or constipation

Chronic stress can deplete the body of many chemicals needed for proper functioning, and we can develop various diseases as a result. Stress can negatively affect our immune system, health, and pain levels, as well as every system in our bodies. Research also shows that we can take steps to change the way we respond to stress to create a healing atmosphere for our bodies. Individuals need to identify the major stressors in their lives, realize how those stressors are affecting them psychologically and physically, and, above all, to determine what methods to use to alleviate stress.

One of the reasons fibromyalgia can be such a difficult condition to live with is its unpredictability. This in itself is very stressful. If only someone could tell you how you are going to feel in six months, one year, or ten years from now, you could at least alleviate some of the uncertainty of living with an illness whose symptoms catch us by surprise day to day, week to week, or even hour to hour! We may wonder what we did wrong to cause our flare-up or what we did right to reduce our symptoms. Our days, weeks, and months can be up and down, like a roller coaster, and we may find ourselves hanging on for dear life, wondering when the next flare-up will send us racing head first to the bottom of the roller coaster. We need to learn to deal with the physical and emotional stresses of that ride. People who have an easier time accepting this uncertainty seem to do better overall than those who cannot handle the flare-up and remissions of FMS. Other people (the lucky ones) who have a milder form of FMS find that the ups and downs are less severe and less frequent, therefore less stressful. Others say that just as they manage to have a good spell, FMS ambushes them again, and they find it difficult to control all the emotional and painful effects of this new attack. This pattern is not easy to cope with, but you need to learn how to handle the flare-ups both physically and emotionally. Accepting the fact that flare-ups will happen and are part of the illness can be a healthy step toward dealing with the ups and downs of living with FMS.

Chronic Stress Can Lead to Severe Illness: Chronic Illness Is Severely Stressing

Everyone with fibromyalgia agrees that stress aggravates symptoms. As fibromyalgia patients, we must identify what our own stressors are and learn how to cope with them to enhance our self-esteem and reduce our painful symptoms.

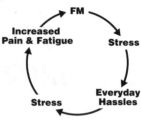

Everyone reacts differently to stress. What is perceived as stressful to one person may go unnoticed by another. Locate the sources of your personal stress factors, so you can reduce them or learn effective ways of coping or controlling them. It is not always the big things in life that create stress for us, but often stress can be caused by the little things that pile up on a day-to-day basis and send our nervous system into overload.

Possible sources of stress:

▲ Marital relations
▲ Work
▲ Friends
▲ Lack of support system
▲ Guilt
▲ Loneliness
▲ Depression
▲ Sexual difficulties
▲ Inadequate nutrition
▲ Commitments

▲ Everyday hassles
▲ Finances
▲ Hurriedness
▲ Perfectionism
▲ Anger
▲ FMS
▲ Anxiety
▲ Holidays
▲ Alcohol, nicotine & caffeine
▲ Worry

Reduce, Eliminate, Negotiate: Balance Is Necessary to Reduce Stress

Look over your life for possible stressors; check the list above and mark any that affect you. These can aggravate your fibromyalgia. You might even have more to add! Try to rid yourself of toxic friends, too many committee meetings, or a job that is giving you little satisfaction and aggravates your fibromyalgia symptoms. Learn to let go of guilt, anger, perfectionism, hurriedness, and obsessive-compulsive behavior. This is easier said than done! Some people may need professional help in overcoming self-defeating behaviors. Social workers, therapists, or psychiatrists may help you sort out these problems. Finding a qualified therapist who relates well with you is important. Anxiety and depression may decrease, as well as some of your fibromyalgia symptoms. Working out problems with your boss or in-laws can help you feel better. Talk to your children and spouse about your fibromyalgia and ask for help and their support. Above all, surround yourself with supportive people, including members of your family, circle of friends, and healthcare team. Setting aside 20 minutes each day for "worry time" to write down your worries can reduce worrying when you are trying to fall asleep. This is also a good time to make a list of things you need to do the next day.

There is evidence that everyday hassles are just as stressful, if not more so, than major events. Simplifying your living space, as well as your life, can help reduce your stress level. Throw out, organize, unclutter, redefine, and simplify, simplify, simplify. If you can afford it, get psychological counseling to help you identify and cope with your sources of stress. If the stressors are reduced in your life, your body can take time to heal. This might be a difficult task for some of you, but well worth the effort. There are many books available on stress management, as well as community educational classes or therapists who can help you reduce stress and cope more effectively. Try to achieve a balance in your life. If your life is balanced, your body can become balanced. Renowned psychologist C.J. Jung noted that primitive people interpreted illness not as a negative, but as the unconscious coming forth to transform a person into someone better. Use this illness as a time to transform your life! Take charge of your fibromyalgia and your life!

Cognitive Behavioral Therapy (CBT)

The following techniques are useful for reducing the negative effects of stress. With continued practice, these techniques can produce positive changes in how your body and mind react to stress.

Self-Talk: What We Say to Ourselves Affects How We Feel.

Researchers trying to help people with fibromyalgia have turned to cognitive behavioral therapy as an additional method of alleviating painful symptoms. A therapist using this technique can teach you how to control disturbing emotional reactions by suggesting more effective ways of interpreting and thinking about your experiences. For example, if you make a mistake at work, you might say to yourself, *I am the most stupid person in the world! I always make mistakes!* The therapist would point out that you do not always make mistakes and that everyone makes mistakes and feels foolish at one time or another. The behavioral aspect of this therapy asks you to note your mood or feelings when you are thinking these thoughts. Painful emotions such as guilt, shame, and anxiety can aggravate pain and your fibromyalgia. We are our thoughts. Negative thinking produces negative behavior. Some research suggests negative thinking causes illness. If negative thinking causes illness, can positive thinking create health? There are many researchers who believe this is possible. If this idea sounds foolish to you, and you decide it would never benefit your fibromyalgia symptoms, you are probably feeling skeptical and discouraged or maybe even angry. Your pain level may increase as you are having these thoughts. On the other hand, if this sounds like a great idea to you, you may feel an uplift in your mood. If you pay attention to your body at the same time, you may notice a slight decrease in your pain level. Our bodies react immediately to our emotions. If we can control our thoughts, maybe we can control our bodies.

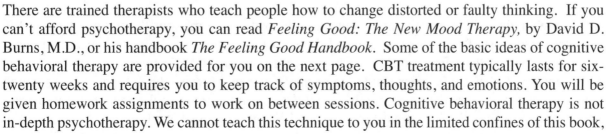

Every day in every way, I'm getting better and better!

There are trained therapists who teach people how to change distorted or faulty thinking. If you can't afford psychotherapy, you can read *Feeling Good: The New Mood Therapy,* by David D. Burns, M.D., or his handbook *The Feeling Good Handbook.* Some of the basic ideas of cognitive behavioral therapy are provided for you on the next page. CBT treatment typically lasts for six-twenty weeks and requires you to keep track of symptoms, thoughts, and emotions. You will be given homework assignments to work on between sessions. Cognitive behavioral therapy is not in-depth psychotherapy. We cannot teach this technique to you in the limited confines of this book, but we want you to have an idea of what it is all about, so you can decide if it is something you should pursue.

During treatment, a cognitive therapist will require you to focus on your negative thoughts and to notice when your thoughts follow any of the following patterns:

▲ **All or nothing thinking.** "I have fibromyalgia, therefore, I can't lead a normal life." Wrong. It would be better to say to yourself, "Many people lead normal lives once they get their fibromyalgia under control, and I can too."

▲ **Overgeneralization**. You see a single negative event as a never-ending pattern of defeat. "My doctor misdiagnosed me; therefore, I can never get better."

▲ **Disqualifying the positive.** Rejecting positive experiences as short-lived and possibly not recurring. "My fibromyalgia symptoms were better this weekend when I rested, but it will never happen again."

▲ **Catastrophizing.** You exaggerate the importance of things. "I can't keep my house as clean as I used to. Therefore, I am a failure." Are you a failure? No, you just cannot do as much as you used to. Ask for help. Learn to live with a messier house!

▲ **Should statements.** "I *should* be able to do all that I did before I had fibromyalgia." You can't, and if you try, you will have a flare-up and frustrate yourself. Be kind to yourself. Treat yourself gently.

▲ **Personalization.** You see yourself as the cause of some negative event for which you were not responsible. "My fibromyalgia must have started because I was not taking care of myself." No one knows why fibromyalgia starts; you are not its cause.

When you experience problems with distorted thinking, your body reacts to your thoughts within milliseconds. Cognitive behavior therapy attempts to change your irrational thought patterns by finding the positive in your negative thinking, stopping self-blame, defusing anger, and reducing feelings of being overwhelmed. Do you say to yourself *I am in pain now and will be forever?* Is that true? Aren't there times when you are free of pain? If you have small amounts of time when you are free from pain, using this technique can increase that time gradually, until you have more time when you are pain-free. Notice how high your pain level is when you are thinking about your pain, when someone has made you angry, or when you are hurrying to accomplish tasks. Notice how low your pain level is when you are engaged in pleasant activities. Researchers know that psychological factors influence the degree of pain we feel. If you develop healthier attitudes, change negative thinking, and learn to be optimistic, your fibromyalgia symptoms can and will decrease when used in conjunction with the other treatments described in this book. It may take many months to benefit from a change in thought patterns, but it is worth trying. You have nothing to lose and everything to gain. **This technique can also reduce the risk of becoming depressed.**

Another technique that is easy to implement is to use positive affirmations throughout the day. We have provided a list of some for you to try. It is better to say these out loud and repeat them on a consistent basis for the affirmations to work. Try repeating to yourself as you exercise or do your daily stretches *Every day in every way, I am getting better and better.* Repeat that ten times three or four times a day, every day for a month. See if it helps you. Some people find it helpful to write down positive affirmations on a card to carry in their purse or pocket. Reading the card a few times during the day can keep your positive thoughts on track and prevent negative thinking from creeping into your mind.

Positive Thoughts for Coping with Fibromyalgia:

- ▲ I am confident of my ability to deal with my health and live a good life.
- ▲ Things are getting better.
- ▲ I am making progress in helping myself feel better.
- ▲ Today I can do what I need to do for my recovery.
- ▲ I can treat myself gently and with the special care I would give a close friend.
- ▲ I am learning what I need to do to take care of my body.
- ▲ I focus on positive actions I can take to advocate for myself.
- ▲ I look for the good this day can bring.
- ▲ I go with the flow of each new day, accepting what I can learn from it.
- ▲ I seek out the positive support I need to live with fibromyalgia.
- ▲ I let go of any muscle tension or problems over which I have no control.
- ▲ I live with positive expectancy: each day I expect to feel better and more relaxed.
- ▲ I counter each stress with techniques I know will reduce negative stress.
- ▲ I can surmount any problem that occurs today with calm, problem-solving skills.
- ▲ I can look for the resources I need to manage any problems.
- ▲ I maintain slow and easy breathing, bringing fresh oxygen to my muscles and taking away muscle waste products.
- ▲ I keep my muscles loose and relaxed throughout the day.
- ▲ I take time during the day to relax and breathe to refresh my muscles.
- ▲ I creatively manage the problems each new day brings.
- ▲ I can do whatever I need to do to take good care of myself.

Changing Negative Self-talk

If you would like to try charting your thoughts on your own, copy the journal page at the end of this chapter and keep track of your thoughts. Write down your negative thoughts and the feelings associated with them. You may be amazed at how often your thoughts are destructive or how quickly you can become pessimistic in your thought patterns. What is important is to become aware of your thoughts, for without awareness of how often your thinking heads downward, your thinking will be impossible to change. Once you notice your thoughts turning negative, determine the emotion that you feel when you are thinking badly about yourself. You may feel worthless, guilty, angry, depressed, sad, or confused. Once you become aware of a destructive thought, turn it into a more positive statement. Some people find it helpful to imagine a stop sign or a red light in their minds to defuse a negative thought. Other techniques are putting a rubber band on your wrist and snapping it every time a negative thought comes up or paying attention to your breathing to deflect your mind away from negative thoughts. You may come up with your own techniques over time. Share them with a friend.

Relaxation Techniques

Relaxation techniques are another useful adjunct to stress management. By relaxation we do not mean the relaxing you do in front of the television with your family at night, although this has its place in reducing stress as well. The relaxation techniques we refer to are those that banish tension from our bodies as well as our minds. Some of these techniques are being used by health professionals for their fibromyalgia patients as an addition to their overall treatment plan. Studies show that those people who practice these techniques regularly had significant reductions in their pain levels, improved daily functioning, and increased their sense of well-being. The regular practice of relaxation can reduce muscle tension, pain, and muscle spasm, as well as improve emotional well-being. Relaxation produces the opposite effect on our bodies than stress does.

Relaxation has Many Advantages:

▲ **Lowers heart rate, blood pressure, and oxygen consumption**

▲ **Reduces the level of blood lactate, a chemical produced in large quantities when we are faced with stress**

▲ **Produces brain EEG wave changes that are of benefit**

▲ **Increases production of serotonin**

▲ **Is psychologically and physiologically more refreshing and energy restoring than deep sleep**

Various Relaxation Techniques Include

▲ **Abdominal or diaphragmatic breathing**
▲ **Meditation**   ▲ **Yoga**
▲ **Relaxation tapes or CDs**   ▲ **Biofeedback**
▲ **Hypnosis or self-hypnosis**   ▲ **T'ai chi and Qigong**

Choose the one best suited to your personality.

Basic Rules for Relaxation

▲ Practice regularly for relaxation to be effective. Aim for five or six times a week for 20 to 30 minutes each session.

▲ Relax in a quiet room, free of distraction. (Sometimes this is hard to find.)

▲ Wear loose, comfortable clothing.

▲ Practice diaphragmatic breathing the entire time you practice relaxing.

▲ Don't get discouraged. Anyone can learn to relax. It's like learning to ride a bicycle!

▲ Don't try to force relaxation; it will come naturally. When you first start practicing, you may find it difficult to stay still for that long. The more you practice, the more effective it will become. Try starting with only five to ten minutes. Gradually increase the length of time as your ability to concentrate increases.

▲ Don't expect results for at least six to eight weeks. Dramatic improvement can occur at this time.

Abdominal or Diaphragmatic Breathing Is

▲ Smooth
▲ Deep
▲ Slow
▲ Gentle

To Practice Diaphragmatic Breathing

▲ Make inhalation and exhalation equal.
▲ Breathe through the nose.
▲ Keep posture straight.
▲ Pay attention to your breathing.

It is impossible to be tense when you are breathing deeply. To breathe abdominally, or diaphragmatically, place your hand on your diaphragm (midway between your navel and your chest) and as you breathe, feel your diaphragm—not your chest—expand and rise. If your chest rises when you breathe, you are breathing too shallowly.

It is also important to pay attention throughout the day to how you are breathing. Are you holding your breath? This creates tension. The body needs the oxygen we breathe in for all of its functions. If you hold your breath, your body is deprived of the "breath of life"! Take time throughout the day to notice if you are breathing shallowly. If you are, take a few minutes to remind yourself to breathe from the abdomen. Breathe deeply! You will be rewarded by less tension!

Meditation

Meditation is a relaxation technique which has been practiced for over 2,000 years. It is simple to learn and cost-effective. All you need is a quiet room, yourself, and 15 to 30 minutes. The object of meditation is to quiet the mind, emptying it of unnecessary "chatter," to achieve a state of profound harmony between body and mind.

Focusing your attention on something specific, such as a word, phrase, thought, breath, object or inspiring idea, can bring a deep calm to your mind and body that is healing and relaxing. Praying the rosary is a form of meditative practice, as are chanting and some forms of prayer.

There are a variety of meditation methods to choose from. Mindfulness meditation, derived from the Buddhist tradition, and transcendental meditation are two better known types. Choose one that suits you and that you enjoy. You can learn how to meditate by reading books on the topic, taking a class, or participating in individual sessions taught by qualified individuals. Meditation is often part of pain management programs and stress management classes. Meditation must be practiced regularly to be most effective. Jon Kabat-Zin, Ph.D., has studied meditation in his pain reduction programs at the University of Massachusetts and has prepared books and tapes on the topic, as well as a training program for health professionals and patients. His contact information is in our resource section at the end of this chapter.

Meditation Suggestions

▲ Sit or lie down in a comfortable position in a quiet environment. Legs should be uncrossed. Wear loose comfortable clothes.

▲ Close your eyes.

▲ Breathe through your nose, practicing diaphragmatic breathing.

▲ Deeply relax your muscles, beginning at your feet, and progressing upward to your face. Pay attention to each body part until it feels relaxed and then move on to the next. Take your time so each body part has a chance to relax. Notice your toes and relax them, then your feet, ankles, calves, knees, thighs, pelvic area, abdomen, buttocks, hips, chest, arms, hands, shoulders, chest, neck, jaw, face, forehead, and back.

▲ Become aware of your breathing after you have relaxed your entire body. Saying a one-syllable word like *one, peace, love,* or any other word sacred and pleasing to you as you exhale is a part of the meditation technique.

▲ It doesn't matter what time of day you practice. You do need to be awake, so try not to fall asleep while meditating.

▲ Continue this for 20 to 30 minutes. Do not use an alarm to time yourself.

▲ When you are done, sit quietly for a few minutes. When you get up you might be amazed by how refreshed you feel.

You might find it difficult at first to concentrate only on your breathing, but that is the object. As thoughts come into your mind, be aware of them and then let them drift away. If you have a painful area, become aware of it, too. Many people find that once they pay attention to their pain while in a meditative state, the pain lessens. The object is not to work on a specific area; the entire body is the focus. Regular meditators have overcome addictions to tranquilizers, high blood pressure, pain, anxiety, and even fibromyalgia.

Relaxation Tapes and CDs

Some people prefer using relaxation tapes or CDs to help them in their relaxation "journey." Some tapes and CDs use guided imagery, which transports you to a peaceful area such as a beach or garden and then guides you through images that produce muscular and mind relaxation. Many tapes have soft background music or ocean sounds that are pleasant and calming. The person guiding you on your "journey" usually has a very soothing voice.

Some tapes are designed for specific needs such as headache relief, stress reduction, insomnia, healing, or pain reduction. The tapes and CDs are not expensive: the price range is between $10 and $20. You can plug these into your tape or CD player and relax. If you have a portable player, you can listen to tapes or CDs on planes, in cars, at the beach, or while you wait for a doctor's appointment. You can buy a few different ones and have a variety to choose from. They are available in specialty stores, or they can be ordered over the phone or the internet. See our list of possible selections at the end of this chapter.

Some psychotherapists, nurses, or hypnotherapists can tailor-make a tape for you. These, of course, may be more expensive. You can tape your own if you like. Like meditation, relaxation must be practiced daily to be effective. These tapes have also been effective for some patients who have trouble sleeping at night. If you cannot find 20 or 30 minutes in your day to listen to a tape or CD, maybe you can find 10 minutes a day to set aside for relaxation.

Hypnosis

Hypnosis is well documented as an effective treatment in reducing anxiety and pain. Controlled studies have proven hypnotherapy effective for the treatment of some fibromyalgia symptoms. A trained hypnotherapist can guide you into a trance-like state similar to deep relaxation. He or she will then guide you through a series of suggestions to reduce pain, eliminate stress and anxiety, and help you sleep. It is not known how hypnosis works. These sessions can be taped so you can practice at home. About 90% of the population can be hypnotized, and hypnosis is safe when done by a properly trained therapist. Most states have a society for hypnotists; many are psychologists or medical doctors who use hypnotism in their practices. Look for one who specializes in relaxation and reduction of pain, stress, and anxiety.

Yoga

Yoga is another relaxation technique that not only relaxes your mind, but also provides stretching and flexibility for your body. Yoga classes, books, and videotapes are available. Be sure to choose a yoga practice that is suited to your physical capabilities. You can learn the stretches and then practice them at home every day or every other day for the most benefit. Fibromyalgia patients need to stretch, and yoga provides some great stretching exercises. Just remember not to strain too much. You don't want to hurt yourself.

Biofeedback

Research and practice have shown that biofeedback can help a person gain some measure of control over many stress-related medical conditions, including chronic pain, headaches, hypertension, Raynaud's phenomenon, and anxiety. Biofeedback therapists have often helped fibromyalgia patients learn how to relax more completely and to decrease their muscle tension, thereby decreasing the patient's level of pain.

When being treated with biofeedback, the patient is hooked up to a sensitive, noninvasive physiological measuring instrument that allows the patient to be aware of changes in his or her body moment by moment. Physiological measurements in the body, such as heart rate, muscle tension, respiration, sweat, and body temperature, are monitored and shown on a computer screen. The biofeedback therapist then helps the patient use this information to relax and regulate body processes that increase tension and pain. Over time, the patient no longer needs the biofeedback equipment to achieve the same results, although a booster session may be required from time to time. Less expensive equipment for home use is also available for rental or purchase.

Biofeedback is one alternative for stress reduction and relaxation and may enhance the effectiveness of your medication.

T'ai Chi and Qigong

T'ai chi and qigong are slow-moving exercises that have been performed for centuries in Asia. They are both moving meditation exercises, that gently exercise joints, help reduce stress, and increase chi energy. Classes on t'ai chi and qigong may be available through local resources such as the Y, yoga centers, or the Arthritis Foundation. Instructional videotapes are available in video stores, libraries, and online, or they can be ordered through *Yoga Journal* or *T'ai Chi* magazines. One online product source is www.tai-chi.com. Dr. Paul Lam has produced a series of excellent videotapes, including, *T'ai Chi for Arthritis*. His videos and DVDs can be ordered from www.taichi-productions.com and are available in several languages.

Any one of these relaxation techniques may help patients who are unable to take medications or for whom medications provide little relief.

Daily Affirmations

Because it takes persistence and motivation to get better with FMS, we have provided you with what we feel are the most important things for you to do on a daily basis. Performing them daily can be difficult because of lack of motivation, fatigue, or just life! We know that if you remind yourself daily about what you could be doing to help yourself, you will be more likely to do it! Here are the top ten things you can do for yourself. You have our permission to photo copy this page, so you can place it in a conspicuous spot where it is readily accessible. Tape it to your bathroom mirror; place it on your bedstand or in your kitchen. Most important, read it daily.

The Most Important Daily Affirmations for Taking Charge of Fibromyalgia

▲ I will practice deep breathing today, because it will reduce my stress level and give my body all the oxygen it requires. This will reduce my anxiety and even out my body chemistry.

▲ I will take all my medications at the appropriate times and in the appropriate dosages today.

▲ I will take all my vitamins today.

▲ I will eat nutritious food today.

▲ I will pace myself today and do only those things necessary for my well-being.

▲ I will do at least one thing today that I really enjoy.

▲ I will exercise today, even if for only two minutes.

▲ I will stretch today.

▲ I will have positive thoughts today.

▲ I will make contact with positive friends or family today.

STRESS MANAGEMENT

Changing Negative Self-talk Journal

Sample:

Negative thoughts: I can not clean the house. My pain is too high.

Negative emotions related to negative thoughts: Anger, sadness, fear, guilt.

Pain level: Pain scale of one-ten with ten being the most pain.

Change negative thought to positive thought: I can wait until tomorrow and see if I feel better or I can do some chores today for 20 minutes and then rest.

Pain level: Use pain scale of one to ten to chart your pain when thinking positively.

NEGATIVE THOUGHT	NEGATIVE EMOTION	PAIN LEVEL	CHANGE TO POSITIVE THOUGHT	PAIN LEVEL

Stress Management Journal

MY STRESSORS	HOW TO MANAGE STRESSORS
(Sample) WORK	*Reduce hours, job training, leave of absence, occupational therapy, massage, hot tubs, medicine, exercise, meditation, sleep*

		Daily Stress Management Chart		
DATE	STRESS (0-10) LEVEL	STRESSORS	SYMPTOMS	COPING METHODS

STRESS MANAGEMENT

		Personal Activity Chart		
TIME	ACTIVITY	SYMPTOMS	STRATEGIES

Stress Management Resources: Tapes, CDs, and Catalogues

Music by Stephen Halpern: www.innerpeacemusic.com 800-909-0707

Enya's music: available at most music outlets and large bookstores

Classical music

New Age music

Imagery Tapes, CDs

Belleruth Naparstek: www.healthjourneys.com; 800-800-8661. She has tapes and CDs specifically for fibromyalgia and CFIDS.

Mary Richards: www. masteryourmind.com; 800-345-8515. We like her *Release Discomfort* and *Relaxing into Sleep* tapes.

Jon Kabat-Zin: www.mindfulnesstapes.com; 508-856-2656. He offers mindfulness meditation practice tapes and book, *Full Catastrophe Living*.

Others can be found at bookstores, music stores, retail outlets such as Target and Wal-Mart or New Age stores.

Catalogues; Other Products

Sounds True, Inc.: www.soundstrue.com; 800-333-9185. This company offers a variety of products, including tapes and books.

Living Arts: www.gaiam.com; 877-989-6321. Provides over 4,500 products for healthy living including organic clothing, household products, massagers, tapes, and books.

TIPS Managing Unavoidable Stress

▲ Counter stress with activities that reduce your stress level.

   Example: Have tea with a friend at a favorite restaurant. Write in your journal every day. Take a walk on your lunch hour. Close your door and put your feet up for ten minutes. Listen to relaxing, soothing music.

▲ Limit other stresses you have control over.

   Example: Postpone dental work. Cancel unnecessary appointments and work tasks. Put off any projects until stress has reduced.

▲ Let go of perfection as a standard for performance for anything that doesn't have to be perfect. We pay an enormous price for perfection in time and energy.

   Example: Try not to judge yourself harshly for work that is less than perfect.

▲ Every hour stand up and stretch, do some relaxed breathing, and repeat to yourself a relaxing thought or phrase.

   Example: "The day is almost over . . . This project is going well."

▲ Take time for yourself. Sleep in late on Saturday. Relax in a bubble bath at night.

▲ Although you may have no control over a current stressful event, you can choose how you react to it. You can choose to stay relaxed and take good care of yourself during difficult periods.

▲ Avoid catastrophic thinking such as *This is awful and terrible*. This type of thinking only makes matters worse and increases your stress level.

▲ Change negative thoughts into positive ones:

Negative Example: "I'm late and the doctor will be angry for having to wait."

Positive Example: "It's not the end of the world that I'm late. I'll give the doctor's office a call and let them know a problem has come up and they can take the next patient who is waiting."

▲ How important is this anyway? Avoid feeling frustrated over details that in the long run aren't going to matter.

▲ Accept the things you cannot change.

▲ Be flexible and try alternatives that may be less than ideal.

Example: Instead of wrapping your relative's gift when you are running late, put it into a gift bag or a brown paper bag with a pretty bow!

▲ Delegate tasks whenever possible to family, friends, and others. We can't do it all.

▲ Treat yourself gently and with the tender, loving care you would give a friend during stressful times.

▲ Exercise regularly during heavy stress periods to avoid muscle tightness and flare-ups. (Make it a priority.)

▲ Pay attention to sleep habits during high stress times. If sleep quality becomes disturbed, a flare-up may occur. Do all you can to get a good night's sleep (e.g., hot bath and relaxation before bed, shut out noise).

▲ Get extra support. Talk and write about what is going on. Look for resources to help you deal with specific problems.

▲ If a stressful situation becomes chronic, get support to make positive changes.

Example: If you have a child who is an alcoholic, try an Al-Anon support group. Find a marriage counselor to help resolve conflicts in a marriage.

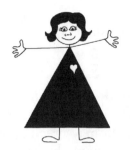

COPING WITH PSYCHOLOGICAL ASPECTS OF FIBROMYALGIA

Recognize Your Feelings

In order to begin to cope with the psychological aspects of FMS, it's important to first accept that it's not "all in your head." Then you can begin to recognize the variety of feelings that you may have about the diagnosis.

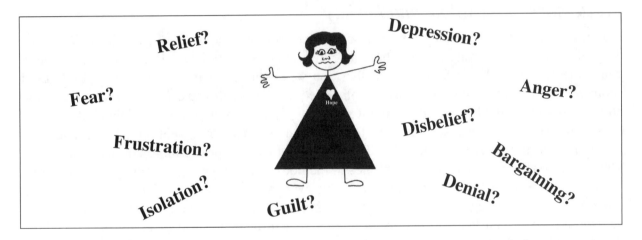

Whatever feelings you have, it's important to recognize them, and to work through them, refocusing your energy on the process of learning to accept or acknowledge your diagnosis. This process takes varying amounts of time for each of us and is often easier said than done. But it's a critical step, because if you stay stuck in the feelings of anger, fear, frustration, or denial of your diagnosis, you forgo the opportunity to move on with your life and learn how to cope successfully.

Feelings

If you have been recently diagnosed with fibromyalgia, you may be relieved that you finally have a name to give all the symptoms you have been experiencing. Some people are relieved initially because uncertainty keeps them feeling fear and anxiety. Once you are diagnosed, you may experience numerous feelings. You may refuse to accept the diagnosis of FMS and wish to continue searching for another cause of your discomfort. If you are confident in your physician's care and diagnostic ability and all other possibilities have been ruled out, it is not useful to continue searching for another reason. It only wastes your time, energy and money. It is better to refocus your energy on getting better. Your feelings may waver from shock, disbelief, and denial to anger, frustration, confusion, and fear. Some people are relieved, while others find themselves locked in a state of alarm, feeling as if their whole world has fallen apart. With the diagnosis of any illness, you may experience significant losses, including loss of your health, and loss of your former capabilities, both physical and mental; possibly loss of friends, family, or your job. Loss causes people to go through a series of emotional reactions that can be overcome with help.

Grief

Research shows that when people are confronted with a significant loss in their lives, they go through certain stages of grieving. When you are diagnosed with an illness such as FMS, you have sustained a loss in your health, which may preclude you from performing tasks that were once easy, prior to developing FMS. You may not be able to work or perform household chores, and you may reduce your social activities because of pain and fatigue. Feelings of grief are one way that nature allows you to turn inward and conserve your energy. You may feel that you want to isolate yourself and not reach out to others, or you may bombard your friends and family with your feelings. Crying and feeling depressed are normal ways of reacting to the loss of your health. It is important to express your feelings at this time, whether with a trusted friend, family member, counselor, or minister. We have mentioned many times throughout this book how journaling your feelings can be helpful. If you are overwhelmed by fear or anxiety, it is important to process your feelings with someone who is supportive and who will not deny or try to diminish your emotional state.

Restlessness, Confusion, and Anxiety

You may feel as if you cannot relax because you feel confused about how your life will be now that you have this diagnosis. You may have anxious thoughts about how you will be able to handle your illness, who will help you, and whether you will ever feel better. You may feel confused about your treatment options. You may be compelled to find out all you can about FMS by reading books or searching the Internet for more information. These activities are beneficial, but they can cause more confusion because so much information and so many treatment options are available. It is important not to overwhelm yourself with details that may create more confusion and fear. The pain of FMS produces physical changes in the body that can generate anxiety or depression. Your thoughts can spiral out of control causing even more anxiety. Anxiety can be managed utilizing the methods suggested in the chapter on stress management and by the use of medication or exercise. You can learn to control your thoughts through the use of cognitive behavioral therapy, which will help calm you and reduce excessive worry.

Helplessness and Fear

Do you feel helpless when trying to cope with your symptoms? If you were previously a strong, physically active person, you may now feel you have lost control over your body and your life. You now have to rely on physicians, physical therapists, medications, and lifestyle changes to help you cope with symptoms. This in itself can upset your emotional state. You may find yourself preoccupied with thoughts of how to cope on a daily basis with the everyday tasks you need to attend to, such as taking care of your family's needs and your own needs.

Some fear is a normal reaction to the loss of your former self. You may be fearful of what the future may bring. You may worry about the illness getting worse or causing death. FMS does not cause death and most studies show it will not become worse with time, if treated properly. You may fear the loss of loved ones who may not understand your illness or be willing to stand by you during this time. Fear can cause much stress and anxiety and at times be overwhelming.

Anger

Anger is a common reaction for people to experience when they are diagnosed with any illness. You may be angry with health professionals if you feel they are not doing enough to improve your symptoms. You may be angry with yourself and wonder what you did to bring this on. Some people are angry with God for their situation. If your FMS is the result of an accident or surgery, you may blame those involved. Taking your anger out on yourself or people close to you will not improve your situation and will only produce more pain. Staying in an angry mode will not help you and it is important to address anger so you can move past it.

Guilt

You may feel guilty because you cannot perform the tasks you used to, such as keeping up your home or working full time. If you cannot work, you may feel guilty over not being able to provide for your family financially. Some people have difficulty asking for help. Now is not the time to berate yourself for things that are outside your control. Ask for help. Often people are willing and glad to help.

Loss of Confidence and Self-esteem

All of the above feelings, coupled with an inability to perform former functions, can make you experience a loss of confidence and lowered self-esteem, especially if you are very disabled by FMS. You may feel as if you are not a productive individual anymore, and you may have problems accepting help from others. You may lose friends or family members due to this illness, which can leave you feeling less empowered.

Many people change careers or search for new hobbies that can take the place of activities formerly enjoyed. You may learn about untapped capabilities within yourself that can be expressed and can make up for any loss of self-esteem or confidence you may experience. You may have to make changes to discover some of your new talents and potential. Many FMS patients have changed careers or found new ways to express themselves by volunteering or mentoring others.

You may use our "Feelings Journal" page at the end of this chapter to help process your feelings. Acknowledging that you have these feelings is the first step toward overcoming them. Some people refuse to admit they have these feelings. This does not help you; it only pushes the feelings down where they can cause havoc. Writing about your feelings can help.

Family Issues

You may find that your family is also experiencing emotional reactions to your illness. Your spouse, significant other, or children may be feeling some or all of the emotions discussed above. It is important to bring these feelings out into the open with effective communication.

Education is very important at this time. Maybe your family members can attend your doctor's appointments, so your physician can clarify and answer their questions about FMS. Your spouse could read this book or other information to give him or her greater insight into your illness and your disability. Attending classes together given by local hospitals, patient conferences with your doctor, or your local support group meetings will also help family members gain greater insight. We allow family members to attend our classes for free and we encourage their participation.

Children do not need to be excluded from learning about fibromyalgia. They can be educated by adults at the child's level of understanding. In your library, you may find some good books to read with children to diminish their fear. A good workbook to use with your children is called *Are You Tired Again? I Understand* by Marilyn W. Deutsch, which provides you with ways to help your child cope with and express feelings about your illness. Sometimes, adults think children cannot or do not need to understand their parent's illness. If children are not educated, they can develop anxiety and fears that can lead to sleep problems, acting out behaviors, and/or depression. Sometimes children's fears are far worse than the reality of the situation. Rosalie and Julie work with many children and know that if children are allowed to discuss their fears, they feel less anxious. Sometimes, parents do not know what questions to ask their children. A trained counselor can help allay children's fears and answer their questions. Being forthright with children is the best policy. They know more than we think.

You and your family may face numerous issues after you are diagnosed with FMS. Your family may want to know how disabled you could become. Could FMS lead to death? Children are extremely frightened by this thought, and it is necessary to reassure them and answer their questions. If you were used to an active social life before FMS, and are now too fatigued and in pain to attend social functions, your spouse may be angry and resentful. If you can no longer work, does your spouse feel burdened by the added financial responsibility?

You may be too tired and in too much pain to perform sexual activities you once enjoyed. This lack of intimacy can be frustrating for both you and your partner. Dr. Pelligrino's book *Inside Fibromyalgia* addresses some of these concerns, with diagrams on positions which are enjoyable and do not increase pain. Some medications, including many of the SSRI antidepressants may reduce sexual desire. Talking about your concerns will help if you can discuss them without anger. Not discussing them will only sabotage your relationship.

You may be unable to perform normal household chores that you once could, which can strain family relationships. Your family may not be used to helping around the home and may be resistant to engaging in household chores. If this is the case, hold a family meeting and arrange a way to have family members help you. Please do not be afraid to ask for help. Even small children can do simple tasks such as emptying the dishwasher or mopping floors. In exchange, you could read them more bedtime stories, let them have a favorite treat, offer more computer time, or in the case of teenagers, more car use, more phone time, later hours or a bigger allowance. Chore charts placed where everyone can see them are useful if everyone has a designated chore to check off when accomplished. Rewards are to be given for completing tasks. They do not necessarily have to be financial rewards. Chore charts can be made in a family meeting or purchased at local drugstores, office supply chains, or discount stores. Some families enjoy using job jars, in which pieces of paper with chores written on them are placed in a jar. Each person picks one chore from the jar, and exchanges can be made by family members if they choose one they don't like.

Do Not Be Afraid to Ask Your Family Members for Help!

Many people do not like to admit they need help. Some may become dependent on others and refuse to try to help themselves. Neither of these methods of dealing with your illness is an effective coping technique. It is preferable to find a middle ground in which you can ask for help when needed, yet do the things you can do. If you lie around feeling sorry for yourself, you will only hinder your ability to get better, and you may not experience all that life does have to offer you, even with FMS as your partner.

Counseling for you and your spouse or family counseling could help your family adjust to any problems that arise. Make sure the counselor has a knowledge of health issues.

Courage to Change

Your life has changed. You don't have a choice about having fibromyalgia, but you do have choices about how you are going to live with it now that it is a part of your life. One step in beginning to cope might include adopting "The Serenity Prayer:"

God grant me the serenity to accept the things I cannot change, the courage to change the things I can, and the wisdom to know the difference.

Reinhold Niebuhr

After being diagnosed with fibromyalgia, you may be faced with changes that you don't want to make, such as pacing your activities, or making time for relaxation, aerobic exercise, stretching—the list could go on and on. Instead of resisting change (which is often our first response), try to look at change as a positive way to make life easier, feel better, and cope more successfully. Sometimes we do need courage to change.

Support

As we make the necessary changes and adjustments, many of us recognize the benefit of having good support. Supportive family members and friends are invaluable and help us to cope. It may be helpful to visualize the layers of support that surround you, as in the diagram on this page. A support journal is also included at the end of this section so that you can write down the people, and organizations that form your layers of support.

First Ring

Identify those family members and friends who can provide some support for you. Many people say that they never would have been able to cope successfully with their fibromyalgia without the support of those closest to them. Do remember, though, to share other parts of your life, even when it seems that your world has narrowed to just yourself and your fibromyalgia.

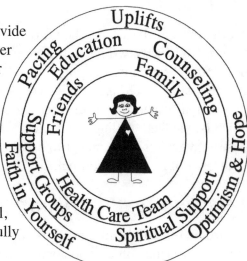

Your healthcare team can be especially supportive during the initial diagnosis and treatment phase. They are available to answer your questions, listen, counsel, educate, and support you in your quest to cope successfully with the many facets of fibromyalgia.

Second Ring

This second layer of support includes the education you receive in the form of classes, individual instruction, articles, videotapes, and books. Counseling and spiritual support can be invaluable in terms of support, and we encourage individuals to pursue them. Support groups are also beneficial for many people, because no matter how much your family and friends love and support you, unless they have fibromyalgia, they really don't know what you're experiencing. Simply the knowledge that you're not alone can make your experience much more bearable. To receive a list of fibromyalgia support groups in your state, contact your local Arthritis Foundation or hospital. National FMS organizations can also supply you with a list of support groups for your state.

Third Ring

Pacing your activities is helpful in managing fatigue and in creating time to "take care of you." Uplifts are those activities that you enjoy, which give you positive energy. For example, having lunch with a close friend, buying yourself some flowers, or going for a walk on a beautiful day. (Further examples of uplifts are found at the end of this section.) By pacing and implementing uplifts, you will create another layer of support for yourself. Being optimistic and having faith in yourself empower you to seek support, feel supported, and extend support to others. These are all part of the process of coping effectively.

Balance

Another method of coping is striving to keep one's life in balance when the pain, fatigue, and limitations of fibromyalgia seem to be weighing you down. We can strive to balance the scale by seeking and developing support (as we just discussed), practicing uplifts, and taking advantage of those resources that can help. Examples are massage, a class in water aerobics, a warm water pool, whirlpool, or a new relaxation tape. Develop your own list of resources that work for you, especially when you need to regain some balance. (Refer to list of uplifts at the end of this section.)

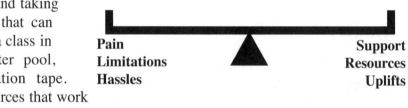

Negative	Positive
Pain	Support
Limitations	Resources
Hassles	Uplifts

Journaling

Journaling can be a very helpful tool in coping with many of the psychological aspects of fibromyalgia. By writing down your thoughts, feelings, fears, hopes, and concerns, you may develop a greater insight, gain a new direction, solve a problem, get in touch with your feelings, or engage in a rich dialog with yourself. Journaling can also provide an outlet for emotional expression, especially when you ensure that only you will see your thoughts. Repressed or unacknowledged feelings can create a lot of stress and are often expressed in unhealthy, destructive ways. Remember to use the various journal pages included in this handbook to start your own fibromyalgia journal.

Learning to "Take Charge"

A chronic illness like fibromyalgia can make patients feel that they lack control over their health. If you experience little or no control, you may come to believe that external factors control your health status—that nothing you initiate or contribute makes a difference. From this perspective, you may feel like a passive player in your treatment.

You'll do better if you adopt an active, "take charge" role in the management of your fibromyalgia. Your healthcare team needs to encourage your active participation and respect your questions, comments, and suggestions. Your willingness to become educated about fibromyalgia and its various medications and treatments is the first step toward becoming actively involved in your care. It is then your responsibility to participate in the various components of your treatment program, to give feedback, and to ask questions of your healthcare team. With this additional input, your treatment program will become more individualized and better suited to your needs.

Ask for Help with Problems That You Can't Handle

Unfortunately, no matter how well we adjust to the changes fibromyalgia may bring to our lives, sometimes problems occur that we just can't seem to handle. We may need help in coping and asking for help. Depression is one of the most common problems the fibromyalgia patients often need help in managing.

The following are signs of depression:

- ▲ **Feelings of sadness that last for too long**
- ▲ **Major changes in sleep habits—sleeping too much or hardly at all**
- ▲ **Listlessness**
- ▲ **Poor concentration**
- ▲ **Major changes in eating habits**
- ▲ **Sense of worthlessness**
- ▲ **Severe feelings of guilt**
- ▲ **Lack of interest in sex**
- ▲ **Thoughts of, or attempts at, suicide**

Depression is a normal part of the grieving process—in this situation, grieving over the loss of health. It is often during this stage that you begin to face the reality of what life is going to be like with fibromyalgia. If you feel unable to arrive gradually at a stage of acceptance or feel stuck in a state of depression, it's very important to discuss this issue with a trusted member of your healthcare team. Depression can lower serotonin and help keep you in a "vicious cycle of pain." It needs to be treated . . . remember to ask for help!

Seasonal affective disorder (SAD) is experienced by some individuals as the days get progressively shorter and they experience less sunlight. Individuals who live in northern climates may be particularly susceptible to this disorder. The deprivation of light, especially during the winter months, may predispose some individuals to depression, fatigue, decreased productivity and motivation, decreased ability to concentrate, and low energy levels. Spending time outside on a sunny day, traveling in midwinter to a southern climate, or using full spectrum bright lights daily can help decrease these symptoms. Apollo Light is one resource for full spectrum lights and features the goLITE which is a small, portable unit that represents the latest in light therapy technology: (www.apollolight.com). Another resource for lights is Light Therapy Products (www.LightTherapyProducts.com). Some insurance companies will pay for a portion of the lights with a doctor's prescription.

Your health professional can suggest how many minutes per day that you should use the light therapy for maximum benefit.

Anxiety and overwhelming stress are additional problems that we often can't handle alone. Consulting a psychologist, counselor, or psychiatrist can be a beneficial and important part of your treatment.

In Review, To Cope Effectively:

▲ **Recognize the feelings you have regarding the diagnosis of fibromyalgia.**

▲ **Refocus your energy on the process of learning to accept or acknowledge your diagnosis.**

▲ **Develop courage to change those things that can make your life easier, help you feel better, and let you cope more successfully.**

▲ **Develop a good support system.**

▲ **Strive to keep your life in balance.**

▲ **Use journaling to express your thoughts, feelings, fears, hopes, and concerns.**

▲ **Learn to take charge of your fibromyalgia.**

▲ **Ask for help with problems that you can't handle, such as depression, anxiety and overwhelming stress.**

Uplifts

Life with chronic pain, fatigue, and other symptoms of fibromyalgia can cause a person to become discouraged or depressed. **Uplifts** are positive experiences, large or small, that can brighten your day and make living with pain easier and more bearable. They are personally chosen and meaningful to the person experiencing them.

Make your own list and keep it handy for times when you are in pain or feeling discouraged. When the scale is weighing on the negative side, balance the scale by injecting an uplift or two into your day to bring the scale to a positive position.

Some examples of uplifting possibilities are:

▲ Take a special coffee or tea break and read a good book.

▲ Take a walk outdoors on a nice day.

▲ Call a friend or family member.

▲ Write in a journal.

▲ Take a nap.

▲ Spend time with a favorite friend or support person.

▲ Go to your favorite floral shop and buy a flower for your desk or table.

▲ Read a good magazine.

▲ Take a hot fragrant bath or shower.

▲ Wear a favorite dress or special soothing perfume.

▲ Go somewhere you've always wanted to go.

▲ Learn something new.

▲ Have a massage or self-massage.

▲ Plan a vacation or other special occasion.

▲ Volunteer for a worthy cause.

▲ Read a book with a child or spouse.

▲ Ask for a hug from a support person.

▲ Buy a special treat or present.

▲ Do some self-care for your pain.

▲ Go to lunch with a special person.

▲ Go to a funny or good movie.

▲ Spend time painting or working on a craft or hobby.

▲ Do a relaxation exercise with music.

▲ Swim in a warm pool.

▲ Have a favorite dinner or other special food.

▲ Write a note to someone expressing how much you care.

▲ Listen to your favorite music station or tape.

▲ Do positive self-talks reminding yourself of your specialness and beauty.

▲ Plan for a goal of something you want to accomplish.

▲ Do some simple stretching exercises or other stress-buster exercises.

▲ Look at a picture book of art, photos, or mementos and reminisce.

Support Journal

Write down the specific people and organizations that form your layers of support. This diagram may give you a better idea of where you can expand your support.

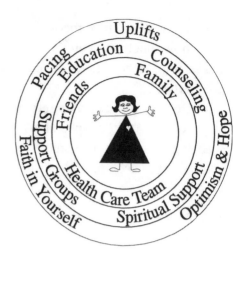

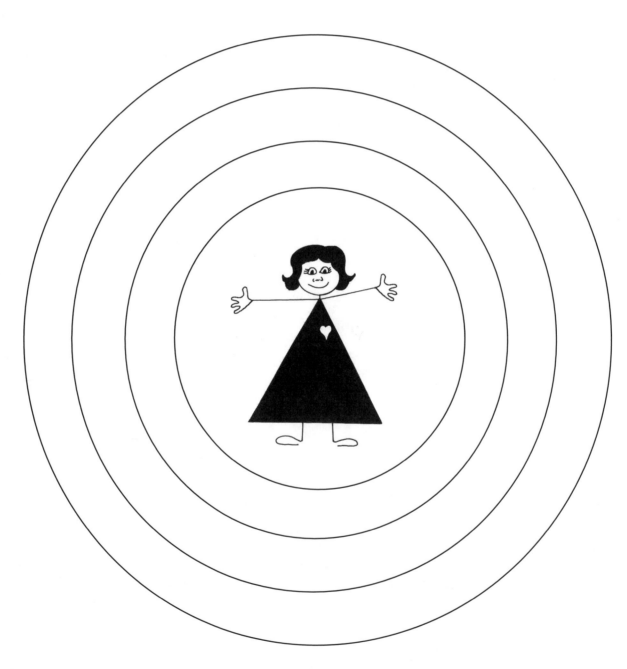

Stress and Coping Resource List

Books

1. *The Big Book of Relaxation* edited by Larry Blumenfeld.

2. *The Book of Stress Survival* by Alix Kirsta

3. *Coping with Stress: A Guide to Living* by Jane Willard Mills

4. *Feeling Good: The New Mood Therapy* by David D. Burns, M.D.

5. *Fire in the Soul* by Joan Borysenko, Ph.D.

6. *Focus on the Positive - The Workbook* by John Roger and Peter McWilliams

7. *Full Catastrophe Living* by Jon Kabat-Zinn, Ph.D.

8. *Healing from Within* by Dennis T. Jaffe, Ph.D.

9. *Healing Words: The Power of Prayer and the Practice of Medicine* by Larry Dossey, M.D.

10. *I Will Live Today! Affirmations for Strength and Healing While Coping with Serious Illness* by Judith Garrett Garrison, M.Ed., L.S.W., and Scott Sheperd, Ph.D.

11. *Is It Worth Dying For?* by Dr. Robert S. Eliot and Dennis L. Breo

12. *Journey into Healing* by Deepak Chopra, M.D.

13. *Successful Living with Chronic Illness* by Kathleen Lewis

14. *Living with It Daily: Meditations for People with Chronic Pain* by Patricia D. Nielsen

15. *Meditations for Healing* by Larry Moen

16. *Mind as Healer, Mind as Slayer* by Kenneth R. Pelletier

17. *Minding the Body, Mending the Mind* by Joan Borysenko

18. *Perfect Health: The Complete Mind/Body Guide* by Deepak Chopra, M.D.

19. *Psychoneuroimmunology: The New Mind/Body Healing Program* by Elliott S. Dacher, M.D.

20. *Quantum Healing* by Deepak Chopra, M.D.

21. *Real Magic* by Dr. Wayne W. Dyer

22. *The Relaxation and Stress Reduction Workbook* by Martha Davis, Ph.D., Elizabeth Robbins Eshelmen, M.S.W., and Matthew McKay, Ph.D.

23. *The Relaxation Response* by Herbert Benson

24. *When Bad Things Happen to Good People* by Harold S. Kushner

25. *Why Me, Why This, Why Now?* by Robin Norwood

26. *You Can Heal Your Life* by Louise L. Hay

27. *You Can't Afford the Luxury of a Negative Thought* by Peter McWilliams

28. *The Chronic Illness Workbook: Strategies for Taking Back Your Life* by Patricia Fennell.

29. *Are You Tired Again...I Understand. An Activities Workbook to Help Children Understand and Live with a Person Who Has a Chronic Illness or Disability* by Marilyn W. Deutsch.

30. *Celebrate Life: New Attitudes for Living with Chronic Illness* by Kathleen Lewis.

Feelings Journal

Feeling	Why Do You Feel This Way?	What Can You Do To Change or Modify the Feeling?
Example: Frustration	I can't do what I want to do, when and how I want to do it. Specific reason: I can't play 18 holes of golf anymore.	Take one day at a time, try a different approach, make small changes. I'll just practice putting or hit a few balls at the driving range. I'll play three holes of golf or watch golf on TV.

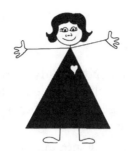

FLARE-UP MANAGEMENT

The course of fibromyalgia varies from one person to another and is characterized by remissions and flare-ups of symptoms. A remission is defined as a period when symptoms are greatly diminished or even absent. Remissions can last for days, weeks, months, and even years, often differing from one time to another. A flare-up of symptoms can often be associated with weather changes, stress, interrupted sleep, depression, postural strain, illness, or even the flu. Sometimes a flare-up can't be attributed to anything we're able to identify, which can contribute to a feeling of frustration and lack of control over our health.

It is extremely important to regain a "take charge" attitude over your fibromyalgia and learn to proactively manage a flare-up. You may feel more anxious, depressed, or hopeless as your symptoms increase, which may contribute to further pain, fatigue, and cognitive problems. When this occurs, some patients may try to cope by frantically calling their physician for help. Others may feel it is useless to try to help themselves and succumb to the flare-up by isolating themselves. It is best to have a plan for dealing with flare-ups before they begin, so you can initiate your flare-up management techniques immediately without having to feel more anxious, depressed, or hopeless about your symptoms. It's also important to understand that the duration, intensity, and type of symptoms often vary and may present you with new challenges.

You may find it helpful to work with your physician or healthcare provider to develop options that you can utilize quickly. You and your physician or other healthcare provider can determine what steps you can take to reduce symptoms or shorten the length of a flare-up. If you determine that extra medication is needed for a short time until symptoms subside, maybe a phone call to the nurse will be all that is needed to get a prescription filled. Or perhaps a few visits to your physical therapist can be arranged, if that works for you. It is important for you, as the patient, to tell your healthcare professional what works for you, as each patient responds differently to different therapies. The following are options that work for many patients, and you can explore these with your healthcare professional:

Remove or change a modulating factor, if possible.
- ▲ Eliminate or reduce repetitive stress (e.g., typing at a keyboard, sitting or standing in one position for extended periods of time, continuous repetition of any muscular movement).
- ▲ Treat other illnesses as they occur; not all symptoms are related to fibromyalgia.
- ▲ Correct posture; change your work height at your desk; consider getting a lumbar pillow.

Evaluate sleep and discuss other medication options with your physician.
- ▲ A different medication or dosage of current medication may be increased.
- ▲ A sleeping medication may be added.
- ▲ Pain medication may be used for a short time to improve sleep quality.

▲ Improve sleep environment; snoring spouses, crying babies, even pets, can interfere with sleep.

Use relaxation or biofeedback.

▲ Use relaxation techniques which can be easily learned from commercially available audiotapes. Some of these tapes include guided imagery that transports you to a peaceful area such as a beach or garden and then guides you through images that produce muscular and mind relaxation.

▲ Use biofeedback techniques to help you relax more quickly, decrease muscle tension, and reduce pain.

▲ Listen to soothing music.

Rest and be gentle to yourself.

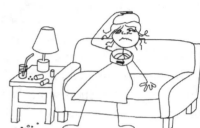

▲ Take frequent breaks from activity.

▲ Cancel unnecessary appointments.

▲ Give yourself permission to take care of your health.

▲ Try to make activities of daily living as easy as possible.

▲ Take a nap and/or try to get more sleep at night.

▲ Refrain from staying in bed for days at a time.

Reduce your stress level.

▲ Identify major stressors and eliminate or modify where you can.

▲ Alter your perception of the stress, whether it is emotional or physical.

▲ Journal your thoughts. By writing down your thoughts, feelings, hopes, fears, and concerns, you may develop greater insight, gain new direction, solve a problem, get in touch with your feelings, and engage in a rich dialogue with yourself.

Use heat or analgesics.

▲ Utilize warm baths, whirlpools, or cold packs.

▲ Use topical creams or gels that reduce pain or those containing prescription pain relievers.

▲ Short-term use of over-the-counter pain relievers can be helpful.

Use massage, acupressure, or acupuncture.

▲ Use self-massage and acupressure tools.

▲ Several sessions of physical therapy may be prescribed.

▲ See a massage therapist.

▲ May be a time to try acupuncture.

Stretch gently.

▲ Increase stretching to ease those kinks and knots. (Try applying heat for 15-20 minutes before.)

Decrease duration and intensity of exercise.

▲ This is not a time to increase exercise; listen to your body for signals.

▲ This is also not a time to stop moving.

Repeat positive messages.

▲ It's easy to feel discouraged, but try repeating these self-affirming messages:
"I am doing everything necessary to feel better."
"This flare-up will be over soon."
"I can cope." "I can cope."

Get extra support during these times from a friend or counselor who understands your illness and listens to you.

Flare-ups ar[...]ing with fibromyalgia. Although they can be frustrating, discouraging, and uncom[...] you can help yourself through them by utilizing these strategies. It is import[...] hat this, too, will pass—as flare-ups always do.

[...]rnal

[...]hurt)

TRIA ORTHOPAEDIC CENTER
8100 NORTHLAND DRIVE
MINNEAPOLIS / MINNESOTA / 55431

For more information visit our website, our state-of-the-science facility at 494 and France, or call 952-831-TRIA (8742). www.tria.com

A state-of-the-science partnership of Park Nicollet Health Services and University of Minnesota Physicians.

[...]ation, etc., may help my discomfort today.

[...]s, unresolved conflict, and postural strain may make my [...]eriencing any of these, I will work on resolving _____

K[...] of the pain is important. When I'm in pain, I will think about (list some ple[...] ghts and memories): _____

_____

What is something special that I can do for myself today? _____

_____

I need to keep my life focused on healthy habits. A healthy habit that I want to work on is

_____

I need to keep connected with my family and friends. They are an important support system for me. I will do _____

_____

Questions and concerns that I want to remember to ask my doctor or nurse: _____

_____

_____

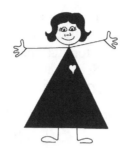

DIET AND NUTRITIONAL SUPPLEMENTS

▲ Researchers have not focused on this area.

▲ Much of this information is taken from anecdotal reports and research prepared by dieticians, nutritionists, holistic physicians, herbalists, and naturopathic doctors.

▲ We cannot guarantee the benefit of any of these treatments.

▲ A well-balanced diet is important in maintaining a healthy body and mind.

▲ Avoid over-processed foods, nicotine, sugar, caffeine, artificial sweeteners, and preservatives.

▲ Good books are available in health food stores and bookstores.

A number of patients in our classes ask how diet or nutritional supplements can help alleviate their FMS symptoms. Although researchers have not focused on this area thus far, some physicians are beginning to assess how vitamin levels, diet changes, and food and chemical sensitivities affect certain individuals with FMS. We would like to provide you with an overview of what we have learned about these topics. We would like to emphasize that much of this information has not been subject to rigorous scientific study specifically for FMS. Much is taken from anecdotal reports and research prepared by dieticians, nutritionists, herbalists, holistic physicians, and naturopathic doctors. We cannot guarantee that any of these nutritional supplements or dietary changes will reduce your symptoms, although more and more FMS sufferers are turning to this form of treatment when all else fails, or are using it in conjunction with other therapies. We cannot emphasize enough that, for many individuals, treating fibromyalgia requires a multitreatment approach, and dietary changes could be one piece of the treatment approach that helps you feel better.

Diet

Remember that a well-balanced diet is an important component of good health. You are what you eat. If you fill your body with poor quality, highly refined, over-processed foods, nicotine, alcohol, sugar, caffeine, artificial sweeteners, and preservatives, your body will suffer. Some FMS and CFIDS patients have benefited from changing their diets to all fresh, organically produced foods and avoiding the ones just mentioned. There are many good books available that discuss healthy eating. A trip to your local book store will help to educate you in this area.

Diet Options

▲ Elimination of MSG & aspartame ▲ Zone Diet

▲ All vegan diet ▲ Antiyeast diet

▲ Low-carbohydrate and high-protein diet

- ▲ Food allergies elimination diet
- ▲ Diet changes for leaky gut syndrome

Always speak to your physician before making any dietary changes.

There have only been a few small studies showing improvement in symptoms by changing diet. When patients are diagnosed with *Candida* and follow the *Candida* diet described in this section, there may be significant improvement in FMS or CFIDS symptoms. There are numerous anecdotal reports of patients' symptoms improving on special diets, or by eliminating specific substances. We provide you with an overview of the diets found helpful.

MSG & Aspartame

There have been a few, very small studies reporting improvement in symptoms when eliminating these substances. MSG (monosodium glutamate) is a flavor enhancer that is used extensively in our food products. It is not only referred to as MSG but also as gelatin, hydrolyzed protein, textured protein, and yeast extract. MSG is broken down into glutamate, an excitatory amino acid that activates the NMDA receptors involved in wind-up sensitization in the central nervous system. It may be difficult to totally eliminate the product if your diet consists of over-refined, highly processed foods or if you eat out often. Aspartame (NutraSweet), which is found in a variety of dietary products, converts, when processed in the body, into the excitatory amino acid aspartate. Aspartate can switch on the pain amplifying receptors. Since scientific evidence shows that FMS patients' NMDA receptors are already activated, eliminating these products from your diet may help symptoms. So many of us, in trying to lose weight, use products containing aspartame, which may be influencing our symptoms. If you cannot give up diet soft drinks, you could try Diet Rite Cola, which has no caffeine or aspartame. Products containing Splenda, another artificial sweetener, are preferable to use. To give up MSG, you will need to look at food labels carefully. There are some books available on this topic, and one good one is *Excitotoxins: The Taste That Kills* by Russell L. Blaylock, M.D.

Vegan Diet

In Finland, a study was performed in which FMS patients ate an all-vegetarian diet consisting of only fresh, cooked foods including fruits, berries, legumes, seeds, vegetables, and nuts. Coffee, tea, alcohol, sugar, and salt were not allowed in this study.

After three months, patients in the vegan group displayed a significant decrease in pain; sleep improved, they experienced less morning stiffness and they felt better overall. When they returned to a "normal" diet, all of their symptoms returned! This is not an easy diet to follow, but it could be worth a try to see if it helps reduce your symptoms. Eating organic foods, which can be expensive, may help rid the body of the toxins found in our food supply.

Low-carbohydrate and High-protein Diet

Some physicians, including Mark Pellegrino, M.D., advocate a high-protein, low-carbohydrate diet for FMS patients. They believe FMS patients may be hypersensitive to insulin. When carbohydrates are consumed in excess, the sugar produced from them quickly enters the bloodstream, causing an increase in insulin levels. Any sugar not needed for energy is stored in the liver and muscles as glycogen or is eventually converted to fat. Potential benefits from this diet could be a decrease in brain fog and a reduction in weight gain, fatigue, IBS symptoms, and problems with yeast. Some patients benefit from a reduction in hypoglycemic reactions, whose symptoms often include irritability, anxiety, and cravings for carbohydrates or sugar. It is interesting to note that this diet also diminishes the intake of some of the foods most commonly found to cause allergic responses, such as wheat or gluten.

Many know about the "Atkins Diet" or the newer less restrictive diet called the "South Beach Diet," popularized by a physician from Florida. While both diets call for restricting carbohydrates for the first two weeks, which helps to reduce cravings, the South Beach Diet allows for more carbohydrates than the Atkins Diet. Weight loss on these diets is due to the body going into ketosis, which is a process that involves burning excess fat for fuel. While the body is burning more fat than carbohydrates, the process of ketosis can produce an unusual breath odor and constipation in some people.

Proponents of these diets recommend that, after the first two more restrictive weeks on the diet, potatoes, bread, pasta, sweets, and alcohol can be slowly added until you begin gaining weight. During the first two weeks, no more than 20 gms of carbohydrates per day are allowed. You will be able to determine how many carbohydrates you can consume in one day by noting when you start to gain weight when you begin to slowly add back carbs. If you find that you feel better on this diet, your level of well-being may determine how many carbohydrates you consume. It is not advisable to stay on the Atkins Diet long term, due to possible negative health consequences.

The Atkins Diet allows few vegetables, while the South Beach diet allows more veggies and complex carbohydrates; it is thought to be a healthier way to diet. This author has used both programs in the past and did feel more energetic and experienced a higher state of well being while on the diets. These may be difficult diets to stick to, particularly if you enjoy bread! These diets have not been studied in FMS patients.

Zone Diet

Some physicians recommend using the Zone Diet popularized by Dr. Barry Sears, who has written a number of books on the topic. This diet consists of eating meals containing properly balanced portions of protein, carbohydrates, and fats. The recommended ratio is 30% protein, 30% fat, and 40% carbohydrates. Snacks as well as meals should include the proportionate ratios. Dr. Sears Web site, www.drsears.com, includes information about this diet.

Reactive Hypoglycemia

The Zone Diet may be helpful in balancing insulin levels, so that your body does not have negative reactions to surges in blood sugar levels when high-carbohydrate meals or snacks are eaten, with the resultant "crashes" or "lows" two-three hours after eating. This is referred to as reactive hypoglycemia and is different from hypoglycemia. Hypoglycemia can be determined by a specialized laboratory test and occurs when your blood sugar crashes if you do not eat regularly. Reactive hypoglycemia is determined by symptoms rather than a laboratory test. Symptoms of reactive hypoglycemia can include shaking, heart palpitations, anxiety, sweating, hunger, fatigue, fibro-fog, hot flashes, irritability, depression, and a craving for sugar and carbohydrates. Eating well-balanced meals, evenly spaced throughout the day, can even out your insulin levels and symptoms. Dr. Mark Pelligrino's low-carbohydrate and high-protein diet discussed earlier also helps control insulin levels. Eating this way may not take your pain away, but it may help decrease the symptoms related to insulin irregularities, such as fatigue, anxiety, or irritability.

Antiyeast Diet

Some physicians and holistic practitioners believe that an underlying yeast problem contributes to FMS and CFIDS symptoms. The most common yeast, *Candida albicans*, is thought to be the culprit. Finding a physician to treat yeast problems can be difficult, however. Many holistic doctors treat for *Candida*, as do many nutritionists and Chinese medicine doctors. Nutritionists cannot prescribe antifungal or antiyeast medications but they will use various herbs, vitamin supplements, and changes in diet to help alleviate yeast overgrowth. Some physicians, such as

Jacob Teitelbaum, M.D., and Michael McNett, M.D. use all of these treatments to rid patients of yeast overgrowth.

Our bodies naturally have yeast living in harmony with friendly bacteria inside our bodies. Yeast are there to help our bodies in various ways, but sometimes the yeast overpower the "good bacteria" and cause a yeast invasion. This can occur after repeated courses of antibiotics. Yeast also thrive on sugar and yeast-laden foods such as cheese, bread, and wine. Giving up sugar and all sugar-containing products, including corn syrup, jelly, and honey, is the recommended treatment for controlling a *Candida* overgrowth. Some practitioners recommend giving up all yeast-containing foods such as cheese, beer, wine, and bread. Others feel that giving up sugar only is sufficient. Your body will most likely go through a withdrawal period in the first seven to ten days of a diet like this; you may even feel worse as the yeast die off because their source of "food" has been removed. Many people are amazed how their craving for sugar decreases if they can abstain from sugar for just ten days. Believe it or not, you may not even want sugar anymore! Doctors recommend replacing the friendly bacteria that have been lost by taking acidophilus supplements or eating plain yogurt (without sugar) that contains live acidophilus cultures.

It is very important to read labels on all foods you buy if you choose to eliminate sugar. Many foods we buy today include sugar disguised as high fructose corn syrup, dextrose, and maltose. Many cereals are loaded with sugar, as are some breads. Shop in a health food store or buy bread from a bread maker who uses only stone-ground grains and adds no sugar. Some grocery store chains are offering more sugar-free selections as consumers are becoming more health conscious. Remember, just because a label says "all natural" or "no artificial ingredients" does not mean the product hasn't been sweetened with fruit juices, which you may need to avoid, too. Because fruits and fruit juices contain naturally occurring sugars, some health practitioners recommend giving these up for a time, as well. You may need six to twelve months on this diet to take care of the yeast overgrowth. That may sound like a long time, but it can be well worth the trouble if you feel better in the future.

Laboratory tests for detecting yeast overgrowth are not thought to be conclusive, so many practitioners use symptoms and questionnaires to determine whether problems are yeast related. Your physician can prescribe antifungal medications for you, and you may also refer to Dr. Teitelbaum's book or his protocol at the end of this book in using this type of therapy. The medications commonly used to treat fungal overgrowth are Diflucan, Sporanox, and nystatin. William Crook, M.D., wrote the Yeast Connection and Women's Health as well as a cookbook for use in the anti-yeast diet available at www.yeastconnection.com.

Food Allergies Elimination Diet

▲ **Many FMS patients report sensitivities to foods, drugs, and chemicals.**

▲ **Sensitivities can make you feel tired, spacey, flulike, and moody.**

▲ **Laboratory tests are often inconclusive for food allergies.**

▲ **A standard elimination diet is effective for detecting food allergies; it can be time consuming and restrictive.**

▲ **Try eliminating the most common allergy-producing foods.**

Many people with FMS feel they have allergies or sensitivities to different foods, drugs, and chemicals found in our environment. Some individuals feel so terrible every day, they cannot distinguish which food or chemical could be a potential problem. It might be wise to find a caring physician who can help you determine which, if any, substances you are allergic to. Sensitivities to various substances can make you feel tired, spacey, achy, flu-like, irritable, or depressed. They can even be life threatening to some sensitive individuals. It may take some time to sort through which substances you are sensitive to, but the results could be well worth your effort. National sources for physician referrals are listed at the back of this book. Another good place to find a physician in your area is at your local support group.

Standard procedures for detecting food allergies are laboratory tests and the elimination diet method. Because laboratory tests are often not conclusive, some practitioners prefer to use the elimination diet for detecting which food(s) you may be sensitive to. The standard elimination diet consists of lamb, chicken, potatoes, rice, bananas, apples, and a cabbage family vegetable. Eat only those foods for two weeks. If some of your symptoms disappear, then it is possible that your symptoms are related to a food sensitivity. If the symptoms do not disappear, it could be that a reaction to one of the foods on the elimination diet is the culprit, and you will have to restrict your diet further. Once symptoms have disappeared, specific foods are re-introduced every four days, one at a time. Symptoms arise if an allergic response occurs. You must be diligent with this method, as it is time consuming and restrictive. An easier approach for the faint-hearted or those not willing to give up so much is to eliminate the most common allergy-producing foods (and usually the ones we like the most) such as milk, wheat, eggs, citrus, sugar, alcohol, chocolate, coffee, and artificial sweeteners such as aspartame (NutraSweet). It is important to note that if you are allergic to these foods, you may feel worse when you give them up before you feel better (usually a week), because your body goes through a withdrawal period. Some people say they experience a dramatic improvement in the way they feel when they eliminate substances to which they have an allergy. Before beginning an elimination diet, it is important to consult a physician or health professional.

We have found—at the Fibromyalgia Treatment Centers of America Clinic in Chicago, run by Dr. Michael McNett and where Rosalie Devonshire, MSW, LCSW, coauthor of this book works—that diet changes can be an important component of improving some symptoms when combined with other treatments. You and your physician can choose which diet works best for you.

Diet Changes for Leaky Gut Syndrome

Some physicians believe this syndrome exists when the protective lining of the intestines develops holes and no longer keeps harmful toxins, bacteria, and inflammatory waste products inside the intestines. Other physicians believe that this is not a syndrome at all and simply does not exist. We will leave this to the researchers to decide. Some physicians believe that toxic substances from what we ingest leak into the bloodstream and cause pain in the intestinal area and muscular pain elsewhere. Leaky gut syndrome can produce fatigue symptoms, as well, by activating inflammatory cytokines. This process may also produce a yeast overgrowth and irritable bowel syndrome.

Treatment consists of using antibiotics to reduce bacteria, adding acidophilus (friendly bacteria) to the diet, and changing the diet to eat less toxic foods, limit alcohol, increase fiber and magnesium. NSAIDs make this condition worse. Zinc supplementation may help.

Many holistic doctors believe that you must clear up your intestinal problems before you can get well. It is, after all, where we break down our food so nutrients can be absorbed into our bodies. Olive leaf extract may help rid your intestines of parasites and yeast.

PMS Fibromyalgia Flare-up

▲ **Treating PMS or menopausal symptoms may help you feel better.**

▲ **Balancing hormones is important.**

▲ **Using prescribed treatments or natural ones can help.**

For those FMS patients whose symptoms flare-up premenstrually, treating premenstrual symptoms might help them feel better at this time of the month. Serotonin and estrogen are found naturally in reduced levels after ovulation, and some women are especially sensitive to this change in their monthly cycles. Also, women who are premenopausal or experiencing menopause may feel a little better if their hormones can be balanced through proper treatment, either with prescribed hormones or natural treatments. Consult your physician for help in this area. There are many good books on this subject. This may be a good time to steer clear of sugar, overly processed foods, and alcohol and to increase your intake of nutritious foods.

Nutritional Supplements

▲ **Limited research is being done in this area.**

▲ **Magnesium, malic acid, and amino acids were discussed in the "Research" chapter.**

▲ **FMS and CFIDS newsletters are good sources of information.**

▲ **It is important to work with a knowledgeable person in this area.**

▲ **Resources are listed in this book.**

Many of our class participants inquire about which nutritional supplements are beneficial for their FMS. There are some anecdotal reports that certain supplements seem to alleviate some people's symptoms. Relief varies from individual to individual, and if supplements help, they often require weeks or months of supplementation. We have already covered magnesium, malic acid, and amino acids in the "Research" chapter.

FMS and CFIDS newsletters can be useful sources for news about nutritional supplementation. Research studies have been few in this area, and so much of the available information is experimental. Thomas Romano, M.D., and a few other researchers are finding vitamin deficiencies in some patients and an overabundance of vitamins in others. The B vitamins seem to be the ones found in low levels, while Dr. Romano has found high levels of vitamin A in some of his patients. Other researchers are just beginning to look at vitamin deficiencies; their studies may produce yet another clue to the mysterious puzzle of the FMS syndrome. Dr. Romano has noted that vitamins can be used to correct a nutritional deficiency or imbalance, or they can be used as pharmacologic agents. Discuss with your physician whether you need your vitamin levels checked and dosages modified. There are blood tests specifically designed to determine vitamin levels, which your physician can order for you. Because many physicians are not trained in nutritional therapies, you might have to look for someone knowledgeable in this area, such as a dietician, nutritionist, naturopathic doctor, or holistic physician. Vitamins and herbs can be harmful if not used properly and can counteract or interfere with prescribed medications, so it is very important to work with someone who is educated and experienced in this area.

Water-soluble vitamins, such as the C and B vitamins, are easily eliminated from the body; therefore it is almost impossible for you to accumulate toxic levels from one or more of these preparations. However, fat-soluble vitamins, such as vitamins A, D, E, and K, can accumulate in the body and exert toxic or untoward effects for many months, even after the excess is noted and the dose modified. For example, it is known that high levels of Vitamin A in cells can be toxic and can cause muscle pain—a situation that we need to avoid!

A good book that covers diet, vitamins, herbs, and other natural methods is *Chronic Fatigue Syndrome* by Michael T. Murray, N.D., a naturopathic physician who is well known and who has published many books on health and healing. Although his book is about CFIDS, many of the remedies relate to FMS, too. Dr. Jacob Teitelbaum also suggests various vitamins, that he uses in his practice for FMS and CFIDS in his book *From Fatigued to Fantastic!* A good book on herbal therapies is *Tyler's Honest Herbal: A Sensible Guide to the Use of Herb and Related Remedies* by Steven Foster and Varro Tyler, Ph.D.

Vitamins

Naturopathic physicians and some holistic physicians use nutritional supplements in their practice. To find a qualified physician, contact the American Association of Naturopathic Physicians or the American Holistic Medical Association listed in the "Resources" chapter. The *Prescription for Nutritional Healing* by Phyllis Balch, C.N.C., and James Balch, M.D., is another resource for supplements useful in treating fibromyalgia symptoms.

Although we have included a list of suggested supplements for you to refer to, we need to remind you that there are other resources that may suggest different vitamins for fibromyalgia than this list includes. This can be very confusing for FMS patients. Until research is carried out on exactly which specific vitamins are helpful in treating FMS, it is up to you and your physician to use good judgment when making decisions about supplementation.

Low levels of vitamins, minerals, and amino acids have been found. Some of them are

▲ Calcium	▲ Glutathione	▲ Potassium
▲ Isoleucine	▲ Vitamins D and C	▲ Histamine
▲ Zinc	▲ Tryptophan	▲ Vitamin E
▲ Taurine	▲ Folate	▲ Serine
▲ B12	▲ Leucine	▲ Carnitine
▲ Methionine	▲ Phosphocreatine	▲ Valine

Researchers have found low levels of numerous vitamins, minerals, and amino acids in the blood of FMS patients. Specific laboratory tests can be performed to test for nutritional deficiencies; speak to your physician about these tests. When you know what your specific nutritional deficiencies are, you can then have a nutritional program tailored to your needs.

Common Supplements

Please remember to discuss any supplements you take with your physician. When vitamins are taken in large amounts, they become more like drugs and should be treated as such.

The following is a report on some of the supplements mentioned most often for FMS patients. These are to be considered in addition to the basic supplements. We cannot possibly report on all supplements mentioned for FMS, but here we provide you with a brief summary on each of the following:

▲ Acidophilus	▲ Digestive enzymes	▲ 5-HTP
▲ Caprylic acid	▲ Essential fatty acids	▲ Jamaica dogwood
▲ Carnitine	▲ GABA	▲ Licorice (*Glycyrrhiza glabra*)
▲ Coenzyme Q$_{10}$	▲ Gingko	▲ L-theanine
▲ Colostrum & transfer factor	▲ Glucosamine & chondroitin	▲ L-tyrosine
▲ Creatine	▲ Glutathione	▲ Magnesium

▲ Malic acid	▲ NADH	▲ SAM-e
▲ Milk thistle	▲ Oil of oregano	▲ Valerian root extract
▲ Monolaurin	▲ Olive leaf extract	▲ Wild lettuce
▲ MSM	▲ Relaxin	
▲ N-acetyl-cysteine	▲ Relora	

Acidophilus

Friendly bacteria found in the intestinal tract can become out of balance due to yeast overgrowth. These friendly bacteria are found naturally in yogurt or in supplements that can help create a healthier intestinal tract. They may also improve immune system function and irritable bowel syndrome. Among the best-known are *Lactobacillus acidophilus* and *Bifidobacterium bifidum*. You may want to purchase a supplement that includes a number of different strains. If you have intestinal problems, you may consider adding this supplement. People who have taken numerous series of antibiotics often need to replenish their beneficial flora with supplements, as the antibiotics kill not only the "bad bacteria" but also the "good bacteria" our bodies need.

Caprylic Acid

This is a fatty acid produced by the body in small amounts. Caprylic acid has antifungal properties and is commonly recommended by naturopathic physicians for use in *Candida* control. It is quickly absorbed through the intestines, so it is best to take it in a timed-release supplement. It may be necessary to take it for three-four months before you see its benefits. Mild stomach upsets and headaches may occur, and practitioners feel this is related to die-off of the *Candida*. Do not use this if you have inflammatory bowel conditions.

Carnitine or Acetyl-L-Carnitine

Carnitine is related to the B vitamins, although it is usually considered an amino acid because it has a chemical structure similar to the amino acids. Its main function in the body is to help transport long-chain fatty acids, which provide energy for cells. It may lower blood triglyceride levels, aid in weight loss, and improve strength in people with neuromuscular disorders. It is found in lower amounts in FMS and CFIDS patients. Carnitine can be manufactured in the body if iron, B1, B6 and the amino acids lysine and methionine are present in sufficient amounts. Vegetarians are more likely to be deficient in carnitine as it is found primarily in meats and not vegetable sources. Many cases of a deficiency are genetic in origin. Acetyl-L-Carnitine is often recommended for FMS, but L-carnitine can be used and is less costly. It can be helpful for mitral valve prolapse.

Coenzyme Q$_{10}$

This is a fat-soluble quinine that is an antioxidant. It facilitates the oxygen consumption of the body and is crucial for making ATP. It is not made by the body. Its level decreases with age. It can be found in sardines, salmon, mackerel, and beef heart. It is used to treat cardiovascular problems, enhance immune function, and improve athletic performance, treat gingivitis, and promote increased energy.

Colostrum and Transfer Factor

Transfer factors are small protein molecules produced by immune cells called T-cells. They are being used by holistic physicians treating FMS and CFIDS patients when they feel a virus, bacterial infection, or parasite is part of the problem.

Colostrum is a mother's first breast milk. It transfers immunity to various diseases from mother to infant. Colostrum supplements are derived from chicken and cow colostrum. Nonspecific colostrum is available for everyday attacks by viruses, allergies, and fungi. There are also colostrums formulated to target specific viruses such as EBV, HHV-6, cytomegalovirus, and others. Colostrum may also increase growth hormone levels. Some of these supplements are expensive, particularly the ones targeted for specific viruses. They are available through vitamin companies.

Creatine

Phosphocreatine levels were found in lower amounts in FMS patient's muscles, along with ATP. It is used to produce energy in the muscles and reacts with ATP. It is produced by the actions of amino acids also found in short supply in FMS patients in some studies. Supplementing with creatine powder, which endurance athletes use to enhance their performance, may boost levels of phosphocreatine in the muscles and provide more energy for you. You need to take this on an empty stomach with a lot of water. Use the amounts recommended on the package. Creatine absorption is optimized when balanced with vitamin C, E and magnesium. Caffeine blocks absorption of creatine.

Digestive Enzymes

Enzymes are various proteins found in the largest amounts in raw or lightly cooked foods. When foods are cooked, many of the enzymes are destroyed. As we age, our ability to produce enzymes naturally decreases. They are utilized by the body in numerous biochemical processes, and have been found to be especially effective in treating sports-related injuries and aid in the digestion of food. Some researchers believe they may enhance healing in sports-related injuries and reduce pain levels.

Essential Fatty Acids

Essential fatty acids are not produced by the body and must be obtained from foods we eat. The two most important types of essential fatty acids are omega-3 and omega-6. Omega-3 acids are found in fish oil and flaxseed oil. Omega-6 fatty acids are found in many plant oils. They are essential to a number of physiological processes in the body, including regulating cholesterol levels, keeping the skin moist, producing prostaglandins, and helping to maintain the structure and function of cell membranes. These are very important supplements for patients with FMS.

GABA (Gamma-aminobutyric Acid)

GABA is an amino acid that acts as a neurotransmitter in the central nervous system. Together with inositol and niacinamide, it prevents stress and anxiety-related messages from reaching the brain. Many of the prescription medications used for FMS work on the GABA receptors. Taking GABA may help you sleep or feel calmer. GABA is often found in combination with other supplements for sleep and anxiety.

Gingko Biloba

This herb increases blood flow to the brain. It aids in improving memory, and is used to treat tinnitus, vertigo, and depression. It is generally used to improve cognitive function.

Glucosamine and Chondroitin

Studies show that these two compounds help support joint function by stimulating the production of cartilage. These compounds are often found together in one supplement, and they help with arthritis.

Glutathione

This is a molecule that consists of three amino-acids: L-glutamate, L-cysteine, and L-glycine. It is a potent antioxidant. Vitamins C and E are dependent on glycine for their effectiveness. It plays a role in the body's detoxification processes, as well as virus repression. It is concentrated in the liver, and many toxins are eliminated from our bodies through glutathione's pathways. It also aids in the manufacture of new muscle mass, the healing of wounds, and the removal of toxic metals from the body.

5-HTP

5-HTP (5-hydroxy-L-tryptophan) is the natural precursor to tryptophan and serotonin. It is a supplement derived from the West African shrub, *Griffonia simplicifolia*. There have been a few studies supplementing this in FMS patients. In a study done by Dr. Caruso of Italy, 50% of patients showed a good or fair improvement in pain levels when they were supplemented with 5-HTP. Side effects are low. 5-HTP works on the serotonin pathway in a way similar to the action of antidepressants. It also improves sleep quality, controls carbohydrate craving, and enhances mood. If you are on antidepressants, speak with your physician before adding this supplement. People who have a problem synthesizing 5-HTP may feel worse with this supplement.

Jamaica Dogwood

This herb has been found to have sedative and antianxiety properties.

Licorice Root

This herb has beneficial effects on the endocrine system, adrenal glands, and liver. It has an anti-inflammatory effect as well. When it is metabolized in the body, its molecules have a similar structure to the adrenal cortex hormones. Overworked adrenals are particularly noted in CFIDS and may also be present in some FMS patents. It may be useful for those who have low blood pressure or an autonomic nervous system dysfunction. It inhibits the growth of some viruses, including herpes simplex, and it is useful for coughs and digestive problems such as gastritis. It is not wise to use this herb long-term due its effects on electrolyte balance, including retention of sodium. Do not use during pregnancy or if you have hypertension or kidney disease. Be certain that you use licorice root which contains glycyrrhizic and glycyrrhetinic acids.

L-theanine

L-theanine is one of the main components of green tea. Research shows that it can increase levels of GABA, a neurotransmitter known for its calming effects, and dopamine, which can help with mood enhancement. Studies in Japan show that it increases alpha waves in the brain, which are known to produce feelings of alertness. It is nondrowsy and may help improve anxiety and mood. L-theanine is marketed heavily in Japan for stress reduction and is available there in gum as well as in food supplements. It is available in our country in health food stores.

L-tyrosine

This is a precursor of the neurotransmitters norepinephrine and dopamine, which regulate mood. It suppresses appetite, helps reduce body fat, aids in the production of melanin, and helps the adrenal, pituitary, and thyroid glands to function properly. A tyrosine deficiency can produce symptoms such as low blood pressure, low body temperature (cold hands and feet), and restless legs syndrome. It is used for stress reduction, as well as depression, anxiety, allergies, and headaches. It may improve cognitive function and benefit chronic fatigue. It is best taken at night or with a high-carbohydrate meal.

Magnesium

Discussed in our "Research" chapter.

Malic Acid

This is a naturally occurring compound that plays a role in converting food into energy for proper muscle function. It allows the body to produce ATP efficiently. It is found naturally in apples and other fruits and vegetables. For pain reduction and increased levels of energy, malic acid combined with magnesium is suggested for fibromyalgia. No adverse side effects or drug interactions are noted.

Milk Thistle

This herb is said to have an amazing effect on the liver. It stimulates liver cells to regenerate and aids in ridding the liver of toxins.

Monolaurin

Monolaurin is a monoglyceride comprised of lauric acid and glycerol. It possesses antiviral activity against several viruses that reside in cell membranes. It may be useful in treating herpes simplex, coronaviruses, and the flu. It may help reduce the outbreak and reoccurrence of EBV or mononucleosis.

MSM

Is a naturally occurring sulfur compound found in our bodies and in many common beverages and foods, including milk, coffee, tea, and green vegetables. This sulfur compound does not affect people who are normally allergic to sulfites. It is supposed to help with arthritis pain and inflammation. MSM is often found in supplements combined with glucosamine and chondroitin.

N-acetyl-cysteine

This is an amino acid precursor to the production of glutathione. It is an effective antiviral and helps break up mucus.

NADH

NADH, found in all living cells, is required for the conversion of tryptophan to serotonin. NADH also facilitates ATP production, which is necessary for energy production in cells. Some studies have shown that it helps mental fatigue and improves alertness in normal, healthy controls. When CFIDS patients took NADH for four weeks, an increase in overall sense of well-being and energy levels was noted in a small percentage of patients in the study. At 18 months of supplementation, over 83% of study participants showed improvement.

Joseph Bellanti, M.D., conducted a small trial with CFIDS patients by supplementing 10 mg per day. Modest improvements in energy levels were found in a subset of patients. This therapy seemed to work only if 5-HIAA urinary levels were elevated (discussed in the research section). Some researchers have theorized that malic acid should be taken indefinitely by some FMS patients, because it converts to NADH in the body and may be all that is necessary.

Oil of Oregano

Oil of oregano is an herbal product used for centuries for medicinal purposes. It is a potent antiseptic, and it is effective for killing yeast, fungi, bacteria, and parasites. It is often used for *Candida* control. The type you take should be enteric-coated in order to reach the intestinal tract where it will do its work. If it is not enteric-coated, it may cause stomach upset.

Olive Leaf Extract

Olive leaf extract has potent antiviral, antifungal, and antibacterial capabilities. It may be useful in treating EBV, *Candida*, herpes I, II, 6, & 7, CFIDS, malaria, Hepatitis B, AIDS, urinary tract infections, flu, and the common cold. It may prevent colds for those who have them frequently due to stress. Olive leaf extract may help normalize heart beat irregularities and provide relief of aching joints. The extract oleuropein is the important substance derived from the olive leaf plant that provides the antimicrobial effects. The supplement you take should contain at least 20% of this extract to be effective.

Relaxin

Some physicians noted that some FMS patients felt better during pregnancy and theorized the improvement might be due to a hormone called relaxin that is secreted during pregnancy. Relaxin is a polypeptide hormone that supports the growth of collagen and elastin in muscles, ligaments, and nerve vessels. It also helps increase blood vessel dilation and benefits kidney function. Dr. Samuel Yue, from Minnesota, found that patients' blood levels of relaxin surge during pregnancy. He believes that a deficiency of this hormone causes symptoms similar to FMS symptoms. This hormone was also used in the 1950's and 1960's during labor and delivery to shorten the length of the birthing process. You can purchase it in health food stores if you'd like to give it a try.

Relora

Relora is a natural plant extract of magnolia and philodendron, which in clinical studies helped reduce stress-induced obesity, anxiety, and irritability. In one study, Relora decreased cortisol levels by 37% and increased DHEA by 227%. Cortisol is a hormone that has been shown to be related to an increase in irritability, food cravings, poor sleep, tense muscles, fatigue and concentration problems. In another study, eight out of ten stressed individuals felt more relaxed, seven out of ten slept better, and nine out of ten had no stomach problems while on Relora. It does not produce drowsiness. None of the study participant were on antidepressants, but most had tried St. Johns Wort for anxiety.

SAM-e (S-adenosyl-methionine)

SAM-e has been shown to reduce morning stiffness, fatigue, and pain and to improve mental outlook in FMS patients. SAM-e is a natural compound found in every human cell; it is involved in over 35 biochemical processes. Animal studies show it increases production of cartilage-building cells in joints and may help provide the necessary chemicals to improve joint lubrication as well. One study proved that it was more effective than NSAIDs in helping relieve the pain of osteoarthritis—and with fewer side effects. Reports show SAM-e can help reduce depression by increasing levels of dopamine and serotonin. It helps produce glutathione, which is found in low levels in FMS and CFIDS patients. It is also a potent liver detoxifier.

SAM-e is being studied to determine its ability to boost the effectiveness of other antidepressants such as Prozac and Zoloft. There are over 40 published studies on its effectiveness in treating depression, and it is widely used in Europe. SAM-e is not to be used by individuals who have bipolar illness. It should be taken in the morning on an empty stomach with plenty of water and with the cofactors B6, B12, and folic acid. More than 400 mg per day can cause restlessness and gastric disturbances. It is important to speak with your doctor if you decide to try this and are already on other antidepressants.

Valerian Root Extract

This herb improves circulation, decreases mucus from colds, and acts as a sedative. It has been used in Europe for many years to improve anxiety, help with sleep, reduce muscle cramps, and diminish pain. It should be at least an 0.8% valernic acid content and come from the root, not the leaf.

Wild Lettuce

This herb has sedating properties.

Supplement Possibilities

A review of supplements most often mentioned for FMS or CFIDS. Each person should review his or her symptoms with a physician to determine which, if any, of these supplements will help. In some cases, you can find supplements that are formulated specifically for FMS or CFIDS.

Essential or Basic vitamins	*Sleep*
One-a-day multiple	5-HTP
Amino acid combination	Tryptophan
Magnesium	Melatonin
Malic acid	Valerian root extract
Essential fatty acids	GABA
Calcium	Passion flower
Vitamins C, D, E	Chamomile
Folate	L-theanine
B-complex vitamins	Wild lettuce
Zinc	Jamaican dogwood
Immune Enhancers	*Antiparasite/Antiviral*
Transfer factors	Olive leaf extract
Colostrum	Oregano oil
Thymic protein	Caprylic acid
Zinc	Echinacea
Astragulus	Monolaurin
Ginseng	Transfer factors
Glutathione	Licorice root
Licorice root	
Olive leaf extract	
Mood	*Energy*
NADH	Ginseng
5-HTP	Licorice root
Tryptophan	DHEA
St. John's Wort	NADH
SAM-e	Coenzyme Q_{10}
L-tyrosine	Creatine
GABA	N-acetyl-cysteine
L-theanine	B-vitamins
Relora	Malic acid
	Magnesium
Others	
Acidophilus or	FOS (Fructo Oligo Saccharides)
Digestive enzymes	Ginkgo bilboa

Adverse Effects of Herbs

The effects of herbs vary according to their potency and the weight, gender, biochemistry, and age of the individual. They also can interact with prescription medications and over-the-counter medications like cough and cold remedies. Herbs are used widely in Europe for medicinal purposes and are fairly safe when taken in appropriate doses. The problem for Americans is that many of our health professionals are not trained in the use of herbs, so we rely on health food store personnel to advise us. Sometimes, these people are not properly trained. So be careful and consult with a knowledgeable practitioner.

Some herbs that are known to be dangerous to take are kava kava, comfrey, borage, colt's foot, crotalaria, senecio, chaparral, germander, jin bu huon (Chinese), ma huang (ephedra), margosa oil, mate tea, mistletoe, pennyroyal, and tung shueh.

Hormonal Supplements

▲ **Melatonin helps induce sleep.**

▲ **DHEA might improve energy.**

▲ **Some can be purchased over the counter.**

▲ **You must be careful because these are potent substances and over-the-counter products are not regulated.**

Melatonin

Melatonin is a hormone manufactured from serotonin and secreted by the pineal gland. It is involved in the synchronization of hormonal secretions relating to our sleep-wake cycles. It is stimulated by darkness and suppressed by light. Some people use it as a sleep aid and to help relieve jet-lag. A study in 1973 reported that melatonin supplementation worsened depression in some cases, so if you have trouble with depression, speak to your physician before trying this remedy. It appears that the sleep-enhancing effects of melatonin happen only when melatonin levels are low. It is not like taking a sleeping pill. So, if you have trouble sleeping, do not have depression, and have low melatonin levels, melatonin taken before bedtime might help you fall asleep and stay asleep. The exact dosage to help your sleep is not known, but 3 mg is more than enough, and some people benefit from dosages as low as 0.1 mg. Because melatonin is a hormone, it can have very strong effects in the body and should not be used indiscriminately. Just because it is available without a prescription does not mean it is safe, or even that all the uses of it are known. Please be careful when using melatonin and, as always, speak to your physician before using this supplement.

DHEA

Many patients with chronic musculoskeletal problems have low DHEA levels. DHEA (dehydroepiandrosterone sulfate) is an adrenal hormone, which was discussed in the "Research" chapter. It's been available only by prescription until recently. Now it can be purchased in many health food stores and some pharmacies. When fibromyalgia patients' DHEA levels were tested, many were found to be low. Supplementing with this hormone has helped some people with FMS feel more energetic. Studies are currently underway to assess DHEA treatment in FMS patients. Consult your physician for the results of these studies.

There is a test available to determine your blood level of DHEA. It can help guide your physician in determining what dosage might be best for you. Dr. Thomas Romano states, "If you have a relatively low DHEA level, then DHEA could be used to bring your blood level into the appropriate range. In this example, the use of DHEA would be the same as using thyroid hormone if someone has a low blood level of thyroid hormone. However, if one wishes to use DHEA if a blood level is not drawn or if the DHEA hormone level is found to be normal, then DHEA is no longer being used as a replacement. In this example, it is being used as a pharmacologic agent to exert specific effects on the human body. Side effects of acne, facial hair growth, and oily skin have been reported, but appear to be less common in those patients who have low DHEA levels and are taking this hormone in amounts necessary to replace the body's store of DHEA." Some people report higher levels of energy when taking this supplement; and it is being touted as an antiaging miracle in magazines and books. Remember, although DHEA is now available without a prescription, it is a potent medication with unknown long-term effects. Discuss with your physician what dosage of DHEA is most appropriate for you.

Important Note
- ▲ **Do not waste your money on "magic cures."**
- ▲ **Work with a qualified person.**
- ▲ **Discuss all supplements you take with your physician.**

Many people have tried various supplements and have spent a lot of money on cures that do not benefit them. Please be mindful of this and make wise choices for yourself when using vitamins or herbs, as they can help or cause harm. Working with a physician or another qualified person may help alleviate problems that could arise when taking nutritional supplements and/or restricting your diet. Discuss any supplements you decide to take with your physician before taking them. If others tell you that they have a particular supplement that will cure you, please beware and do not expect any one supplement to totally resolve your symptoms. If we had found that one supplement, we would all be taking it and be cured! A list of referral resources is given in the back of this book.

Increasing Serotonin Naturally

Much research has been done on increasing serotonin naturally. There are a few good books available on the subject. These are listed in the resource section at the end of this chapter.

Some Methods of Increasing Serotonin Naturally Are
- ▲ **Relaxation, meditation, feeling calm**
- ▲ **Reducing anxiety**
- ▲ **Reducing perfectionism and compulsivity**
- ▲ **Adequate sunlight**
- ▲ **Adequate exercise: too much depletes serotonin**
- ▲ **Laughter—having fun!**

I'm Confused. Which Supplements Do I Take?
- ▲ **Speak to a knowledgeable physician or dietician.**
- ▲ **Ask for tests to determine which nutrient you may be deficient in.**
- ▲ **Refer to physician protocols in this book.**

You may be thinking, *This is all so confusing. Which supplement do I take and when?* The reason there are so many supplements recommended for fibromyalgia is that many of these treatments address underlying medical problems which are contributing to fibromyalgia symptoms such as metabolic disturbances, immune system problems, hormonal dysregulations, viral or parasitic infections, psychological symptoms, sleep problems, or gastrointestinal problems. Finding a physician or dietician knowledgeable in treating all of these areas, who can design a nutritional program tailored to your particular needs, is the best way to address nutritional deficiencies.

At the very least, make sure you take a high quality multivitamin, extra B vitamins, magnesium, malic acid, and calcium, as well as the essential fatty acids found in fish oil, and vitamins C and E and iron (if you need it). An amino acid complex is often suggested. All other supplements can be a decision you make with your health professional or after careful evaluation. If it's determined that you have *Candida*, you can then try some of the supplements recommended for ridding your body of yeast and try the special *Candida* diet. You can try some of the immune boosting supplements if you get frequent infections. Supplements to help with your sleep are also worth consideration.

Margy and David Squires of To Your Health have put together a program designed to take the guesswork out of vitamin supplementation, and we have included it in our book for your convenience. They have developed *Get With the Program*, which may take some of the confusion and guesswork out of which supplements to take. They include in this program the basic and most effective supplements found so far for FMS patients. You may want to try their supplements and or contact them at 800-801-1406 or on the Web at www.e-tyh.com. Their address is To Your Health, Inc., 17007 E. Colony Drive, Suite 107, Fountain Hills, Az 85268.

Fibromyalgia Educational Systems, Inc. cannot guarantee the efficacy of their program and supplements, but we do feel that it may be helpful for some FMS patients. Remember to contact your physician before starting any nutritional supplements.

When beginning their program, you will note that part of it includes treatment for *Candida* or bowel problems. Please refer to our information on the *Candida* or antiyeast diet, as you may want to consider following those recommendations at the same time for optimal results. Continuing to ingest yeast or sugar-related items will help the yeast or *Candida* to grow. This will be detrimental to you in the long run and is self-defeating to the program.

GET WITH THE PROGRAM!

Reprinted with permission from TyH Publications, Inc. All rights reserved.

Research has established many nutritional deficiencies and imbalances in chronic disease. As owners of supplements specifically for the fibromyalgia and chronic fatigue market, we hear from many people who are overwhelmed with the choices available. Isn't there a simple supplement program that I can follow that eliminates the guesswork but still gives me results? Thus, we outlined a basic nutritional program that addresses the common FMS/CFS issues of pain, sleep, fatigue and the gut which we called Get With the Program. Additionally, the beauty of the program is that the supplements are designed to work together to increase the overall symptom relief. Having said that, please note that we ask you to share any supplements you take with your doctor or healthcare professional before beginning this or any program, as you may have individual health problems that we can neither advise on nor address in this general program.

Take a multiple daily.

A multiple is the basis of your program. Make it a good one! Most comprehensive formulas require you to take four-six tablets or capsules a day. Anything less, and there's probably not enough in it to be therapeutic or correct deficiencies that are a given in most chronic diseases. Research studies suggest it takes six-eight months to show blood level changes and make a difference in how you feel. The Foundation Formula™ powder is the easiest option and most complete, replacing 30-40 different nutrients in a single dose, plus it includes scFOS for the gut. Multi-Gold™ is our high potency multiple in a traditional capsule form, and it also contains malic acid for energy and scFOS for the gut. TyH Products: Multi-Gold™ or Foundation Formula™, take as directed on the label.

Take extra magnesium, preferably glycinate.

Thomas Romano, M.D., suggests getting a serum RBC level to start. Muscle biopsies show decreased magnesium levels, and leading physician researchers suggest 400-1,200 mg of magnesium a day. Most multiples contain very little magnesium. Magnesium can help with irritable bowel, migraines, tight and painful muscles, and a host of other FMS complaints. Studies show that malic acid with the right form of magnesium (glycinate) is even more effective in relieving muscle pain and increasing energy. TyH Products: Fibro-Care™ amd/or Fibro-Care Cal™ (Cal-Mag). Take as directed on the label.

Boost serotonin with 5-HTP.

If you have increased pain, disrupted sleep, and/or a "sad" feeling, chances are you have low serotonin levels. Your doctor may suggest Zoloft, Prozac, or other serotonin reuptake medications (SSRIs) which do not really increase serotonin but only control what you already have. 5-HTP actually adds serotonin and is a good substitute for those who don't want SSRI's side effects, one of which may be a 25-50 pound weight gain! TyH Product: 5-HTP (50-100 mg, two-three times a day).

Add cold-pressed flaxseed oil.

Although the omega oils in flaxseed are known anti-inflammatory fighters and FMS/CFS are not inflammatory in nature, the health benefits of these oils cannot be understated for brain cognition, the heart, weight control, and so forth. The liquid oil is the easiest way to get your daily dose in 1-2 tablespoons. Capsules are usually gel-caps to protect the oil from oxygenation. Flaxseed oil is sensitive to heat, light, and air, so make sure the oil is cold-pressed, like Barlean's, to preserve the oil's intrinsic nutrient value. TyH Products: Barlean's Flaxseed Oil.

Get to sleep.

You cannot even begin to get well without sleep. Besides resting, the body also repairs, especially in REM stage IV. While some people may require pharmaceutical assistance to help themselves "remember" how to stay asleep, it doesn't always get you into REM. Natural remedies work without the rebound effect or playing the "drug tolerance game" of changing meds as the effect wears off with use. Adding 5-HTP to the night program (which converts to melatonin) is also helpful. TyH Product: Valerian Rest™ or Sleep Formula™.

Help the mitochondria to increase energy.

The mitochondria are the energy powerhouses of every cell, and studies suggest a malfunction in the Krebs energy cycle. While magnesium is critical to the Krebs, Coenzyme Q_{10} is fuel for the mitochondria. Just don't take it too close to bedtime as it can keep you awake! Malic acid also is an energy booster, and is found in TyH's Fibro-Care™ and both multiple products. TyH Product: Q-Caps 100 mg (two-three times a day in a divided dose).

Heal the gut of Candida and/or bowel problems.

If you suspect you have *Candida* or other bowel problems based on symptoms of bloating, diarrhea, constipation, multiple food allergies, rashes, and inability to take vitamins in any form, do not start this program without clearing up those issues first! You need your stomach and bowels in "proper" working order or your ability to absorb nutrients to effectively reduce FMS/CFS symptoms is severely handicapped. Work with your doctor or do the pre-program *Clear & Replenish™*, using Olive Leaf ES™ and Acidophilus ES™. After 2-3 weeks or when gut symptoms improve, then *"get with the program!"*

It's best to start with one product at a time, adding to the program slowly, especially if you've never supplemented before. Many find relief taking a multiple along with magnesium and malic acid, then adding other supplements as symptoms warrant. For more information on supplements mentioned, go to the TyH website at www.e-tyh.com. You can also talk to anyone at TyH by calling 800-801-1406 with any questions or comments.

The Pre-Program, Clear & Replenish™

You cannot get well if you have a gut problem. This may sound like a bold statement, but it is a biological truth. An estimated 75% of people with FMS and CFS have *Candida* overgrowth, leaky gut, irritable bowel syndrome (IBS), and digestive dysfunction. While gut is not a glamorous word (and usually not a topic for discussion), a healthy gut or gastrointestinal (GI) tract is fundamental to good health. If you are supplementing to alleviate symptoms of a chronic disorder, *a healthy gut is critical to the absorption of the nutrients*. Without a healthy gut, you cannot absorb nutrients. If you can't absorb the nutrients, how can you get well? That's why holistic doctors assess and treat any gut problems first before prescribing any other therapies.

This six-week pre-program, therefore, is designed to first detox and then replenish your GI system for optimum absorption of the supplements in *Get With the Program*.

The GI system can be explained simply: it's the process that food or nutrients go through from the time they enter your mouth to their final exit as waste products. At any point (mouth, esophagus, stomach, small and large intestines) where there's a malfunction, your health will be affected. The pre-program focuses on one of the number one problems facing FMS and CFS: *Candida* overgrowth (candidiasis). Some researchers suggest that 30-50% of the world may have a yeast problem; it's as high as 75% in FMS/CFS!

It Takes Two

Many people make the mistake of treating candidiasis by taking either product alone. While olive leaf is effective in eliminating yeast overgrowth (along with parasites), it's only half the story. Others take acidophilus to replenish the good bacteria, but there's no place for acidophilus to "live" if the yeast is not eliminated first. You must do both: "clear and replenish." Take olive leaf extract to clear your intestine of unwanted visitors like parasites and excessive yeast. Follow with acidophilus to replenish the friendly bacteria necessary to digest food and absorb nutrients. New studies indicate that a pre/probiotic blend restores faster than a probiotic alone, such as in our Acidophilus ES™. You'll start seeing changes in about six weeks, including lessening of fatigue and brain fog. You may need to be on the pre-program longer than 28 days if your yeast infestation is long standing. Once you start feeling better again, you will recognize the need to do a "clear and replenish" on a regular basis, two-three times a year.

PRE-PROGRAM - Clear & Replenish (28 Days)*

Clear

Days 1-14. Olive Leaf ES™ will clear your intestines of unwanted visitors like parasites and excessive yeast. The patented scFOS in Olive Leaf ES™ helps to prepare the environment and is available as food for acidophilus in the next step. **Dosage:** two caps three times per day in divided dose.

Days 15-28. Continue on Olive Leaf ES™ while taking Acidophilus ES™. Take at last one hour apart.

Replenish

Days 15-28. Acidophilus ES™ will replenish the friendly bacteria that are necessary to digest food and absorb nutrients, as well as balance the ratio of good bacteria to bad in the small intestines. Again, the scFOS provides both food and a beneficial environment (remember the ecology!) for the friendly bacteria (acidophilous) to flourish and stay in control. **Dosage:** Acidophilus ES™, three caps three times per day, at least one hour before or after Olive Leaf ES™ dose, preferably on an empty stomach.

Please keep the following in mind:

- You will feel worse the first two-three days on the program, because toxins are released during yeast die-off. This is known as the Hexheimer's Reaction. You may feel achy, flulike, and miserable. Diarrhea is also possible as the body cleans out the infected environment.

- Drink plenty of water to help flush out the toxins.

- Add a buffered vitamin C (500 mg) throughout the day to counteract toxic effect.

- Add a proteolytic enzyme (Fibro-Enzymes™ one-two tablets) two-three times a day to help relieve achiness and clear out toxic debris which interferes with healing.

  You'll start seeing and feeling changes in about six weeks, e.g. less fatigue and brain fog.

- Repeat the *Clear & Replenish*™ program two-three times a year as a preventive measure.

- You may want to stay on a daily dose of two caps of Olive Leaf ES™ and two caps of Acidophilus ES™, taken at least one-two hours apart to maintain a friendly ecology.

  Remember, 28 days is not a magic number! You may need to stay on the pre-program longer if your yeast infestation is long-standing. If you stop too soon, you may give yeast another chance to regain control.

*Dosage recommendations by TyH Advisor, Kelly Hannigan, N.M.D.

Medical Disclaimer: These statements have not been reviewed by the FDA. For informational purposes only. Not intended to diagnose, cure, treat, or prevent any medical condition, nor substitute for professional medical advice.

DIET AND NUTRITION

Dr. Teitelbaum, Dr. Romano, and Dr. Flechas have also identified some supplements they find useful in their practices. These are described in the back of this book in their treatment protocols. Dr. Teitelbaum has developed a line of vitamins tailored specifically for FMS/CFIDS with Enzymatic Therapy. Many of these products can be purchased online at his Web site or in health food stores. See his protocol for suggestions.

Some physicians use intravenous vitamin therapy, which is believed to be better absorbed. When intravenous therapy of vitamins is used, your physician may include a number of different vitamins, depending on your needs.

Vitamins are also available by injection, particularly B-12. You can learn to give yourself B-12 injections so you do not have to go into the doctor's office all the time.

Remember that laboratory tests can be utilized to determine which vitamin deficiencies you have.

The following supplement companies are reliable, and they provide quality vitamins. You may also find supplements made specifically for FMS and CFIDS in your local health food store.

To Your Health   800-801-1406   www.e-tyh.com

Integrative Therapeutics   800-931-1709   www.integrativeinc.com

Prohealth   800-366-6056   www.immunesupport.com

Dr. Jacob Teitelbaum's supplements   www.endfatigue.com (Click on Orders)

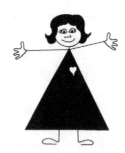

ALTERNATIVE TREATMENTS: AN OVERVIEW

Alternative medicine emphasizes wellness and prevention. Practitioners may use natural substances to heal and support the body. They look for causes for health problems in a patient's lifestyle or habits, such as diet, nutritional deficiencies, poor stress management, exposure to toxic substances, lack of exercise, and others. Alternative medicine may also be referred to as complementary medicine. Because many insurance companies do not reimburse for alternative treatments, patients must pay out-of-pocket, which can sometimes prove to be very expensive. Vitamin supplements alone can cost well over $100 per month. Carefully research your alternative treatments and practitioners to make sure you are not wasting your time and money.

In the past, many U.S. physicians claimed that much of the research on alternative medicine was not up to their scientific standards and have dismissed the merits of many alternative treatments. Much of the research for these therapies has come from Europe where alternative treatments are more commonly used. At this time, new research is being carried out in American facilities on some alternative treatments. The government has opened the National Center for Complementary and Alternative Medicine at the NIH (National Institutes of Health) http://nccam.nih.gov. One of the major problems with researching alternative therapies is that natural substances are not patentable, so pharmaceutical companies do not want to waste their time and money on something they cannot patent and profit from financially.

Some insurance companies are beginning to pay for alternative therapies, because they are finding them to be cost effective. Chiropractic therapy is now covered by most insurance carriers. The FDA recently ruled that acupuncture needles are an approved medical device, so more healthcare plans will be covering acupuncture as well. A few plans, mainly on the West Coast, are starting to cover homeopathy, herbs, massage, and aromatherapy when referred by an M.D. The state of Washington became the first state to require that health insurance companies cover licensed alternative healthcare practitioners.

Integrated or holistic healthcare centers have opened up in many American cities which offer both allopathic (Western M.D.s) physicians and alternative therapists. A Harvard study found that one-third of Americans routinely used alternative therapies, calculating that $14 billion was spent on these therapies in 1990. Physicians were surprised by this report, because many patients did not tell their doctors they were using alternative treatments. In recent years, the American Medical Association passed a resolution encouraging its members to become better informed regarding the technique and practice of alternative care. Many medical schools are now offering classes in alternative therapies, and more research is being carried out in major medical centers, universities, and research laboratories.

One of the complaints about alternative therapists is that many are unlicensed. We need stringent licensing procedures and qualified schools for these therapists, because Americans are undoubtedly going to continue to see these practitioners. Public interest in alternative therapies is gaining momentum, and licensing would help legitimize these therapists.

FMS Patients Seeking Alternative Therapies

Many FMS patients seek out alternative healthcare practitioners. Why? Because they have a chronic condition with no known cure, and they hope to find a cure somewhere. Often, patients simply do not like to take drugs and want to use more natural methods to heal their illness. FMS patients' sensitivity to drugs makes them likely candidates for natural substances. Many alternative therapies have been around for centuries, long before Western medicine. Although a substantial number of FMS patients try these therapies, we do not have extensive hard data on which therapies work for which symptoms or how much they help. It is up to you to become better educated in this area. Some patients like the individual attention they receive from alternative practitioners, who often have more time to spend with each patient than M.D.s who are struggling under time restrictions from managed healthcare companies. Many people prefer the holistic approach taken by some M.D.s who have blended traditional and alternative treatments.

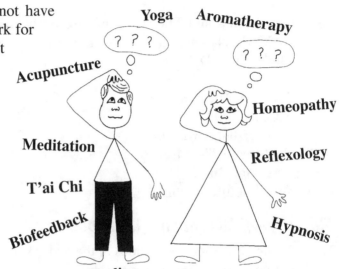

Frustrated with their pain and fatigue and with the years of research and development that are often necessary for FMS treatments to be approved for traditional care, some patients are trying remedies which are unproven for FMS. Some people swear that a particular treatment cured them. Because FMS is an individual illness, however, what works for you may not work for others. This variation is true even for the regularly prescribed medications for FMS. Also, be reminded that if a particular supplement truly was the cure for FMS, we would not need to read this book. We would all be cured! Most research shows that FMS sufferers need to change many aspects of their lives and try a variety of treatments in order to feel better. This treatment plan might include dietary changes, exercise, massage, stress management, nutritional supplements, and the use of conventional medicines. Most studies show that one change is not enough to produce benefits.

Be a Wise Consumer

When trying new treatments, be aware that quacks and charlatans do exist. There are people just waiting to collect money from desperate people, and FMS patients are sometimes desperate! Some will try anything to alleviate their pain. We must be careful and know that some substances are dangerous even though they are natural and sold over the counter. Some alternative treatments lack credentialing organizations and accredited or recognized training institutions. Treatments can range from beneficial to harmless to outright dangerous. They can also be very expensive. Let the buyer beware. Educate yourself before you try any remedy.

Conventional drugs, surgeries, and treatments can also be dangerous. Some drugs work for some FMS patients, alleviating their pain in varying degrees, improving sleep, and lifting mood. Some do not help at all, make us feel worse, or produce intolerable side effects. Just ask any FMS patient who has experienced tricyclic hangover, heart palpitations, increased pain, weight gain, ulcers, insomnia, or depression from one of the medications commonly prescribed for FMS. How many people have had needless surgery or expensive diagnostic tests for back pain that continued after surgery? Conventional medicine is also not 100%.

If the American public continues to use alternative therapies, more will be available, more and better research will be conducted, and allopathic and alternative therapists will discontinue their cold war and work together in improving our health.

For information about The Office of Alternative Medicine, write:
> NCCAM/National Institutes of Health
> Bethesda, MD 20892

OR

> NCCAM Clearinghouse
> P.O. Box 7923
> Gaithersburg, MD 20898
> Toll-free: 888-644-6226
> Fax: 866-464-3616
> email: info@nccam.nih.gov

Glossary of Alternative Therapies

The following are brief descriptions of the better known alternative therapies, along with national numbers to call for information on each.

Acupressure – Manual application of pressure with fingertips or acupressure tools at points where acupuncture needles would be inserted. American Massage Therapy Association, 500 Davis Street, Evanston, IL 60201; 847-864-0123. www.amtamassage.org

Acupuncture – Ancient Chinese medical treatment based on the belief that the body has a number of meridians that conduct energy throughout the body. Symptoms result from a blockage in these meridians. The treatment consists of inserting fine needles, sometimes along with heat, electricity, herbs, oils or lasers, at various points along the body's meridians, chosen to alleviate blockages for specific symptoms. Its mechanism of action is not completely understood, but it is believed to stimulate endorphins (painkillers) and serotonin. The FDA has recently approved acupuncture needles as safe medical devices. American Academy of Medical Acupuncture; 800-521-2262. www.medicalacupuncture.org

Applied Kinesiology – A system developed by chiropractors to test muscle strength. An applied kinesiologist uses procedures that strengthen weak muscles and relax tense muscles. This helps rebalance an out-of-balance body. Allergies and vitamin deficiencies are also detected and treated using this method. International College of Applied Kinesiology; 913-384-5336. www.icakusa.com

Aromatherapy – A holistic treatment that uses essential oils derived from plants to restore the body's health through the sense of smell. These oils are either inhaled, put in bath water, massaged into the skin, or diffused into the air. National Association for Holistic Aromatherapy; 888-ASKNAHA. www.naha.org

Ayurveda – Ancient system of Indian holistic medicine based on the Hindu scriptures. It is based on the three doshas called vata, pitta, and kapha. Each person has a predominant dosha or combination. Imbalances in these can cause ill health. The Ayurvedic practitioner uses foods, herbs, meditation, and exercise to correct imbalances. National Ayurvedic Medical Association; 941-929-0999. www.ayurveda-nama.org

Chiropractic – Illness is believed to stem from misaligned joints or vertebrae, preventing transmission of signals between the brain and the rest of the body. Chiropractic physicians manually manipulate the spine and joints to improve alignment. It is the second most prevalent form of therapy after conventional medicine. Many chiropractors offer nutritional counseling as well as kinesiology, craniosacral work, and massage therapies as adjuncts to manual manipulation. American Chiropractic Association; 800-986-4636. www.amerchiro.org

Hands-on Healing – Any treatment using a laying on of hands (although there does not actually have to be touching) by healers who act as channels to harness spiritual, God-given or universal healing energy. The American Holistic Nurse's Association has performed studies in this area and found evidence that some form of healing does take place in the patient's body when this technique is employed. There are many branches of this therapy: Reiki, Healing Touch, Omega Healing, followers of Barbara Brennan (a healer and former NASA physicist), Renewal Therapy, Polarity, Mari-El, Shiatsu, and others. Reiki Alliance; 208-783-3535. www.reikialliance.com. Healing Touch; 303-989-7982. www.healingtouch.net

Holistic Medicine – Any practice of medicine that considers the whole person—physically, mentally, and emotionally. It not only treats the diseased area, but also strives to heal underlying causes. American Holistic Medical Association; 505-292-7788. www.holisticmedicine.org

Homeopathy – Samuel Hahnemann developed homeopathic medicine over 200 years ago in Germany. He coined the phrase, "Let like be treated by likes," or the Law of Similars. It is based on the assumption that a substance that provokes symptoms in a healthy person cures those same symptoms in a sick person, and the more diluted the dose, the greater its efficiency in helping the body heal itself. The remedies, as they are called, are inexpensive and can often be found in local health food stores. There are homeopathic physicians in some areas of the U.S., although many more are found in Europe. National Center for Homeopathy; 703-548-7790. www.homeopathic.org

Magnetic Therapy – The use of magnets to improve energy and blood flow in the body. Our bodies are surrounded by magnetic fields, which affect us according to weather changes, the earth's magnetic fields, power lines, and electrical appliances. There are magnetic strips, pillows, mattresses, and shoe inserts. These are placed on the body in areas where there is pain and are believed to improve blood flow to that area. Some physicians are beginning to use them in their practices. You can purchase magnets through catalogs, in drug stores, or from one of the multilevel marketing organizations. For a catalog go to www.midamericamarketing.com.

Naturopathy – Uses the body's self-healing system to repair itself. Only natural therapies are employed: fasting, organic foods, water therapy, aromatherapy, massage, osteopathy, and supplements. American Association of Naturopathic Physicians; 866-538-2267. www.naturopathic.org

Reflexology – Restoring health through the massaging of specific areas in the feet and hands. Certain points on the feet are thought to correspond to organs and other areas of the body. Reflexology Association of America; 978-779-0255. www.reflexology-usa.org

More alternative resources are listed in the "Resources" chapter of this book.

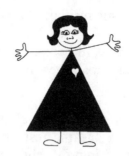

PIONEERING TREATMENTS

▲ **Some physicians have been using treatments not yet thoroughly researched.**

▲ **Try these treatments with extreme caution.**

▲ **These physicians use a variety of tests, medications, vitamins, and hormones.**

▲ **Many of their patients do well.**

▲ **Read about their treatments in our book, their books, in FMS newsletters, or in the *CFIDS Chronicle*.**

▲ **Share this information with your physician.**

▲ **Contact pioneering physicians personally.**

Some physicians have been treating FMS patients with "experimental" therapies. Some of these treatments have not been subjected to scientific study at this time, although many are in the process of being researched and others will be studied in the future. We would like to share with you a few of the more widely recognized physicians performing this type of pioneering work, because we feel that this information should be freely accessible to all FMS sufferers. If you choose to try some of these therapies, you may have to find a physician in your area willing to accommodate you. Remember to try a novel therapy with extreme caution. The authors of this book are not providing all the necessary information needed to undergo these treatments, but are giving an overview of the main points of these treatments. The physician protocols are listed in the Appendix at the back of this book. Those interested in using their treatments should purchase the physician's book or contact the doctor personally to acquire the correct protocol. Many of the physicians have useful information on their Web sites.

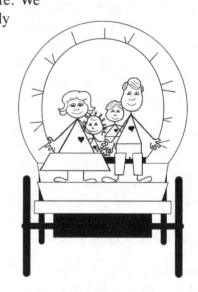

Dr. Jacob Teitelbaum is one such physician. He has experienced CFIDS and FMS and knows firsthand how it affects people. We have already made reference to his book which describes in accurate detail his treatment protocol for FMS and CFIDS. Dr. Teitelbaum has provided a synopsis of his protocol in the Appendix. He uses various laboratory diagnostic tests to assess a number of problems he feels contribute to FMS and CFIDS. After he takes a complete history, he may treat a patient with some or all of the

following: synthroid or armour thyroid to boost a low thyroid level, corte[...]
insufficiency, DHEA to boost DHEA levels, medications to treat neu[...]
hypotension which causes dizziness, oxytocin (a female hormone), estrogen an[...]
various vitamins, antidepressants, herbals for sleep aids, antiyeast treatments[...]
therapies, homeopathics, and various other medications.

Dr. Teitelbaum's treatment program has benefited many patients and takes into ac[...]
that FMS symptoms may be caused by a combination of factors. You may want to[...]
book and share it with your own physician who might be interested in trying these tr[...]nents. He
also offers a newsletter. Ordering information is listed in the "Resources" chapter.

Dr. Jay Goldstein is another physician and researcher whom we have mentioned previously
in the "Research" chapter. He recently retired after treating FMS and CFIDS patients for over
15 years and has written a book geared for the physician called *Betrayal by the Brain: The
Neurologic Basis of Chronic Fatigue Syndrome, Fibromyalgia Syndrome and Related Neural
Network Disorders*. He also offers a companion book written by a patient, for patients, which
you can also order, called *A Companion Volume to Dr. Jay A. Goldstein's Betrayal By the
Brain*, by Katie Courmel. His treatment protocol differs substantially from those who use
medications to alleviate only specific symptoms, such as low serotonin levels. He believes
FMS and CFIDS patients suffer from problems in the way their brains process sensory input
from noise, lights, odors, pain, food, medications, and chemicals. By a complex mechanism
involving various brain chemicals, our brain interprets information it receives from our
environment, filters out appropriate and inappropriate information, and tells our body how to
handle the input. Dr. Goldstein felt a decade ago that our brains are misinterpreting the
information, resulting in an amplification of pain signals, odors, and other sensations. Just
going to the local mall bombards our senses with so many stimuli that the trip can prove
exhausting. This "wears out" the brain and can contribute to the cognitive problems many
experience. Although he has recently retired from practice, his books are worth reading.

Dr. Goldstein believes FMS and CFIDS patients have a genetic predisposition for developing
these syndromes. Developmental issues, in which one feels unsafe for a period of time causing a
hypervigilant attitude, can change the way the brain responds to stimuli; exposure to viruses,
severe emotional stress, and exposure to environmental stressors contribute to the development of
these syndromes. Some people may be particularly strong in their genetic predisposition and may
develop these syndromes no matter what their stressors may be, while others need a variety of
stressors before they will develop FMS or CFIDS.

Dr. Thomas Romano, M.D., editor of this book, offers his treatment protocol in the Appendix. Dr.
Jorge Flechas also utilizes an interesting protocol in his practice and Dr. Michael McNett has
included an overview of his treament for FMS. The Web site www.immunesupport.com, has
articles reprinted by a number of physicians who are having excellent results with their treatment
protocols.

Specific Treatments

- ▲ Oxytocin • DHEA • Nitroglycerin
- ▲ Atenolol • Florinef • Increase salt and water
- ▲ Guaifenesin
- ▲ Ketamine
- ▲ Xyrem (GHB)
- ▲ Heavy metal toxicity
- ▲ Mercury toxicity
- ▲ Alpha-Stim
- ▲ Decompression surgery
- ▲ Neurofeedback
- ▲ sEMG electromyography
- ▲ Prolotherapy
- ▲ Pioneering physicians'
  treatments overview

tocin • DHEA • Nitroglycerin

Another therapy that has proven beneficial to some patients, in conjunction with other treatments described, is that used by Jorge Flechas, M.D., Jay Goldstein, M.D., and Jacob Teitelbaum, M.D. We have already mentioned that DHEA levels were found to be low in FMS patients. By carefully listening to his patients' complaints, Dr. Flechas decided that the hormone oxytocin, along with DHEA supplementation, might help alleviate some of his patients' symptoms. He first runs a blood test to determine baseline DHEA levels, then adds supplements to bring levels up to what they should be at around age 30. Dosages need to be determined by a physician, as DHEA has side effects, and the risks of long-term usage have not yet been determined. Checking estrogen and testosterone levels is also recommended.

Once the DHEA is up to optimal levels, Dr. Flechas tries his patients on a 10-ml injection of oxytocin. Often patients notice a flushed feeling in their hands or face immediately after the injection, which may last for a few minutes. Positive effects take approximately two weeks. Dr. Flechas recommends taking supplements of choline and inositol to increase the effectiveness of the oxytocin. Nitroglycerin is another medication he adds to his regime to enhance pain relief. Patients who benefit from this treatment often have cold hands and feet and are pale. Daily injections of oxytocin can be given, or there is a capsule available from the pharmacies listed in the Appendix. Dr. Goldstein believes injections are more effective.

Not much has been written about oxytocin, but it is known to have a role in inducing labor in pregnant women, facilitating the let-down response in lactating women, and regulating blood circulation in the small vessels of the body. It also has an analgesic effect, raises sex-drive levels, affects concentration, and performs a host of other functions. It is released during orgasm. This hormone works within a complex network of other chemicals in our bodies that have been found to be dysregulated in FMS patients, such as neuropeptide Y, corticotropin-releasing hormone (CRH), thyroid hormone, estrogen, DHEA, and others.

Two of the side effects of this treatment are weight gain and water retention.

Atenolol • Florinef • Increase Salt and Water Intake for Neurally Mediated Hypotension

If you are troubled by dizziness and/or fainting spells, you might want to speak to your physician about having a cardiologist perform a tilt table test. During the test you are strapped to a table and turned 70 degrees so that your legs are close to the floor but do not touch it. Normally, when you get up from a sitting position, your brain signals your blood pressure to perform properly when your feet touch the ground. Researchers have found that CFIDS patients and some FMS patients have a dysfunction in the regulation of this system, and their blood pressure drops significantly, causing improper blood flow to the brain. This dysfunction can lead to feelings of fatigue and other symptoms associated with FMS/CFIDS. These tests were originally performed by Johns Hopkins University researchers and replicated by Daniel Clauw, M.D., of the University of Michigan. A natural treatment for this problem consists of increasing salt intake and drinking lots of water. Some physicians prescribe atenolol (Tenormin), a beta-blocker, or Florinef (fludrocortisone), an adrenal steroid. These drugs have side effects that can be explained by your physician.

You could have this condition even if you do not have low blood pressure or a history of fainting or dizziness. This treatment is well worth pursuing and might be a good addition to your overall program.

Guaifenesin

Dr. St. Amand of Marina Del Ray, California, has been using guaifenesin, an ingredient found in the cough medicine Robitussin. Theorizing that FMS patients have a genetically inherited defect in how their bodies excrete phosphates, Dr. St. Amand found that pure guaifenesin works on the kidneys to increase removal of phosphates through the urine. He has treated over 3,000 patients in this manner and claims to have had good results. But, when Dr. Robert Bennett performed a year-long placebo-controlled trial of guaifenesin, guaifenesin proved to be ineffective. In his study, 20 FMS patients were given 600 mg of guaifenesin twice a day and another 20 patients were given a placebo twice daily. None of the 40 patients knew if they were taking guaifenesin or the placebo. All were instructed not to take salicylates, because they interfere with the functioning of guaifenesin. Dr. Bennett found that none of his study variables changed significantly over the year and that the response to guaifenesin was the same as that for the placebo. Obviously, Dr. St. Amand and Dr. Bennett disagree on the usefulness of this compound. Dr. St. Amand believes Dr. Bennett's results were not positive because salicylates, a common ingredient in cosmetics, aspirin, and herbal medications, were not totally excluded from the study and rendered the guaifenesin treatment ineffective.

The guaifenesin controversy has intrigued many and may be further studied in the future. At this time, its effectiveness is certainly questioned. Many patients try this treatment, some have good results. Dr. St. Amand's Web site is www.guaidoc.com.

Ketamine

One study using intravenous morphine, lidocaine, and ketamine showed that ketamine proved to be the most effective in reducing pain levels. Morphine, an opioid, did not help at all in this study; lidocaine, an anaesthetic used in trigger point injections, was somewhat helpful; and ketamine, an NMDA pain receptor antagonist, decreased pain and had a longer lasting effect than the others. With its promising results, this study could help lead researchers to other drugs which affect the NMDA receptors and possibly help alleviate pain for FMS patients. Ketamine also comes in a liquid and is used to change the perception of pain. It was originally created for use as an anesthetic. It's abused on the streets as "Special K".

Xyrem (GHB or gamma hydroxybutyrate)

Dr. Martin Scharf, a sleep specialist of the Tri-State Sleep Disorders Clinic in Cincinnati, has been studying Xyrem and its effectiveness in treating various sleep disorders. Xyrem has been abused on the streets where it is known as the "date rape drug." It has been approved by the FDA for narcolepsy (a sleep disorder which causes uncontrollable sleeping during the day), and Dr. Scharf has found it to be helpful in solving some of the sleep problems associated with FMS. It increases slow-wave sleep as well as growth hormone levels. In studies, it produced improvement in sleep quality, reducing pain and fatigue. When patients discontinued using the medication, they did not experience any rebound effect as occurs with some of the other sleeping medications. At this time, further research is being conducted on GHB in FMS patients. Dr. Scharf hopes to have the drug approved for FMS in the future.

Heavy Metal Toxicity

Numerous metals can cause toxicity due to occupational or residential exposure. They include arsenic, cadmium, copper, lead, iron, manganese, mercury, nickel, gold, silver, zinc, and others. Most metals are not toxic in small amounts, and many are required by our bodies for optimal physical functioning. When a person is exposed to large amounts of a metal due to a workplace accident or has had long-term exposure to these metals, serious symptoms or illness can result.

Poisoning can cause impairments in the functioning of our central nervous system, fatigue, and damage to blood, lungs, liver, kidneys and other organs in the body. It is believed by researchers that long-term exposure can result in slow, progressive, physical, neurological, and degenerative diseases that may mimic Alzheimer's disease, Parkinson's, muscular dystrophy, or multiple sclerosis. Many of you have heard about the difficulties that arise when children ingest lead from paint chips or from chronic exposure from its use in pipes or drains in homes built before 1940. It's been found to cause learning disabilities and emotional problems.

Symptoms are not difficult to recognize when someone has an acute exposure to any of these toxic substances. They may include cramping, nausea, vomiting, pain, sweating, headaches, difficulty breathing, and convulsions. When exposure is long-term and in smaller amounts, symptoms of learning difficulties, impaired cognitive, motor and language skills, emotional difficulties, insomnia and general feelings of ill-health are difficult to associate with their cause. The diagnosis is made from observation of symptoms, history of possible exposure, and the results of laboratory tests. Tests include blood tests, liver and renal function, urinalysis, fecal tests, X-rays, and hair and fingernail analysis.

Some physicians test for metal poisoning when treating a patient for FMS or CFIDS if symptoms warrant and if past history suggests that exposure has taken place. If you think you may have been exposed to any of these substances, you need to discuss the situation with your physician.

Mercury Toxicity

Many people have had mercury silver fillings placed in their teeth, and some may have symptoms related to the mercury in their fillings. Mercury is a known toxin that exerts a variety of toxic effects in the body. Today there is no single test that can diagnose mercury poisoning. When there has been no acute exposure, the medical profession relies on symptoms to determine if there is a need to investigate further. Over 200 symptoms can result from mercury exposure. Most of them relate to industrial exposures, accidental spills, or chronic exposure. Since mercury has been in use in dental amalgams (fillings in your teeth) for decades, there has been a significant amount of controversy among dentists over the possibility of poisoning due to long-term exposure to the vapors released from the dental fillings.

Symptoms of mercury toxicity can include irritability, anxiety, restlessness, emotional instability, loss of memory, concentration problems, fatigue, depression, antisocial behavior, suicidal tendencies, muscle weakness, loss of coordination, bleeding gums and loosening of teeth, abdominal cramps, chronic diarrhea or constipation, abnormal heart rhythms, abnormal blood pressure, unexplained elevations of cholesterol and triglycerides, repeated infections, cancer, headaches, ringing in the ears, joint and muscle pain, unusual numbness or burning sensations, unsteady gait, allergies, excessive perspiration, and sinus congestion.

If you have mercury fillings, you may want to find a physician who will test you for mercury toxicity. Urine is collected over a 24-hour period and is then sent to a special lab for analysis. If the levels of mercury are toxic, a chelation treatment may be recommended. In chelation, the chelating substance binds to the toxin and removes it from the body via the urine. There are a variety of substances used in chelation, depending on the type of metal exposure. Physicians must be trained in this treatment.

If it is determined that you have mercury toxicity, you will want to have your mercury fillings removed and replaced by a dentist who is trained in removing your old fillings. This must be done carefully so as not to expose you to the mercury vapors that are released when the fillings are removed.

Natural therapies can be utilized for chelation, detoxification, and protection of toxic substances. Many supplements have also been found useful in alleviating symptoms of FMS and CFIDS. These supplements include vitamins C, E, A, glutathione, selenium, zinc, lactoferrin, cilantro, green tea, calcium, l-cysteine, N-acetyl-cysteine, alfalfa sprouts, MSM, chlorella, SAM-e and silymarin.

Resources:

The Chelation Way, Morton Walker, D.P.M., Avery Publishing.

Silver Dental Fillings: The Toxic Timebomb: Can the Mercury in Your Dental Fillings Poison You? Sam Ziff.

American Board of Clinical Metal Toxicology
1407 1/2 N. Wells St.
Chicago, Illinois, 60610
800-356-2228 Fax:312-266-3685
www.abct.info

American Dental Association
211 East Chicago Ave.
Chicago, Illinois, 60611
312-440-2500
www.ada.org

American College for Advancement in Medicine
23121 Verdugo Drive, Suite 204
Laguna Hills, California, 92653
800-532-3688 Fax 949-455-9679
www.acam.org

Consumers for Dental Choice
1725 K Street NW, Suite 511
Washington, D.C. 20006
202-822-6307
www.toxicteeth.org

Alpha-Stim

The Alpha-Stim is an FDA recognized drug-free treatment for anxiety, depression, and insomnia. This device passes microcurrent levels of electrical stimulation across the head by clip electrodes attached to one's earlobes. This process is called cranial electrical stimulation (CES). Depending on the disorder being treated, CES may be recommended for 20 minutes to an hour each day, for days, weeks, or longer. When used to treat localized pain, specialized probes or self adhesive electrodes are placed around the painful area. When the Alpha-Stim is turned on, a microcurrent that is similar to the electricity that's naturally found in the body passes through the area being treated. The Alpha-Stim works by moving electrons through the body at a variety of frequencies, affecting the cell's electrical charge.

The unit is the size of a portable tape player and is very easy to carry. Insurance will often cover the treatment in a clinic setting, if it is prescribed. The Alpha-Stim may be purchased for home use if prescribed by a physician or nurse practitioner. Many insurance companies have full or partial coverage for the Alpha-Stim 100. Side effects are minimal, with very few individuals having experienced a headache, dizziness, skin irritation or burn where the electrode is attached.

There have been over 125 studies performed on the use of the Alpha-Stim in providing relief for anxiety, depression, and sleep problems since 1981. A study at the Robert Wood Johnson Medical School in New Jersey on Alpha-Stim's effectiveness in FMS patients was published in the *Journal of Clinical Rheumatology* in 2001. FMS patients used the unit at a low level for one hour per day over a three-week period. Improvement in tender point score, pain, quality of sleep, feeling of well-being, mood, and quality of life were reported at significant levels. Pain levels were decreased by 27%. Sleep was improved in over 90% of patients. Scores were improved in the anxiety and anger area by more than 40%, and fatigue was reduced by 25%. After the study, clients who used the Alpha-Stim at higher levels for longer periods of time showed more improvements than the study participants. It is interesting to note that in other diseases it is used for longer periods of time. More research is needed on FMS patients to determine how long to use it and when. Currently, there are a few studies being conducted in various centers. Alpha-Stim was developed by neurobiologist Dr. Daniel L. Kirsch, who has been a leading pioneer in the field of electromedicine since 1972.

If you decide to try this treatment, you will need a physician or nurse practitioner's prescription. You can purchase the units directly from the manufacturer: Electromedical Products International, Inc. 800-367-7246 or www.alpha-stim.com.

Alpha-Stim 100: combined microcurrent and cranial stimulator for pain, anxiety, depression and insomnia.

Alpha-Stim SCS: for anxiety, depression insomnia and stress.

Decompression Surgery of Craniovertebral Stenosis

Michael J. Rosner, M.D., who is a neurosurgeon in North Carolina, found that some patients with FMS or CFIDS also have cervical spinal stenosis or Chiari malformation. These two neurological abnormalities cause cervical cord or nerve root compression. Symptoms associated with these abnormalities are similar to FMS/CFIDS symptoms and may include headaches, neck pain, upper and lower extremity pain, burning, a feeling of tightness, numbness, clumsy hands, stiffness, spasticity, atrophy, flushing, sweating, urinary frequency, irritable bowel, burning feet, dizziness, sore throats, blurred vision, and cognitive problems. Spinal cord compression can occur from a congenital cervical stenosis, from an accident where the neck is hyperextended, after surgery, or after a viral infection. Abnormal findings in a neurological exam may indicate this condition; an MRI is needed to confirm it. Numbness, weakness, and imbalance are particularly important symptoms to note in evaluating this condition.

Other physicians have found that a number of patients with FMS or CFIDS who are also diagnosed with cervical spinal stenosis and/or Chiari malformation respond favorably to decompression surgery. The surgical procedures to correct these abnormalities relieve the pressure from the spinal cord, improving the flow of spinal fluid. Over 50% of Dr. Rosner's patients reported that many of their symptoms improved from these surgical procedures and included the following:

▲ Headache	88%		▲ Memory	62%
▲ Sore throat	72%		▲ Bowel	57%
▲ Joint pain	82%		▲ Bladder	70%
▲ Muscle pain	80%		▲ Balance	78%
▲ Grip strength	75%			

Conservative treatment for this condition consists of limiting neck hyperextension and flexion by wearing a cervical collar. Supporting the neck during the night with proper cervical pillows may also be helpful, along with physical therapy and improving posture.

This is yet another potential problem that may be contributing to some patients' symptoms. A careful neurological exam and MRI may be indicated for some people with FMS, so that a potentially treatable neurological abnormality is not overlooked. You may want to discuss this possibility with your physician. The National Fibromyalgia Research Association is a resource for additional information: 503-588-1411. There are a few surgeons performing this surgery, and this organization can give you information and provide written materials for your physician.

Neurofeedback

Stuart Donaldson, Ph.D., of Calgary, Alberta, Canada, has been treating patients with a combination of biofeedback and EEG brain wave therapy, which is drug-free and has shown to be helpful in reducing symptoms. EEG brain wave therapy or EEG biofeedback is also called neurotherapy. It is a form of biofeedback which helps an individual take voluntary control of brain wave activity. It is a relatively new technique, and there are not many practitioners trained in it. Physicians, psychologists, nurses, and social workers may be trained in this therapy. Neurotherapy may help treat subgroups of FMS patients who have suffered from various forms of trauma that have affected the central nervous system or brain.

Following a traumatic injury to the central nervous system or brain due to whiplash, a fall, surgery, infection, toxic exposure, or psychological trauma, a condition known as EEG slowing can occur. This can produce symptoms found in FMS and other conditions such as postconcussion syndrome and posttraumatic stress disorder. It can affect pain, memory, and mood among other things. Stuart Donaldson, Ph.D., conducted a research study on FMS patients and found that people with a past history of traumatic injury to the central nervous system typically show an excess of slow brain waves. This occurs when theta or delta brain wave patterns are present when people are awake. The slower the frequency and the more often slow brain waves appear, the greater the degree of abnormality. These abnormal brain waves appear when brain cells are damaged, regardless of the cause of injury.

Researchers at the NIH have found that EEG slowing of brain waves can be treated using EEG stimulation. In these studies, people who had functioned at a high level prior to developing FMS responded very well to treatment.

During a treatment, painless electrodes are placed on the scalp to record brain wave activity. The sensors pick up brain wave patterns and a computer analyzes the data from the sensors. This information is displayed on the computer screen. The patient can then retrain the brain to produce favorable brain waves. Clinicians determine which brain wave patterns to change.

The brain produces waves that are known as

Delta- slow frequency waves seen most often during deep sleep
Theta - slightly faster brain wave found in a drowsy, relaxed state
Alpha - found in relaxed and meditative states
Beta - produced when a person is alert and focused
High Beta - produced when a person is anxious

Studies have shown neurotherapy produces significant improvement in many areas for FMS patients including pain, sleep, fatigue, cognition, depression, and anxiety. Neurotherapy also reduced patients' need for medications.

At least 20-50 sessions may be needed for improvement to occur. It is expensive; the total cost can be up to $3,500-$4,000, although some insurance companies will pay for the treatment. Neurotherapy is also being used for Attention Deficit Disorder, seizure disorder, brain injuries, migraines, anxiety, and depression. You might want to try this treatment if you can find a practitioner in your area.

sEMG Electromyography

This technique is used to help retrain the muscles by placing biofeedback sensors on specific muscles to measure their electrical activity. This allows the clinician to identify and correct muscle imbalances. Computer software displays the results on a video screen. The clinician uses this information to prescribe individualized exercises for the patient to perform at home to aid in retraining the muscles. This treatment facilitates lasting improvement in other therapies such as massage, relaxation biofeedback, acupuncture, and stress management. sEMG treatment may require fewer sessions than EEG neurofeedback. Researchers have found that, when combined with EEG neurofeedback, patients see greater improvement than when either treatment is performed alone.

EEG neurofeedback and sEMG feedback help facilitate myofascial treatment, which focuses on loosening up the connective tissue of the body and is discussed in the "Pain Management" chapter. Researchers feel these treatments used in combination may produce greater improvement in symptoms. Not all patients with FMS will experience good results, particularly if there has been significant structural damage or neurological damage from long-standing infections or toxic exposure.

For information contact

Mary Lee Esty, Ph.D., L.C.S.W. at the Neurotherapy Centers in Washington, D.C. at www.neurotherapycenters.com.

Stuart Donaldson, Ph.D. has a center in Canada and can be reached at www.myosymmetires.ca/index.html

Prolotherapy

For those who experience localized back or neck pain, a treatment called prolotherapy may be beneficial in reducing pain to those portions of the body. Prolotherapy involves a series of injections into the ligaments and muscle-tendon attachments in affected regions. It can also be performed in other areas of the body, such as the shoulder, neck, knees, or feet. The injection consists of a benign solution of dextrose (sugar molecule used by tissues for growth) with a mild anesthetic. The injection produces an inflammatory response that sends chemicals to repair the injected areas. During this process, collagen fibers are produced which aid in providing support to the area that was torn or stretched due to a whiplash, accident, or fall. The function of ligaments and tendons can increase by as much as 35-40% in the treated areas. It is an effective treatment for chronic low back pain in some patients, helping in some cases by as much as 75%.

Prolotherapy was developed in the 1940s. It requires multiple injections, spaced two-four weeks apart. If the physician is well practiced, the injections can be surprisingly painless, although there will be soreness or stiffness at the injection site for a day or two after the treatment. This is not a cure for FMS, but if you have an area of localized pain or have not recovered from a whiplash injury, it may help that area feel less painful. When you are in pain, any little bit helps! Improvement in pain reduction should be noted by the fourth treatment. Insurance may not cover the cost of treatment.

Important Note

We believe these novel treatments are exciting to report on because they add to the treatment options that may reduce your symptoms. Some physicians may not be familiar with these therapies, so it might be up to you to educate them. In most cases, because these treatments are so new, it is not known whether they are beneficial when prescribed singly or in conjunction with other treatments. In general, these treatments have not been subjected to rigorous research, and using them may be risky. They might be something to look into, however, if you have tried the other, more researched treatments described in this book and you still do not feel better. Many physicians feel a multidisciplinary treatment approach is necessary to control FMS, which means using all, many, or some of the treatment options described in this book. At this time, we still do not have a "magic" pill which cures all the symptoms of FMS, but at least we have more treatment options to choose from than we did previously. We, the authors, feel we have covered the major new treatments available at this time, although we do not claim to have knowledge of all treatments that are being carried out at this point in time. Please call or write to us if you know of any treatments you feel are worth reporting.

Pioneering Physicians' Treatments Overview

Many holistic physicians believe that FMS and CFIDS symptoms are caused by a variety of factors including

- ▲ Dysfunctional immune system
- ▲ Spinal cord compression
- ▲ Toxic substances
- ▲ Hormonal problems
- ▲ Metabolic problems
- ▲ Infections/parasites/viruses
- ▲ Physical trauma
- ▲ Nutritional deficiencies
- ▲ Sleep disorders

Treatment may be as follows:

1. Rule out other illnesses.

2. Treat sleep disorders.

3. Uncover perpetuating factors.
- ▲ Test for infectious agents - HHV-6, Cytomegalovirus, EBV, Mycoplasma
- ▲ Test for parasites
- ▲ Test for fungal growth (*Candida*)
- ▲ Test for nutritional deficiencies - vitamins, amino acids, minerals
- ▲ Test hormone levels - adrenal, thyroid, cortisol, growth hormone, estrogen, testosterone, progesterone, DHEA
- ▲ Look for physical problems - spinal decompression, chiari malformation
- ▲ Treat trigger points, myofascial pain, disc problems
- ▲ Test for toxic metals

4. Treat with
- ▲ Antivirals/antibiotics
- ▲ Intravenous/injectable vitamin therapy
- ▲ Modifications of diet
- ▲ Antiparasite medications and supplements
- ▲ Hormonal supplementation

- ▲ **Treatments for metal toxicity**
- ▲ **Oral supplements**
- ▲ **Modifications of lifestyle**
- ▲ **Physical therapy, myofascial release or trigger point therapy**
- ▲ **Specific medications for symptom reduction**
- ▲ **Neurofeedback, biofeedback, or relaxation techniques**
- ▲ **Psychological counseling**

This is an outline of treatments utilized by many physicians who are having good success with patients who do not respond to more conservative treatments. You may wish to share this information with your physician. Dr. Teitelbaum, Dr. Romano, Dr. Flechas, and Dr. McNett, whose protocols are in this book, use many of the treatments suggested in this outline. For information on other physicians who utilize these methods, go to www.immunesupport.com for articles by physicians who explain their treatment protocols. Members of a local FMS, CFIDS, or chronic pain support group may recommend a doctor in your area who is practicing in this manner.

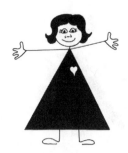

TAKING CHARGE OF FIBROMYALGIA: A SUMMARY

Because we have given you so much information on how to take charge of your FMS, we realize you are probably feeling quite overwhelmed with your newfound knowledge. To help you feel less overwhelmed, we've highlighted the main steps so you can quickly see what you need to do in order to **Take Charge of Your Fibromyalgia!**

1. Find a sympathetic and knowledgeable physician.

2. Acknowledge or accept your diagnosis.

3. Educate yourself, your friends, family and co-workers.

4. Begin a fibromyalgia journal.

5. Discuss the need for appropriate medications with your physician.

6. Improve sleep quality.

7. Learn appropriate pain management techniques which you can do yourself at home or at work.

8. Exercise.

9. Eat foods that are high in nutritional value.

10. Learn stress management techniques.

11. Learn to cope with the psychological aspects of living with a chronic illness.

12. Pursue counseling, if necessary.

13. Treat flare-ups quickly.

14. Be assertive in your health care.

15. Use all resources available to you.

16. Pace and balance.

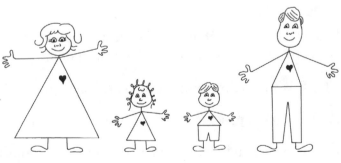

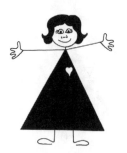

HOPE

Healing begins with hope.

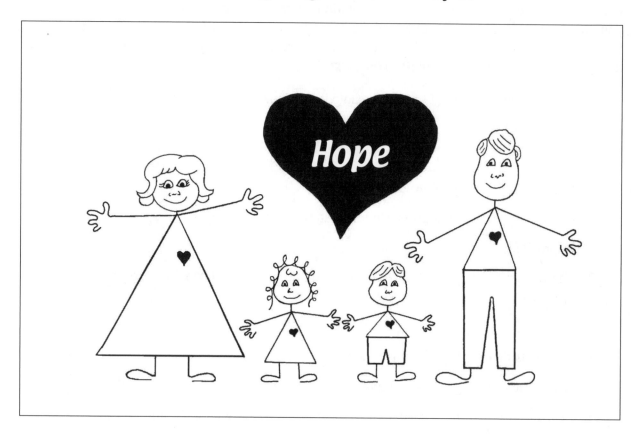

Hope Conclusion

When we live with fibromyalgia, we can feel isolated, misunderstood and diminished by illness and a myriad of losses. We may be fearful of those things we don't understand and can't predict.

HOPE is what allows us to hang on for one more day as we muster the courage to try again.

HOPE is putting one foot in front of the other; it's the victory of the human spirit over adversity.

HOPE enables our bodies to begin healing and helps to carry us through the days that we feel alone and overwhelmed.

May each and every one of you who is living with fibromyalgia have HOPE of taking charge of this condition.

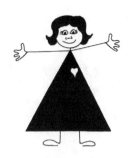

RESOURCES

Books

Backstrom, Gayle. *I'd Rather Be Working: A Step-by-Step Guide to Financial Self-Support for People with Chronic Illness.* American Management Association, 2002.

Backstrom, Gayle and Dr. Bernard Rubin. *When Muscle Pain Won't Go Away: The Relief Handbook for Fibromyalgia and Chronic Muscle Pain.* Taylor Trade Publishing, 1998.

Barrett, Marilyn, Ph.D., Ed. *The Handbook of Clinically Tested Herbal Remedies.* Haworth Medical Press, 2004.

Berne, Katrina, Ph.D. *Chronic Fatigue Syndrome, Fibromyalgia and Other Invisible Illnesses.* Third Edition. Hunter House, 2001.

Bigelow, Stacie, M.A. *Fibromyalgia: Simple Relief through Movement.* John Wiley & Sons, 2000.

Birkhoff, Brent. *Seasons of Fibromyalgia.* Self-published, 2004.

Burton, Gail and Rosenbaum, M.D., Michael. *Candida Control Cookbook: What You Should Know and What You Should Eat to Manage Yeast Infections.* Aslan Publishing, 2002.

Catalano, Ellen Mohr, M.A. and Kimeron N. Hardin, Ph.D. *The Chronic Pain Control Workbook: A Step-by-Step Guide for Coping with and Overcoming Pain.* New Harbinger Publications, Inc., 1996.

Caudill-Slosberg, Margaret, M.D., Ph.D. *Managing Pain Before It Manages You.* The Guilford Press, 2001.

Chaitow, Leon, N.D., D.O. *Fibromyalgia Syndrome: A Practitioner's Guide to Treatment.* Churchill Livingstone, 2000.

Davies, Clair, N.C.M.T. *The Trigger Point Therapy Workbook: Your Self-Treatment Guide for Pain Relief.* New Harbinger Publications, 2001.

Donoghue, Paul, Ph.D. and Mary Siegel, Ph.D. *Sick and Tired of Feeling Sick and Tired: Living with Invisible Chronic Illness.* W.W. Norton and Company, 2000.

Emmal, Marline, Ph.D. *Fibromyalgia and Female Sexuality.* Trafford Publishing, 2001.

Fennell, Patricia, M.S.W, C.S.W-R. ***The Chronic Illness Workbook: Strategies and Solutions for Taking Back Your Life.*** Hew Harbinger Publications, Inc, 2001.

Foster, Steven and Varro Tyler, Ph.D. ***Tyler's Honest Herbal: A Sensible Guide to the Use of Herbs and Related Remedies.*** Haworth Press, 1999.

Fransen, Jenny, R.N. and I. Jon Russell, M.D., Ph.D. ***The Fibromyalgia Help Book.*** Smith House Press, 1997.

Gardiser, Kit. ***We Laughed, We Cried: Life With Fibromyalgia.*** KMK Associates, 1995.

Goldberg, Burton and Ed. of Alternative Medicine Digest. ***Alternative Medicine Guide To Chronic Fatigue, Fibromyalgia, and Environmental Illness.*** Alternative Medicine.com Books, 1998.

Goldberg, Burton and Larry Trivieri, Jr. ***Chronic Fatigue, Fibromyalgia, and Lyme Disease.*** Celestial Arts, 2nd Edition, 2004.

Goldenberg, Don, M.D. ***Fibromyalgia: A Leading Expert's Guide To Understanding And Getting Relief From The Pain That Won't Go Away.*** Perigee Books, 2002.

Goldstein, Jay A., M.D. ***Betrayal by the Brain: The Neurological Basis of Chronic Fatigue Syndrome, Fibromyalgia Syndrome and Related Neural Network Disorders.*** Haworth Medical Press, 1996.

Hanner, Linda, John Witek, M.D. and Robert Clift. ***When You're Sick and Don't Know Why: Coping with Your Undiagnosed Illness.*** DCI Publishing, 1991.

Hutchinson, Jennifer, Cynthia Still and Bill Still. ***The Truth about TMJ: How to Help Yourself.*** Reinhardt and Still Publishers, 1994.

Inkeles, Gordon and Iris Schencke. ***Ergonomic Living: How to Create a User-Friendly Home and Office.*** Fireside Publishing, 1994.

Lewis, Kathleen. ***Celebrate Life: New Attitudes for Living with Chronic Illness.*** The Arthritis Foundation, 2000.

Lewis, Kathleen. ***Successful Living with Chronic Illness: Celebrating the Joys of Life.*** Avery Publishing Group, 1985.

Natelson, Benjamin, M.D. ***Facing & Fighting Fatigue: A Practical Approach.*** Yale University Press, 1998.

O'Brien, Mary, M.D. ***Chronic Fatigue Syndrome: Charting Your Course to Recovery.*** Anadem Publishing, 1997.

McCall, Timothy B., M.D. ***Examining Your Doctor: A Patient's Guide to Avoiding Harmful Medical Care.*** Citadel Trade Publisher, 1996.

St. Marie, Barbara, M.A., A.N.P., G.N.P. and Susan Arnold, B.A., R.N., C.H.T.P., Editors. ***When Your Pain Flares Up.*** Fairview Press, 2002.

Pelligrino, Mark, M.D. ***A Sunnier Tomorrow.*** Anadem Publishing, 1998.

Pelligrino, Mark, M.D. *Fibromyalgia: Up Close & Personal with Mark J. Pellegrino, M.D.* Anadem Publishing, 2005.

Pelligrino, Mark, M.D. *Inside Fibromyalgia.* Anadem Publishing, 2001.

Pelligrino, Mark, M.D. *Laugh At Your Muscles. Volume I and II.* Anadem Publishing, 1995 and 1997.

Pelligrino, Mark, M.D. *The Fibromyalgia Supporter.* Anadem Publishing, 1997.

Pelligrino, Mark, M.D. *Understanding Post Traumatic Fibromyalgia.* Anadem Publishing, 1996.

Register, Cheri. *The Chronic Illness Experience: Embracing the Imperfect Life.* Hazelden Publishing and Educational Services, 1999.

Russell, I. Jon, M.D. Ed. *The Fibromyalgia Syndrome: A Clinical Case Definition For Practitioners.* Haworth Medical Press, 2004.

Salt, William II, M.D. and Edwin Weason, M.D. **Fibromyalgia and the MindBodySpirit** *Connection: 7 Steps for Living A Healthy Life with Widespread Muscular Pain and Fatigue.* Parkview Publishing, 2000.

Shankland, Wesley, D.D.S., M.S. *TMJ: Its Many Faces.* Anadem Publishing, 1996.

Shomon, Mary. *Living Well with Chronic Fatigue Syndrome & Fibromyalgia: What Your Doctor Doesn't Tell You......That You Need To Know.* Harper Resource, 2004.

Simmons, Kenna. *Natural Treatments for Fibromyalgia.* The Arthritis Foundation, 2003.

Starlanyl, Devin, M.D. *The Fibromyalgia Advocate.* New Harbinger Publications, 1998.

Starlanyl, Devin, M.D. and Mary Ellen Copeland, M.S., M.A. *Fibromyalgia and Chronic Myofascial Pain Syndrome: A Survival Manual.* New Harbinger Publications, 2001.

The Arthritis Foundation. *The Arthritis Foundation's Guide to Good Living with Fibromyalgia.* Longstreet Press, 2001.

Teitelbaum, Jacob, M.D. *From Fatigued to Fantastic!* Avery Publishing Group, 2001.

Teitelbaum, Jacob, M.D. *Pain Free 1-2-3! A Proven Program to Get YOU Pain Free Now.* Deva Press, 2005.

Teitelbaum, Jacob, M.D. *Three Steps to Happiness! Healing Through Joy.* Deva Press, 2003.

Wallace, Daniel, M.D. and Janice Wallace. *All About Fibromyalgia.* Oxford University Press, 2002.

Wallace, Daniel, M.D. and Janice Wallace. *Fibromyalgia: An Essential Guide for Patients and Their Families.* Oxford University Press, 2003.

Wallace, Daniel, M.D. and Janice Wallace. *Making Sense of Your Fibromyalgia: A Guide for Patients and Their Families.* Anadem Publishing, 1999.

RESOURCES

Wells, Susan Milstrey. *A Delicate Balance: Living Successfully with Chronic Illness.* Perseus Publishing, 2000.

Williamson, Miryam. *Fibromyalgia: A Comprehensive Approach.* Walker and Company, 1996.

Williamson, Miryam. *The Fibromyalgia Relief Book: 213 Ideas for Improving Your Quality of Life.* Walker & Company, 1998.

Disability Resources

Disability Workbook for Social Security Applicants: Managing Your Application for Social Security Disability Insurance Benefits 5th edition. Douglas M. Smith, Atty. at Law. Physician's Disability Services, Inc., 2001; 410-431-5279.

Overview of the Social Security Disability Process. Brochure, The CFIDS Association of America, PO Box 220398, Charlotte, NC 28222-0398; 704-365-2343. www.cfids.org

Physician's Disability Services, Inc. Books, products, services, resources for disability applicants. Physician's Disability Services, Inc., PO Box 822, Severna Park, MD 21146; 410-431-5279. www.disabilityfacts.com

Social Security Disability Benefits Information. Pamphlet, National Chronic Fatigue Syndrome and Fibromyalgia Assn., PO Box 18426, Kansas City, M.O. 64133; 816-313-2000. www.ncfsfa.org

Understanding Social Security and Disability Evaluation Under Social Security. Social Security Administration, Baltimore, MD 21235; 800-772-1213. www.socialsecurity.gov

Internet Resources

This is just a partial listing of the thousands of Web sites available on the subject. These are the ones we have utilized and feel provide quality information. There are many more we cannot include.

American Academy of Pain Management	www.aapainmanage.org
American Academy of Osteopathic Physicians	www.osteopathic.org
American Academy of Physical Medicine & Rehabilitation	www.aapmr.org
American Physical Therapy Association	www.apta.org
American Fibromyalgia Syndrome Association	www.afsafund.org
Arthritis Foundation	www.arthritis.org
Assoc. of Myofascial Trigger Point Therapists	www.myofascialtherapy.org
British Columbia Fibromyalgia Society	www.mefm.bc.ca/bcfm/
Center for Disease Control	www.cdc.gov
Chronic Fatigue & Immune Dysfunction Syndrome of America	www.cfids.org
Chronic Neurotoxins	www.chronicneurotoxins.com
CFS Research	www.cfsresearch.org
Clinical Trials Funded by NIH	www.clinicaltrials.gov
Colorado Health Site	www.coloradohealthsite.org/fibro
Co-Cure Message Board	www.co-cure.org

Consumers for Dental Choice	www.toxicteeth.org
Dr. Lowe's Web site (thyroid disorders)	www.drlowe.com
FMS Doctor Locator	www.beatcfsandfms.org
Fibro Hugs	www.fibrohugs.com
Fibrom-L Email Discussion Group	www.fmscommunity.org
Fibromyalgia Educational Systems	www.fmsedsys.com
Fibromyalgia Information	www.ncf.carleton.ca/fibromyalgia/
Fibromyalgia Network	www.fmnetnews.com
Fibromyalgia Patient Support Center	www.fmpsc.org
Fibromyalgia Treatment Centers of America	www.fmtcoa.com
Fibromyalgia Support	www.fibromyalgiasupport.com
Food and Drug Administration	www.fda.gov
Internat'l Academy of Compounding Pharmacies	www.iacprx.org
International Myopain Society	www.myopain.org
Village Health	www.ivillagehealth.com/boards
Jacob Teitelbaum, M.D.	www.endfatigue.com
John Hopkins Univ Med Center Health Info	www.intelihealth.com
Kent Holtorf, M.D.	www.chronicfatigue.about.com
MediConsult (drug info)	www.mediconsult.com
Medline Plus	www.nlm.nil.gov
ME-NET (International resources)	www.me-net.dds.nl
Men with Fibromyalgia	www.menwithfibro.com
National Council for Reliable Health Info	www.ncrhi.org
National Fibromyalgia Association	www.Fmaware.org
National Fibromyalgia Partnership	www.fmpartnership.org
National Fibromyalgia Research Assoc.	www.nfra.net
National Institutes of Health	www.nih.gov
National Women's Health Info Center	www.4woman.org
Oregon Fibromyalgia Foundation	www.myalgia.com
Paragon Clinic /FTCOA	www.paragonclinic.com
Paul StAmand, M.D. (guaifenison)	www.guaidoc.com
Pro Health, Inc.	www.immunesupport.com
PubMed Database-Nat'l Library of Medicine	www.ncbi.nlm.nih.gov
Quack Watch	www.quackwatch.com
Restless Legs Syndrome Foundation	www.rls.org
Remedy Find	www.remedyfind.com
Social Security Advisory Service	www.ssas.com
Social Security Online	www.ssa.gov
Spine Universe (pain info)	www.spineuniverse.com
Thyroid Foundation of America	www.allthyroid.org
The American Pain Foundation	www.painfoundation.org

The Chronic Syndrome Support Association	www.cssa-inc.org
The Fibromyalgia Community	www.fmscommunity.org
The Pediatric Network	www.pediatricnetwork.org
To Your Health (vitamins/supplements)	www.e-tyh.com
TMJ Association	www.tmj.org
WebMD	www.my.webmd.com
World Arnold Chiari Malformation Assoc.	www.pressenter.com/~wacma/

RESOURCES

Medical Journals

American Journal of Pain Management - This is the official journal of the American Academy of Pain Management. This peer-reviewed journal is dedicated to the transmission of knowledge related to the study and practice of pain management; www.aapainmanage.org.

Arthritis & Rheumatism/Arthritis Care & Research - The official journal of The American College of Rheumatology and the Association of Rheumatology Health Professionals. Peer-reviewed journal that publishes both original research and review articles that promote excellence in the clinical practice of rheumatology; www.arthritisrheum.org.

Journal of Musculoskeletal Pain - Peer-reviewed medical journal containing FMS scientific abstract information. Appropriate for lay people as well as medical professionals; www.haworthpress.com.

Journal of the Chronic Fatigue Syndrome - Peer-reviewed medical journal containing CFIDS scientific abstract information. Appropriate for patients and health professionals; www.haworthpress.com.

PAIN - This is the official journal of the International Association for the Study of Pain. It is a peer-reviewed journal that publishes original research on the nature, mechanisms and treatment of pain; www.iasp-pain.org.

Patient Organizations/Newsletters

Many of these organizations provide information regarding support groups, physician referrals and links to other organizations.

American Association for Chronic Fatigue Syndrome - For health professionals as well as support groups, institutions, individuals or organizations interested in furthering research, information, ideas and treatment for CFIDS/FMS. Membership for health professionals is $75.00. Provides scientific information, and a speakers bureau of health professionals. It is made up of research scientists, physicians, licensed medical professionals and other institutions. 27 N Wacker Drive. Suite 416, Chicago, IL 60606; 847-258-7248, fax: 847-748-8288; www.aacfs.org.

American Fibromyalgia Syndrome Association AFSA - A non-profit organization that provides educational information, including updates on research funding activities for FMS and CFIDS. 6380 E. Tanque Verde Rd., Suite D. Tucson, AZ 85715-3822; Phone: 520-733-1570; www.afsafund.org.

Arthritis Foundation - Publishes and distributes pamphlets, books, brochures and other printed material regarding rheumatoid arthritis, osteoarthritis, lupus, FMS and other arthritic – related illnesses. Chapters located in many U.S. cities. Some offer self-help classes, educational conferences, support groups and seminars for patients. Contact your local chapter for the name of a support group in your area. P.O. Box 7669, Atlanta, GA 30357; 800-283-7800; www.arthritis.org.

CFIDS Association of America - National organization dedicated to CFS research, advocacy and patient support. Membership fee includes a subscription to 2 newsletters: *The CFIDS Chronicle* and *The CFS Research Review*. P.O. Box 220398, Charlotte, NC 28222-0398; 800-44203437, resource line 704-365-2343, fax: 704-365-9755; www.cfids.org.

CFIDS and Fibromyalgia Health Resource - Offers high-quality supplements and publishes a newsletter called *Health Watch*. They provide one of the best internet sites for information on FMS and CFIDS. 1187 Coast Village Road, Suite 1-280, Santa Barbara, CA 93108; 800-366-6056, fax: 805-965-0042; www.immunesupport.com.

Fibromyalgia Network - The *Fibromyalgia Network* is a quarterly newsletter that provides patients and health care professionals with the latest information on FMS, CFS, and related conditions. Each issue contains articles on new research, drugs, and advice on coping. P.O. Box 31750, Tucson, AZ 85751; 800-853-2929; www.fmnetnews.com.

National CFIDS Foundation - A volunteer, non-profit organization, providing a quarterly newsletter. Dues are $35.00. Primary focus is in providing information and funding for research. 103 Aletha Rd. Needham, MA 02492; 781-449-3535, fax: 781-449-8606; www.mcf-net.org.

National Dysautonomia Research Foundation - Provides information, printed materials, and a patient education newsletter. 1407 W. Fourth Street Suite 160, Red Wing, MN 55066; 651-267-0525, fax: 651-267-0524; www.NDRF.org.

National Fibromyalgia Association - Non-profit founded to promote awareness of fibromyalgia to patients and the public. They publish a triannual publication called *Fibromyalgia Aware* and educate through conferences and its Web site. 2200 N. Glassell St. Suite A, Orange, CA 92863; 714-921-0150, fax: 714-921-6920; www.fmaware.org.

National Fibromyalgia Partnership - Non-profit organization dedicated to providing high quality information to patients via their newsletter, *Fibromyalgia Frontiers,* as well as patient conferences in and around the Washington, DC area. They are also involved in patient advocacy at NIH. 140 Zinn Way, Linden, VA 22642; 866-725-4404, fax: 866-666-2727; www.fmpartnership.org.

National Fibromyalgia Research Association - A non-profit organization dedicated to education, treatment and finding a cure for FMS. NFRA funds research, travels to health-care professional conferences and supplies educational materials to physicians, patients and also helps raise public awareness. P.O. Box 500, Salem, OR 97308; 503-588-1411; www.NFRA.net.

National ME/FM Action Network - Goal is to provide information and help patients with issues ranging from insurance problems, government issues, children with the illness, schools, the media, physician and attorney referrals and lack of proper medical testing. 3836 Carling Avenue, Hwy 17 B, Nepean, Ontario K2H 7V2, Canada. Phone and fax: 613-829-6667; www.mefmaction.net.

Restless Legs Syndrome Foundation - 819 Second Street, SW, Rochester, MN 55902; 507-287-6465; www.rls.org.

The M.E. Association of Canada - Publishes a monthly newsletter, *The Messenger,* which is available in Canada, England, and Australia. It provides physician and support group information in English as well as French. 246 Queen Street, Suite 400, Ottawa, Ontario KIP 5E4, Canada; 613-563-1565, fax: 613-567-0614; www.mecan.ca/.

The Nightingale Research Foundation - Publishes a quarterly magazine on new medical information about CFIDS. It conducts research and sponsors public education programs for the international CFIDS community. Its goal is to provide patients and medical professionals with information on the illnesses. 383 Danforth Avenue, Ottawa, Ontario K2A OE1, Canada; 613-728-9643, fax: 613-729-0825; www.nightingale.ca/.

Thyroid Foundation of America - One Longfellow Place, Suite 1518, Boston, MA 02114; 800-832-8321; www.allthyroid.org.

TMJ Association, LTD. - PO Box 26770, Milwaukee, WI 53226; 414-259-3223; www.tmj.org.

To Your Health - Nutritional company founded by Margie and David Squires offers a free resource catalogue and newsletter, *Healthpoints,* for FMS, CFIDS, arthritis and chronic pain. Their information focuses on nutrition. 17007 East Colony Drive, Suite 105, Fountain Hills, AZ 85268; 800-801-1406; www.etyh.com.

Vulvar Pain Foundation - Non-profit foundation that provides information on vulvodynia and offers a newsletter for members. 203 North Main Street, Suite 203, Graham, NC 27253; 336-226-0704; www.vulvarpainfoundation.org.

There are many other organizations that are dedicated to providing help, support and education to patients who suffer from FMS or CFIDS. Many of these groups are locally based and can be found by contacting some of the above mentioned organizations who provide links to the local sites or phone numbers. We apologize if we have not included your group in this publication. Please contact us if you would like to be included in future editions.

Pharmacies for Special Prescriptions

International Academy of Compounding Pharmacists, P.O. Box 1365, Sugar Land, TX 77487; Phone 800-927-4227, Fax: 281-495-0602; www.iacprx.org. They will be able to find a compounding pharmacy to fit your needs.

Belmar Pharmacy - Lakewood, CO; 800-525-9473; www.belmarpharmacy.com.

Professional Arts Pharmacy - 800-832-9285.

Women's International Pharmacy - 800-279-5708; www.womensinternational.com.

Professional Organizations

American Academy of Pain Medicine (AAPM)
4700 W. Lake Avenue
Glenview, IL 60025
847-375-4731,fax: 877-734-8750
www.painmed.org

American Academy of Pain Management
13947 Mono Way #A
Sonora, CA 95370
209-533-9744
www.aapainmanage.org

American Academy of Physical Medicine and Rehabilitation
One IBM Place, Suite 2500
Chicago, IL 60611
312-464-9700
www.aapmr.org

American Academy of Sleep Medicine
One Westbrook Corporate Center, Suite 920
Westchester, IL 60154
708-492-0930
www.aasmnet.org

American Board of Clinical Metal Toxicology
14071/2 N. Wells Street
Chicago, IL 60610
800-356-2228
www.abct.info

American Chiropractic Association
1701 Clarendon Blvd.
Arlington, VA 22209
703-276-8800
www.acatoday.com

American Chronic Pain Association
PO Box 850
Rocklin, CA 95677
916-632-0922
www.theacpa.org

American College of Advancement in Medicine
23121 Verdugo Drive, Suite 204
Laguna Hills, CA 92653
800-532-3688
www.acam.org

American College of Rheumatology
1800 Century Pl, Ste. 250
Atlanta, GA 30345
404-633-3777, fax:404-633-1870
www.rheumatology.org

American Massage Therapy Association
500 Davis St. 9th floor
Evanston, IL 60201
888-843-2682
www.amtamassage.org

American Occupational Therapy Association
4720 Montgomery Lane
PO Box 31220
Bethesda, MD 20824
301-652-2682
www.aota.org

American Osteopathic Association
142 E. Ontario St.
Chicago, IL 60611
800-621-1773
www.Osteopathic.org

American Physical Therapy Association
111 North Fairfax Street
Alexandria, VA 22314-1488
800-999-2782
www.apta.org

Arthritis Foundation
1330 W. Peachtree St.
Atlanta, GA 30309
800-283-7800
www.arthritis.org

International Myopain Society
PO Box 6904092
San Antonio, TX 78269
210-567-4661, fax: 210-567-6669
www.myopain.org

National Association of Myofascial Trigger Point Therapists
1541 Summit Hills Drive, N.E.
Albuquerque, NM 87112
www.myofascialtherapy.org

Professional Organizations for Alternative Therapies

American Association of Naturopathic Physicians
3201 New Mexico Avenue NW Suite 350
Washington, D.C., 20016
866-538-2267, fax: 202-274-1992

American Botanical Council
6200 Manor Rd.
Austin, TX 78723
512-926-4900, fax: 512-926-2345
www.herbalgram.org

American Herbalists Guild
1931 Gaffis Road
Canton, GA 30115
770-751-6021, fax: 770-751-7472
www.americanherbalistsguild.com

American Holistic Medical Association
12101 Menaul Blvd., NE Suite C
Albuquerque, NM 87112
505-292-7788, fax: 505-293-7582
www.holisiticmedicine.org

American Holistic Nurses Association
P.O. Box 2130
Flagstaff, AZ 86003
800-278-2426
www.ahna.org

American Society of Clinical Hypnosis
140 N. Bloomingdale Rd.
Bloomingdale, IL 60108
630-980-4740, fax: 630-351-8490
www.asch.net

Applied Kinesiology
6405 Metcalf Ave. Suite 503
Shawnee Mission, KS 66202
913-384-5337, fax: 913-385-5112
www.icakusa.com

Aromatherapy
4509 Interlake Ave N #233
Seattle, WA 98103
888-ASK-NAHA, fax: 206-547-2680
www.naha.org

Association for Applied Psychophysiology and Biofeedback
10200 West 44th Ave., Suite 304
Wheat Ridge, CO 80033
303-422-8436, fax: 303-422-8894
www.aapb.org

Healing Touch
445 Union Blvd. Suite 105
Lakewood, CO 80228
303-989-7982, fax: 208-783-4848
www.healingtouch.net

National Center for Homeopathy
801 North Fairfax Street, Suite 306
Alexandria, VA 22314
703-548-7790, fax: 703-548-7792
www.homeopathic.org

National Certification Commission for Acupuncture and Oriental Medicine
11 Canal Center Plaza, Suite 300
Alexandria, VA 22314
703-548-9004, fax: 703-548-9079
www.nccaom.org

National Ayurvedic Medical Association
2017 Fiesta Drive
Sarasota, FL 34231
941-929-0999
www.ayurveda-nama.org

Reflexology Association of America
4012 Rainbow Ste. K-pmb #585
Las Vegas, N. 89103
978-779-0255, fax: 978-779-0855
www.reflexology-usa.org

Reiki Alliance
204 N. Chestnut St.
Kellogg, IO 83837
208-783-3535, fax: 208-783-4848
www.reikialliance.com

Tapes/CDs/Catalogues

Master Your Mind Tapes and CDs
Mary Richards
881 Hawthorne Creek
Walnut, CA 94596
800-345-8515
www.masteryourmind.com

Health Journeys
Resources for Mind, Body and Spirit
Guided imagery/stress reduction/conferences
Belleruth Naperstak, MSW, LISW
891 Moe Dr., Suite C
Akron, OH 44310
800-800-8661
www.healthjourneys.com

Sounds True Catalogue
800-333-9185
www.soundstrue.com

Testing Resources

AAL Reference Laboratories, Inc.
1715 E. Wilshire #715
Santa Ana, CA 92705
800-522-2611
www.antibodyassay.com

Elisa-ACT Biotechnologies
14 Pidgeon Hill #300
Sterling, VA 22181
800-553-5472
www.elisaact.com

Great Smokies Diagnostic Laboratory
63 Zillicoa St.
Asheville, NC 28801
800-522-4762
www.gsdl.com

Hemex Laboratories
2505 West Baryl Avenue
Phoenix, AZ 85021
800-999-2568
www.hemex.com

Immunosciences Lab, Inc.
8730 Wilshire Blvd. Suite 305
Beverly Hills, CA 90211
800-950-4686
www.immuno-sci-lab.com

Medical Diagnostic Laboratories
133 Gaither Dr. Suite C
Mt. Laurel, NJ 08054
877-269-0090
www.mdlab.com

Vitamin Diagnostic/European Laboratories of Nutrients
Industrial Drive and Route 35
Cliffwood Beach, NJ 07735
732-583-7773
Email: vitamindia@aol.com

FMS Awareness Bracelet

Attractive pink and red bracelets made of soft durable silicone. All funds will go to support FMS research. $1.00 each. Discounts for multiple orders available.

To order contact the **National Fibromyalgia Association**, www.nfranet.com or call 503-588-1411.

Videos

Candida video by Michael McNett, MD. Excellent video that explains how *Candida* and FMS interact and appropriate treatments. Available at: Fibromyalgia Treatment Centers of America, 4332 N. Elston, Chicago, IL 60641; 773-604-5321; www.ftcoa.com.

Chronic Myofascial Pain Syndrome: A Guide to the Trigger Points by Devin Starlanyl. Two hour video; 800-748-6273; www.newharbinger.com.

Fibromyalgia Exercise Video by Patty Bourne, Kinesiologist. 30 minute video of warm-up and stretching, aerobics and cool down movements. OYM Hospital, Physiotherapy Dept., 327 Re Street, Oakville, Ontario, L6J3L7; www.directquest.com/Fibromyalgia/videos/.

Fibromyalgia Exercise Videos by Sharon Clark, Ph.D. Three videos are available: Stretching, Aerobic Exercise and Toning and Strengthening. Ordering information available at Oregon Fibromyalgia Foundation, 1221 S. W. Yamhill, Suite 303, Portland, OR 97205; www.myalgia.com.

Fibromyalgia and You Video by I. Jon Russell, M.D., Ph.D. This video features fibromyalgia patients and leading FMS experts who discuss fibromyalgia and how it affects people's lives. It also includes a discussion of current research, treatment and strategies for coping. Ordering information is available from Fibromyalgia Information Resources, PO Box 690402, San Antonio, TX 78269.

Myofascial Pain Syndromes: The Travell Trigger Point Tapes. 6 part tape series explaining the Travell method of treating trigger points. Wolters Kluwer Health, 16522 Hunters Green Parkway, Hagerstown, MD 21740; 800-527-5597; www.lww.com.

Myofascial Release Vidoes by John Barnes. Explains how to perform myofascial release. Suitable for professionals as well as patients who wish to learn more about this technique. 222 West Lancaster Avenue, Paoli, PA 19301; 800-FASCIAL; www.myofascialrelease.com.

Physician Referral Resource

Fibromyalgia Resources Group, Ltd., Betsy Jacobson. Founded in 1991, an international service which recommends fibro-literate doctors who have been referred by satisfied patients. Email requests to: kindness@fibrobetsy.com and include your exact location. You will also receive lists of treatment modalities, coping suggestions, resources, and FM research abstracts. New recommendations are welcome but no self referrals.

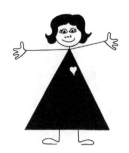

REFERENCES

History

Reilly, P., Littlejohn, G. History of Fibromyalgia. *Journal of Musculoskeletal Pain*, 1(2), 1993.

Diagnosis and Symptoms

Anthony, KK., et al. Juvenile primary fibromyalgia syndrome. *Current Rheumatology Rep,* 2001 April; 3(2): 165-171.

Arthritis Foundation, Atlanta, Georgia, 30326. *Fibromyalgia (Fibrositis),* 1992.

Bonafide, R.P., Downey, D.C., Bennett, R.M. An association of fibromyalgia with primary Sjogren's syndrome: a prospective study of 72 patients. *Journal of Rheumatology*, 22(1), 133-136, January 1995.

Buchwald, D., Garrity, D. Comparison of patients with chronic fatigue syndrome, fibromyalgia, and multiple chemical sensitivities. *Arch Intern. Med.,* 154(18), 2049-53, September 26, 1994.

Buskila D, Neumann L, Alhoashle A, et al. Fibromyalgia Syndrome in Men. *Semin Arthritis Rheum (US),* 2000 August; 30(1), 47-51.

Calabro, J. Fibromyalgia (Fibrositis) in children. *The American Journal of Medicine,* 81 (Suppl. 3A), 1986, September 29.

Citera G, Arias MA, Maldonado-Cocco JA, et al. The effect of melatonin in patients with fibromyalgia – a pilot study. *Clin Rheum* 2000;19:9-13.

Clauw, D. New insights into fibromyalgia. *Fibromyalgia Frontiers,* 2(4), Fall 1994.

Clauw DJ, Schmidt M, et al. The relationship between fibromyalgia and interstitial cystitis. *J Psychiatr Res.* 1997; 31(125).

Conte, PM, Walco, GA, and Kimura Y. Temperament and stress response in children with juvenile primary fibromyalgia syndrome. *Arthritis and Rheumatology,* 2003 October; 48(10): 2923-30.

C. Kennedy M, Felson Dt, A prospective long-term study of fibromyalgia syndrome. *Arthritis Rheum.* 1996 Apr; 39(4):682-5.

D. Mengshoel AM, Haugen M. Health Status in fibromyalgia—a follow-up study. *J Rheumatol.* 2001 Sep; 28(9):2085-9.

G. Park DC, Glass JM, Minear M, Crofford LJ. Cognitive function in fibromyalgia patients. *Arthritis Rheum.* 2001 Sep; 44(9):2125-33.

Goldenberg, D.L., et al. High frequency of fibromyalgia in patients with chronic fatigue seen in a primary care practice. *Arthritis Rheum,* 33(3), 381-387, 1990.

Goldenberg, D.L., Diagnostic and therapeutic challenges of fibromyalgia. *Hospital Practice,* 1989, September 30.

Hashkes, PJ, Friedland, O, Jaber L, Cohen, HA, Wolach, B, Uziel, Y. Decreased pain threshold in children with growing pains. *Journal of Rheumatology,* 2004 March;31(3): 610-613.

Imbierowicz, K and Egle, UT. Childhood adversities in patients with fibromyalgia and somatoform pain disorder. *Eur J Pain,* 2003; 7(2): 113-119.

J. Al-Allaf AW, Ottewell L, Pullar T, The prevalence and significance of positive antinuclear antibodies in patients with fibromyalgia syndrome:2-4 years' follow-up. *Clinical Rheumatology* 2002 Nov; 21(6):472-477.

Kashikar-Zuck, S, Graham, TB, Huenefeld, MD et al. A review of biobehavioral research in juvenile primary fibromyalgia syndrome. *Arthritis Care Res.* Dec 2000; 13(6), 388-97.

Kashikar-Zuck, S., Vaught, MH, Goldschneider, KR, Graham, TB, and Miller, JC. Depression, coping and functional disability in juvenile primary fibromyalgia syndrome. *PAIN,* 2002 October; 3(5): 412-419.

Krilou, L. Chronic fatigue syndrome. *Pediatric Annals,* 24(6), 290-294, June 1995.

Lehman, Thomas, MD. Growing pains or fibromyalgia: diagnosing and helping teens with FM. *Fibromyalgia Aware,* August-November 2004 (7), 68-69.

Lehman, Thomas, MD. *It's Not Just Growing Pains: A Guide to Childhood Muscle, Bone and Joint Pain,* Rheumatic Diseases and the Latest Treatments. Oxford Press, 2004.

Moldofsky, H. Nonrestorative sleep and symptoms after a febrile illness in patients with FMS and CFIDS. *Journal of Rheumatology,* 16(Suppl 19), 150-153, 1989.

Nishikai, Nasahiko. Primary fibromyalgia and chronic fatigue syndrome: are these diseases identical? *Journal of Musculoskeletal Pain*, 3(1), 40, 1995.

Paulson M, Norberg A and Danielson E. Men living with fibromyalgia-type pain: experiences as patients in the Swedish health care system. *J Adv Nurse (Eng)*, 2002 October; 40(1), 81-95.

Reid, G.J., Lang, B.A., and McGrath, P.J. Primary juvenile fibromyalgia: psychological adjustment, family functioning, coping and functional disability. *Arthritis and Rheumatism*, 40(1), 752-760, 1997.

Romano, T.J. Fibromyalgia in children; diagnosis and treatment. *The West Virginia Medical Journal*, 87, 1991, March.

Tayag-Kier, CE, Keenan, GF, Scalzi, LV, et al. Sleep and periodic limb movements in sleep in juvenile fibromyalgia. *Pediatrics*, Nov 2000; 106(5), E70.

The American College of Rheumatology. Criteria for the classification of fibromyalgia. *Arthritis and Rheumatism*, 33 (2), 1990, February.

U.S. Department of Health and Human Services. CFS definition. *Center for Disease Control Report*, Feb. 2002.

Wallace, Daniel J MD. *All About Fibomyalgia*. Oxford University Press, New York. 2002.

Waylonis, G.W., and Heck, W. Fibromyalgia syndrome. *American Journal of Physical Medicine and Rehabilitation*, 71 (6), 1992, December.

White KP, Harth M, Speechley M et al.; A general population study of fibromyalgia tender points in noninstitutionalized adults with chronic widespread pain. *J Rheumatol* 2000, 27:2677-2682.

White K.P., Carette S., Harth M., Teasell R.W. Trauma and fibromyalgia: is there an association and what does it mean? *Seminars Arthritis Rheum 29*, 2000:200-216.

Wolfe, F., Ross, K., Anderson, J., Russell, I.J., and Hebert. L. The prevalence and characteristics of fibromyalgia in the general population. *Arthritis Rheum*, 38(1), 19-28, 1995.

Yunus, MB. Gender differences in fibromyalgia and other related syndromes. *Journal of Gender Specif Med (US)*, 2002 Mar/April; 5(2), 42-7.

Yunus MB, Inanici F, Aldag JC, et al. Fibromyalgia in men: comparison of clinical features with women. *Journal of Rheumatology*, 2000 Feb; 27(2), 485-90.

Yunus, M.B., and Masi, A.T. Juvenile primary fibromyalgia syndrome: a clinical study of thirty three patients and matched controls. *Arthritis and Rheumatism*, 28, 1985.

Yunus, M.B., del Castillo, L.D., and Aldaq, J.C. Prognosis of regional fibromyalgia (RF). University of Illinois College of Medicine, Peoria, IL 61605. *Poster session at 1994 ACR/ARHP Annual Meeting*, October, 1994.

Medical Conditions

Bennett, R.M., Smythe, H.A., Wolfe. Recognizing fibromyalgia. *Patient Care*, 23: 60-83, July 15, 1989.

Schumacher, R. *Primer on the Rheumatic Diseases*. 9th edition, Atlanta: Arthritis Foundation, 1988.

Research

Abud-Mendoza C, et al. Hypothalamus-hypophysis-thyroid axis dysfunction in patients with refractory fibromyalgia. *Arthritis & Rheumatism, Abstract Supplement* 1997;40(9).

Ahles, T.A., Yunus, M.B. Riley, S.D., Bradley, J.M., and Masi, A.T. Psychological factors associated with primary fibromyalgia syndrome. *Arthritis Rheum*, 27:1101-1106, 1984.

Ahles, T.A., Yunus, M.B., and Masi, A.T. Is chronic pain a variant of depressive disease? The case of primary fibromyalgia syndrome. *Pain*, 29:105-111, 1987.

Arnold LM. Genetic linkage of fibromyalgia to the serotonin receptor 2a region on chromosome 13 and the HLA region on chromosome 6. Abstract #505, presented at the 2003 annual meeting of the American College of Rheumatology, Orlando, FL.

Bengtsson, A., et al. Reduced high energy phosphate levels in the painful muscles of patients with primary fibromyalgia. *Arthritis Rheum*, 29 (7):817-821, 1986.

Bennett, R., et al. Low levels of somatomedin-c in patients with FMS. *Arthritis Rheum*, 35 (10):1113-1116, 1992.

Bennett, R.M. (ed) The fibrositis/fibromyalgia syndrome. Current issues and perspectives. *Am J Med*, 1986:81 (suppl 3A):1-115.

Bennett, R., et al. Aerobic fitness in patients with fibrositis. *Arthritis Rheum*, 32 (4):454-460, 1989.

Bennett, R.M., Clark, S.R., Burckhardt, C.S., Walcz, K.J. A double blind placebo controlled study of growth hormone therapy in FMS. *Journal of Musculoskeletal Pain*, (3)1:110, 1995.

Bonafede, P., Nilson, D., Clark, S., et al. Exercising muscle blood flow in patients with fibrositis: a xenon clearance study. *Arthritis Rheum*, 31 (suppl): S14, 1987.

Bou-Holaigh I, et al. provocation of hypotension and pain during upright tilt table testing in adults with fibromyalgia. *Clinical and Experimental Rheumatology*. 1997;15:239-246.

Buchwald, D., Sarrity, D. Comparison of patients with chronic fatigue syndrome, fibromyalgia, and multiple chemical sensitivities. *AMA Intern Med*, 154(18):2049-53, 1994.

Burckhardt, Carol, et al. FMS and quality of life: A comparative analysis. *J Rheumatology*, 20:(3) 475-479, 1993.

Buskila D, Neumann L: The development of widespread pain after injuries. *J Musculoskel Pain* 2002, 10:261-267.

Buskila D, Shnaider A, Neumann L, et al,: Fibromyalgia in hepatitis C virus infection. Another infectious disease relationship. *Arch Intern Med* 1997, 157-2497-2500.

Buskila D, et al. Increased rates of fibromyalgia following cervical spine injury: a controlled study of 161 cases after traumatic injury. *Arthritis and Rheum* 1997;440(3):446-52.

Campbell, S.M., Clark, S., Tindall, E.A., Forehand, M.E., and Bennett, R.M. Clinical characteristics of fibrositis. A "blinded" controlled study of symptoms and tender points. *Arthritis Rheum,* 26:817, 1983.

Caro, X.J., Kinstad, N.A., Russell, I.J., and Wolfe, F. Increased sensitivity to health related questions in patients with primary fibrositis syndrome. *Arthritis Rheum,* 30:63, 1987 (Abstract).

Caro, X.J., Wolfe, F., Johnston, W.H., and Smith, A.L. A controlled and blinded study of immunoreactant deposition at the dermal-epidermal junction of patients with primary fibromyalgia. *J Rheum,* 13:1086, 1986.

Clark, S., Campbell, S.M., Forehand, M.E., Tindall, E.A., and Bennett, R.M. Clinical characteristics of fibrositis. II. A "blinded," controlled study using standard psychological tests. *Arthritis Rheum,* 28:132-137, 1985.

Clauw, Daniel, et al. Abnormal auditory event: related potentials in FMS. Abstract. ACR Meeting 1994. Minneapolis, Minn.

Clauw, Daniel, Fibromyalgia: More than just a musculoskeletal disease. *Amer Family Physician*, 52(3):843-851, 1995.

Crofford, Leslie J., et al. Analysis of circadian plasma ACTH and cortisol levels in patients with fibromyalgia (FM) and chronic fatigue syndrome (CFIDS). 1487, Scientific abstracts from the American College of Rheumatology Annual Meeting, October 1996.

Crofford LJ: The hypothalamic pituitary adrenal stress axis in fibromyalgia and chronic fatigue syndrome. *Z Rheumatol* 1998, 57:67-71.

Crofford, LJ. Neuroendocrine abnormalities in fibromyalgia and related disorders. *AM J Med Sci* 1998, 315:359-66.

Crofford, LJ, Young EA, Engleberg NC, Korszun A, Brucksch CB, McClure La, Brown MB, Demitrack MA: Basal circadian and pulsatile ACTH and cortisone secretion in patients with fibromyalgia and /or chronic fatigue syndrome. *Brain Behav Immun.* 2004 July;18(4):314-325.

Crofford LJ and Appleton, BE. The treatment of fibromyalgia: a review of clinical trials. *Current Rheum Rep,* 2000 April; 2(2): 101-103.

Dailey, P.A., Bishop, G.D., Russell, I.J., and Fletcher, E.M. Psychological stress and the fibrositis/fibromyalgia syndrome.
J. Rheumatol, 17:1380, 1990.

Daoud KF, Barkhuizen A: Rheumatic mimics and selected triggers of fibromyalgia. *Curr Pain Headache Rep* 2002, 6:284-288.

Ferraccioli, Neuroendocrinologic findings in FMS. *J. Rheumatology,* 17 (7):869-873, 1990.

Fitzcharles MA, Costa DD and Poyhia R. A study of standard care in fibromyalgia syndrome: a favorable outcome. *Journal of Rheumatology,* 2003 January; 30(1), 154-9.

Goldstein, J. *CFIDS*: *The Limbic Hypothesis*. Haworth Medical Press, New York, 1993.

Gracely RH, Petzke F, Wolf JM et al,: Functional magnetic resonance imaging evidence of augmented pain processing in fibromyalgia. *Arthr Rheum* 2002, 46:1333-1343.

Griep, E.N., Boersma, J.W., de Kloet, E.R. Pituitary release of growth hormone and prolactia in the primary fibromyalgia syndrome, *J Rheum,* 21(11):2125-30, November 1994.

Gur A, Cevik R, Nas K, Colpan L, Sarac S: Cortisol and hypothalamic-pituitary-gonadal axis hormones in follicular-phase women with fibromyalgia and chronic fatigue syndrome and effect of depressive symptoms on these hormones. *Arthritis Res Ther,* 2004;6(3):R232-8.

Haddad JJ, Saade Ne, Safieh-Garabedian B: Cytokines and neuro-immune-endocrine interactions: a role for the hypothalamic-pituitary-adrenal revolving axis. *J Neuroimmunol* 2002, 133-1-19.

Hellstrand, K., and Hermodsson, S. Role of serotonin in the regulation of human natural killer cell cytotoxicity. *J Immunology,* 139: 869, 1987.

Hudson, J.I., Hudson, M.S., Pliner, L.F., et al. Fibromyalgia and major affective disorder: A controlled phenomenology and family history study. *Am J Psychiatry,* 142:441-446, 1985.

Jacobsen S., et al. Primary Fibromyalgia: Clinical parameters in relation to serum procollagen type III aminoterminal peptide. *Br J Rheumatology,* 29 (3):174-177, 1990.

Jeschonneck, M., and Sprott, H., et al. Pathological changes in peripheral blood flow in fibromyalgia, 1484, Scientific Abstracts from the ACR annual meeting.

Johansson, G., et al. Cerebral Dysfunction in FMS: evidence from regional blood flow measurements, otoneurological tests and cerebro spinal fluid analysis, *Acta Psychiatr Scand*, 91(2):86-94, 1995.

Jubrias, Bennett & Klug. Increased reasonance in the phosphodiester region of PNMR spectra in the skeletal muscle of FMS patients. *Arthrit Rheum,* 37 (6):801-807, June 1994.

Kirmayer, L.J., Robbins, J.M., and Kapusta, M.A. Somatization and depression in fibromyalgia syndrome. *Am J Psychiatry,* 145:950-954, 1988.

Kwiatek R., Barnden L., Tedman R., Jarrett R., et al. Regional cerebral blood flow in fibromyalgia. *Arthritis Rheum 43,* 2000: 2823-2833.

Larson, A.A., Kitto, K.F. Antagonism of nerve growth factor induced hyperalgesia by the substance PNM2 - terminal meatabolete, SP(1-7). *Journal of Musculoskeletal Pain,* 3(1):1995.

205

REFERENCES

Lund, N., et al. Muscle tissue oxygen pressure in FMS. *Scand J Rheumatology,* 15:165-173, 1986.

Maier SF: Bi-directional immune-brain communication: Implications for understanding stress, pain, and cognition. *Brain Behave immune* 2003. 17-69-85.

Martinez-Lavin M., Hermosillo A.G. Autonomic nervous system dysfunction may explain the multisystem features of fibromyalgia. *Seminars Arthritis Rheum* 29, 2000: 197-99.

McBeth J, Dilman AJ, Macfarlane GJ: Association of widespread body pain with an increased risk of cancer and reduced cancer survival: A prospective, population-based study. *Arthritis Rheum* 2003, 48:1686-1692.

McCain, G. Diurnal hormone variation in FMS. *J. Rheum,* 16 (suppl 19):154-157, 1989.

Mengshoel, A., et al. Muscle strength and aerobic capacity in FMS. *Clin Exp Rheumatology,* 8:475-479, 1990.

Moldofsky, H., and Warsh, J.J. Plasma tryptophan and muskuloskeletal pain in nonarticular rheumatism ("fibrositis syndrome"). *Pain,* 5:65, 1978.

Mountz, J., et al. Regional cerebral blood flow in caudate nuclei is associated with pain thresholds in patients with FMS. *ACR 57th Annual Scientific Abstracts of Arthritis Rheum,* S221, 1993.

Neeck, G., Riedel, W. Thyroid function in patients with FMS. *J. Rheumatology,* 19 (7):1120-2, 1992.

Neeck, G., Riedel, W. Neuromediator and hormonal pertubations in fibromyalgia syndrome: results of chronic stress? *Baillieres Clin Rheumatol.,* 8(4):763-75, November 8, 1994.

Nicolson G. Co –infections in Fibromyalgia and Chronic Fatigue syndrome, and other chronic illnesses. *Fibromyalgia Frontiers* 2002;10(3).

Payne, T.C., Leavitt, F., Garron, D.C., et al. Fibrositis and psychological disturbance. *Arthritis Rheum,* 25:213-217, 1982.

Pellegrino, M., et al. Familial occurrence of primary fibromyalgia. *Arch Phys Med Rehab,* 70:61-63, 1989

Pelligrino, Mark J. MD. *Inside Fibromyalgia.* Anadem Publishing. 2001

Price DD. Staud R, Robinson ME, et al.: Enhanced Temporal summation of second pain and its central modulation in fibromyalgia patients. *Pain* 2002, 99: 49-59.

Quan N, Herkenham M: Connecting cytokines and brain: a review of current issues. *Histol Histopathol* 2002, 17:273-288.

Romano T.J. Brain SPECT findings in FMS patients with headache. *ACR 57th Annual Scientific Abstracts of Arthritis Rheum,* S250, 1993.

Romano, T.J. Magnesium deficiency in fibromyalgia syndrome. *Journal of Nutritional Medicine,* 4:165-167, 1994.

Russell, I., Vaeroy, H., et al. Cerebrospinal fluid (CSF) biogenic amine metabolites in FMS and rheumatoid arthritis. *Arthritis Rheum,* 35 (5):550-556, 1992.

Russell, I.J., Biochemical abnormalities in fibromyalgia syndrome, *J. Musculoskeletal Pain,* 2(3):101-103, 1994.

Russell I.J. Serum amino acids in fibromyalgia syndrome. *J Rheumatology,* 16 (suppl 19):158-163, 1989.

Russell, I.J., Fletcher, E.M., Tsui, J., and Michalek, J.E. Comparisons of RA and fibrositis/fibromyalgia syndrome using functional and psychological outcome measures. 1989 (Un Pub).

Russell, I., et al. Abnormal natural killer cell activity in fibrositis syndrome is responsive In-Vitro to IL-2. *Arthritis Rheum,* 31 (4 suppl.): S24, 1988.

Russell, I.J., et al. Cerebrospinal fluid substance p is elevated in FMS, ACR 57th annual scientific abstracts. *Arthritis Rheum,* S223, 1993.

Russell, I.J., et al. Cerebrospinal fluid biogenic amino metabolites in fibromyalgia/fibrositis syndrome and RA. *Arthritis and Rheum,* 35 (5):550-556.

Russell, I. Jon, et al. Treatment of fibromyalgia syndrome with super malic: A randomized, double-blinded placebo controlled, crossover pilot study. *J. Rheum,* 22(5):953-8, May 1995.

Russell, I. Jon. *Rheum Dis. Clinics NA,* 15 (1):163, 1989.

Russell IJ. Fibromyalgia syndrome sub-groups. Editorial. *Journal of Musculoskeletal Pain* 2002;46(5):1136-7.

Saskin, P., Moldofsky, H., Lue, F.A. Sleep and posttraumatic rheumatic pain modulation disorder (Fibrositis Syndrome). (letter). *Clinical and Experimental Rheumatology,* 2:195, 1984.

Simms, R.W., et al. Lack of association between fibromyalgia syndrome and abnormalities in muscle energy metabolism. *Arthr Rheum,* 37(6):794-800, June 1994.

Sletvold, H., Stiles, T., Landre, N.I. Information processing in primary fibromyalgia, major depression and healthy controls. *J Rheum,* 22(1):137-42, January 1995.

Staud R, Vierck CJ, Cannon RL, et al,: Abnormal sensitization and temporal summation of second pain (wind-up) in patients with fibromyalgia syndrome. *Pain* 2001, 92:165-175.

Staud R. The abnormal central pain processing mechanism in patients with fibromyalgia. *Fibromyalgia Frontiers* 2002;10(3):18.

Tanum, L., Malt, V.F. Sodium lactate infusion in fibromyalgia patients. *Biological Psychiatry,* 38:559-561, 1995.

Thorson, Kristin, ed. *Fibromyalgia Network.* p. 6, April 1994.

Thorson, Kristin. *Advances in Research.* Pamphlet, p. 10-11, 1994.

Thorson, Kristin, ed. *Fibromyalgia Syndrome: Advances in Research.* Pamphlet, p. 11, April 1994.

Thorson, Kristin. *Fibromyalgia Network.* p. 6, July 1993.

Thorson, Kristin. *Fibromyalgia Network.* July 1992.

Thorson, Kristin. *Fibromyalgia Network.* October 1996.

Thorson, Kristin. Looking Into Autonomic Nervous System Dysfunction. *Fibromyalgia Network.* October 1995.

Torpy DJ, Papanicolaou DA, Lotsikas AJ, et al,: Responses of the sympathetic nervous system and the hypothalamic-pituitary-adrenal axis to interleukin-6-A pilot study in fibromyalgia. *Arthritis Rheum* 2000, 43:872-880.

Vaeroy, H., et al. Elevated CSF levels of substance p and high incidence of raynauds phenomenon in patients with fibromyalgia. *Pain,* 32:21-26, 1988.

Vaeroy, H., Merskey, M. Progress in fibromyalgia and myofascial pain. *Pain Research and Clinical Management,* Vol. 6: Elsevier Press, 1993.

Wallace, D. Cytokines and immune regulation in FMS. *Arthritis Rheum,* 32 (10):1334-5, 1989.

Wallace, Daniel J. MD. *All About Fibromyalgia.* Oxford University Press, Inc. New York.

Wallace D. J., Linker-Isreale M., Hallegua D., Silverman S., Silver D., Weisman M.H. Cytokines play an etiopathogenetic role in fibromyalgia: a hypothesis and pilot study. *Rheumatology* (Oxford) 40, 2001: 743-749

Waylonis, G.W., and Heck, W. Fibromyalgia syndrome. *American Journal of Physical Medicine and Rehab,* 71 (6), Dec. 1992.

Wendler, Jorg, Hummel, T., Kramer, O., Kraetsch, H., Kalden, J., Kobal, G. Decreased olfactory performance in patients with fibromyalgia in the presence of an increased estimation of subjective sensibility. 380, Scientific Abstracts ACR Annual Meeting, October 1996.

Wolfe, F., Cathey, M.A., Kleinheksel, S.M., et al. Psychological status in primary fibrositis and fibrositis associated with rheumatoid arthritis. *J Rheumatol,* 11:500-506, 1984.

Yunus, MB. Central sensitivity syndromes: a unified concept for fibromyalgia and other similar maladies. *Fibromyalgia Frontiers,* 2001 (Vol 9, Num 3):3-8.

Yunus, MB, MD. Gender differences in fibromyalgia and other related syndromes. *Journal of Gender-Specific Medicine* 5, no.2 (2002). 42-49.

Yunus, et al. Interrelationships of biochemical parameters in classification of FMS and healthy normal controls. *JMP,* 3(4):15-24, 1995.

Yunus, Muhammad B., Rawlings, Karolyn K., Khan, Muhammad, Green, Jack R. Fibromyalgia syndrome (FMS): evidence of genetic linkage to HLA 1482. Scientific abstracts ACR Annual Meeting., October 1996.

Sleep

Dauvilliers, Y and Touchon J. Sleep in fibromyalgia: review of clinical and polysomnographic data. *Neurophysiology Clinics,* 2001 Feb; 31(1): 18-33.

Drewes, A. M., et al. Sleep intensity in FMS: focus on the microstructure of the sleep process, *Br J Rheum* 34(7):629-35, 1995.

Drewes, A. M., et al. A comparative study of sleep architecture in subjects with rheumatoid arthritis versus subjects with FMS. *J Muskuloskeletal Pain* 3(1):69, 1995.

Fitzcharles MA, Costa DD, Poyhia R. A study of standard care in fibromyalgia syndrome: a favorable outcome. *J Rheumatol* 2003. Jan; 30 (1): 154-159.

Hauri, P., and Linde, S. *No More Sleepless Nights.* New York: John Wiley and Sons. 1990.

Jacobs, GD. Short insomnia therapy beats sleeping pills. *Archives of Internal Medicine,* Sept 27, 2004; (164): 1888-1896.

Leventhal, et al. Controlled study of sleep parameters in patients with FMS. *J Clin Rheumatol,* 1(2):110-113, April 1995.

MacFarlane, J.G., Shahal, B., Mously, C. and Moldofsky, H. Periodic K-alpha sleep EEG activity and periodic limb movements during sleep: comparisons of clinical features of sleep parameters. *Sleep,* 19: 200-204, 1996.

Moldofsky, HK. Disordered sleep in fibromyalgia and related myofascial facial pain conditions. *Dental Clinics of North America,* 2001 October; 45(4): 701-13.

Moldofsky, HK. Management of sleep disorders in fibromyalgia. *Rheum Dis Clin North America,* 2002 May; 28(2): 353-65.

Moore, K. Sleep disturbances and fatigue in women with FMS and CFIDS. *JOGNN* 24(3):229-233, March/April 1995.

Roizenblatt S, Moldofsky H, et al. Alpha sleep characteristics in fibromyalgia. *Arthritis and Rheum* 2001; 44:222-30.

Schaefer, KM. Sleep disturbances linked to fibromyalgia. *Holistic Nursing Practice,* 2003 May-June; 17(3): 120-7.

Thorson, K. *Fibromyalgia Network.* 1989, October.

Thorson, K. *Fibromyalgia Network.* 1990, January.

Thorson, K. *Fibromyalgia Network.* 1997, January.

Yunas, M.B., and Alday, J.C. Restless legs syndrome and leg cramps in fibromyalgia syndrome: a controlled study. *British Medical Journal,* 312: 1339, 1996.

Medications

Abeles, M. Long term effectiveness of orphenadrine citrate in the treatment of fibromyalgia. ACR 56th Annual Scientific Meeting Poster Presentation. A270, Atlanta, 1992.

Arnold LM, Hess EV, Hudson JI, Welge, Berno SE, Keck PE Jr, A randomized, placebo-controlled, double-blind study, flexible-dose study of fluoxetine in the treatment of women with fibromyalgia. *Am J Med* 2002;112(3):191-7.

Barkhuizen A: Rational and targeted pharmacologic treatment of fibromyalgia. *Rheum Dis Clin North AM* 2002, 28: 261-290.

Boissevain, Michael D., McCain, Glenn A. Toward an integrated understanding of fibromyalgia syndrome. *Pain,* 45, 227-238, 1991.

Branco, Jaime C., Martini, Alfredo, Palva, Teresa. Treatment of sleep abnormalities and clinical complaints in fibromyalgia with trazodone. 390, Scientific Abstracts, ACR Annual Meeting, October 1996.

Clauw, Daniel, Gaumond, Ethan, et al. Capsaicin skin tests in fibromyalgia. 382, *Scientific Abstracts,* ACR Annual Meeting, October 1996.

Fisher, Peter. Effect of homeopathic treatment in primary fibrositis. *BMJ,* 229, 365-366, 1989.

Freda B. J., Schwartz M. Treatment of whiplash associated with neck pain with botulinum toxin-A: a pilot study. *J Rheumatol 27,* 2000:481-484.

Gemmell M, et al. Homeopathic Rhus Toxicodendron in treatment of fibromyalgia. *Chiropractic Journal of Australia.* Vol 21; No 1, March 1991, 2-1.

Goldenberg, D.L. A review of the role of tricyclic medications in the treatment of fibromyalgia syndrome. *Journ Rheum,* 19, 137-139, 1989.

Goldenberg, D.L., Felson, O.T., and Dinerman, H. A randomized controlled trial of amitriptyline and naproxen in the treatment of patients with fibromyalgia. *Arthritis Rheum,* 29:1371, 1986.

Hales, Ferguson, Yudofsky. *What You Need to Know About Psychiatric Drugs.* New York: Balantine, 1991.

Henriksson, K.G., Bergtsson. Fibromyalgia - a clinical entity. *Canadian Journal of Physiology and Pharmacology,* 69, 672-677, 1991.

Katy R. S. et al. Pilot study of methylphenidate once daily in cognitively impaired individuals with FMS. ACR conference 2002. abxt # 1657.

Kemple, K MD. Use of opioids in FMS. APS meeting, Nov. 25, 2000. Atlanta, Ga.

Kirsta, Alex. *The Book of Stress Survival.* Great Britain: Simon & Schuster, 1986.

K. Sorenson J, Bengtsson A, Ahler J, et al. Fibromyalgia: are there different mechanisms in the processing of pain? A double blind crossover comparison of analgesic drugs. *J Rheumatol* 1997;24:1615-1621.

Holman A. J., et al. Pramipexole for FMS. ACR conf 2002 abst 189.

McCarty, Daniel J., et al. Treatment of pain due to FMS with topical capsaicin: a pilot study. *Seminars in Arth and Rheum* Vol. 23 (6) Suppl. 3, pp. 41-47, June 1994.

Moldofsky, M. The effect of zolpidem in patients with FMS - a dose ranging, double blind, placebo controlled, modified crossover study, *J Rheumatology,* 23(3):529-33, 1996.

Naschitz J, Dreyfuss D, Yeshurun D, Rosner I. Midodrine treatment for chronic fatigue syndrome. *Postgrad Med J.* 2004 Apr; 80(942):230-232.

O'Malley P. G., Balden E., Tomkins G., et al. Treatment of fibromyalgia with anti-depressants: a meta-analysis. *J Gen Internal Medicine* 15, 2000:659-666.

Popadopouols I. Treatment of fibromyalgia with tropisetron. *Clin Rheum* 2000; 19: 6-8.

Romano, Thomas, and Stiller, John W. Usefulness of topical methyl salicylate, camphor and menthol lotion in relieving pain in FMS patients. *Amer Journal of Pain Management,* Vol. 4, pp. 172-174, Oct. 1994.

Roth, Sanford. Topical NSAID therapy in fibromyalgia symptoms in osteoarthritis (OA) with hyanalgese-D, 391, Scientific Abstracts ACR Annual Meeting, October 1996.

Russell I. J., Kamin M., Bennett R. M., et al. Efficacy of tramadol in treatment of pain in fibromyalgia. *J Clin Rheumatol 6,* 2000:25-257.

Russell, I.J. Therapy with tizandin decreases substance P, and may reduce serum hyaluronic acid as it improves symptoms of FMS. ACR conference 2002. Abstract # 1655.

Russell, I. Jon. Treatment of primary fibrositis syndrome with ibuprofen and alprazolam. *Arthritis Rheum,* 34 (5), 552-560, 1991.

Russell, I. Jon. Fibromyalgia syndrome: approaches to management. *Bulletin on the Rheumatic Diseases,* 45(3), May 1996.

Searle, Ambien Brochure. July 1994.

Smith TA. Type A GABA receptor subunits and benzodiazepine binding; significance to clinical syndromes and their treatments. *Br J Bio Med Sci* 2001; 58:111-211.

Thorson, K. *Fibromyalgia Network.* April 2002.

Thorson, Kristin. *Getting the Most Out of Your Medicines!* p. 7, 1994.

Thorson, Kristin. Combining science, experience and creativity to treat FMS and CFIDS, *Fibromyalgia Network,* 8, July 1996.

Thorson, Kristin. July. *Fibromyalgia Network,* 1991.

Thorson, Kristin. Prozac-Elavil combination therapy, *Fibromyalgia Network,* 5, January 1996.

Yunus, M.B., Masi. Short term effects of ibuprofen in primary fibromyalgia syndrome: a double blind, placebo controlled study. *Journ Rheum,* 16, (4), 527-32, 1989.

Pain Management

Almeida TF, Roizenblatt S, Benedito-Silva AA, Tufik S. The effect of combined therapy(ultrasound and inferential current) on pain and sleep in fibromyalgia. *Pain* 2003 Aug;10 4(3):665-72.

Buskila D, Neumann L: Musculoskeletal injury as a trigger for fibromyalgia/posttraumatic fibromyalgia. *Curr Rheum Rep* 2000, 2:104-108.

Davies, Claire, 2001. *The Trigger Point Therapy Workbook: Your Self-Treatment Guide For Pain Relief*. New Harbinger Publications, Inc.

Elert J, Kendall SA, Larsson B, et al,: Chronic pain and difficulty in relaxing postural muscles in patients with fibromyalgia and chronic whiplash associated disorders. *J Rheumatol* 2001, 28:1361-1368.

L. Richards SC, Scott DL. Prescribed exercise in people with fibromyalgia: parallel group randomized controlled trial. *British Med J* 2002: 325:185.

M. Jones KD, Burckhardt CS, Clark SR, et al. A randomized controlled trial of muscle strengthening versus flexibility in fibromyalgia. *J Rheumatol* 2001;29:1041-1048.

Offenbacher, M and Stucki, G. Physical therapy in the treatment of fibromyalgia. *Scandinavian Journal of Rheumatology Supplement,* 2000; 113: 78-85.

Rooks, D.S., et al. The effects of progressive strength training and aerobic exercise on muscle strength and cardiovascular fitness in women with fibromyalgia: a pilot study. *Arthritis and Rheum* 47(1), Februaru 2002:22-28.

Sim, J and Adams N. Therapeutic approaches to fibromyalgia syndrome in the United Kingdom: a survey of occupational therapists and physical therapists. *Eur J Pain*, 2003; 7(2): 173-180.

Smith M, Gokula RR, and Weismantel A. Does physical therapy improve symptoms of fibromyalgia? *Journal of Family Practice,* Sept 2003; 52(9), 717-9.

Sonkin, L.S.,1994. Myofascial pain due to metabolic disorders. Diagnosis and treatment, Chapter 3. In *Myofascial Pain and Fibromyalgia,* edited by E.S. Rachlin, St. Louis:Mosby-Yearbook, Inc.

Travell, J.G. and D.G. Simons, 1992. *Myofasial Pain and Dysfunction: The Trigger Point Manual.* Vol.II, 2nd ed. Baltimore: Lippincott and Wilkins.

Acupuncture

Blair, James, Mease, Phillip, et al. The use of acupuncture as an intervention in a FMS and CFIDS self-management program. *Journal of Musculoskeletal Pain*, 3(1), 90, 1995.

Deluze, Christophe, Bosia, Lorenzo, Zirbs, Chantraine, Vischer. Electroacupuncture in fibromyalgia: results of a controlled trial. *BMJ* 305:1249-52, Nov. 1992.

Posture

Anderson, B. *Stretching*. Bolinas, California: Shelter Publications, Inc., 1980.

Saunders, H.D. *Self Help Manual for Your Back*. Minneapolis: Educational Opportunities, 1990.

Exercise

Anderson, Bob. *Stretching*. Bolinas, CA: Shelter Publications, Inc., 1980.

Bennett, R.M., et al. Aerobic fitness in patients with fibrositis. *Arthritis and Rheum,* 32, (4), 454-460, 1989.

Cardahl, K. Dyspnea in chronic primary fibromyalgia. *J. Intern Med,* 226, (4), 265-270, 1989.

Clark, S.R., Burckhardt, C.S., Bennett, R.M. FM patients improve oxygen consumption and pain score during a 3 month program of aerobic exercise, *J Musculoskeletal Pain*, 3(1):70, 1995.

Gowans, Susan, Voss, Susan, deHueck, Amy, Richardson, Mary. A Randomized Controlled Trial of Exercise and Education in Fibromyalgia. 387. Scientific Abstracts. ACR Annual Meeting. October, 1996.

Jacobsen, S., Danneskiold-Sams. Dynamic muscular endurance in primary fibromyalgia compared with chronic myofascial pain syndrome. *Archives of Physical Medicine and Rehabilitation,* 73 (2), 170-173, 1992.

Kazyama, H.H.S., et al. Fibromyalgia: Continuous physical therapy program with or without long term medical supervision, *Journal of Musculoskeletal Pain*, 3(1):126, 1995.

McCain, Glenn. A controlled study of the effects of a supervised cardiovascular fitness training program on the manifestations of primary fibromyalgia. *Arth Rheum,* 31, (9), 1135-1141, 1988.

Mengshoel, A.M., Höllestad, N.K., Förre, O. Pain and fatigue induced by exercise in fibromyalgia patients and sedentary health subjects, *Clinical and Experimental Rheumatology,* 13:477-482, 1995.

Novregaard, J., et al. Exercise training in treatment of fibromyalgia, *J Musculoskeletal Pain,* 3(1):105, 1995.

Sternbach, Richard. *Mastering Pain: A Twelve-Step Program for Coping with Chronic Pain*. New York: Ballantine, 1987.

Work-related Issues

Henriksson, C., Burckhardt, C. Impact of fibromyalgia on everyday life: a study of women in the USA and Sweden. *Disability and Rehabilitation*, 18(5):241-8, May 1996.

Waylonis, G.W., Ronan, P.G. and Gordon, C. A profile of fibromyalgia in occupational environments. *American Journal of Physical Medicine and Rehabilitation*, 73(2):112-5, April 1994.

Wolfe, F., Anderson, J., Harkness, D., Bennett, R.M., Caro, X., Goldenberg, D.M., Russell, I.J. and Yunus, M.B. The Work and Disability Status of Persons with Fibromyalgia. Abstract presented at 1995 ACR/ARHP Annual Meeting, October 1995.

Stress Management

Alex, Kirsta. *The Book of Stress Survival.* Great Britain: Simon and Schuster, 1986.

Bennett, R. Group treatment of FMS - a 6 month outpatient program, *J Rheumatology*, 23(3):521-8, 1996.

Burns, David D. *Feeling Good: The New Mood Therapy.* New York: Signet, 1980.

Chopra, Deepak. *Quantum Healing.* New York: Bantam, 1990.

Gaston-Johansson F. A comparative study of feelings, attitudes and behaviors of patients with fibromyalgia and rheumatoid arthritis. *Soc Sci Med,* 31, (8):941-947, 1990.

Hart, Archibald. *The Hidden Link Between Adrenalin and Stress.* Dallas Word Publishing, 1986.

Jaffe, Dennis T. *Healing From Within.* New York: Simon and Schuster, 1980.

Kabat-Zinn, Jon. *Full Catastrophe Living.* New York: Dell, 1991.

Nielson, Warren R., Walker, Cathie, McCain, Glenn. Cognitive behavioral treatment of fibromyalgia syndrome: preliminary findings. *Journal Rheum,* 19, 98-103, 1992.

Shames, Richard., Sterin, Chuck. *Healing with Mind Power.* Emmaus: Rodale Press, 1978.

White, John, and Fadiman, James (Eds.). *Relax.* USA: Confucian Press, 1976.

Wigers, Horven, et al. Effects of aerobic exercise versus stress management treatment in FMS. *Scand J Rheumatology*, 25(2):77-86, 1996.

Coping with Psychological Aspects

Anderburg UM, Marteinsdottir L, Theorell T,et al,: The impact of life events in female patients with fibromyalgia and in female healthy controls. *European Psychiatry* 2000, 15: 295-301.

Arnold LM, Hudson JI, Hess EV, Ware AE, Fritz DA, Auchenbach MB, Starck LO, Keck PE Jr: Family study of fibromyalgia. *Arthritis Rheum.* 2004 March; 50(3):944-52.

Barrows KA, Bradley BP. Mind-body Medicine: An introduction and review of the literature. *Med Clin North Am.* 2002 Jan; 86(1):11-31.

Finset,A, Wigers, SH, Gotestam KG: Depressed mood impedes pain treatment response in patients with fibromyalgia. *J Rheum.* 2004 May;31(5):976-80.

Gupta A, Silman AJ. Psychological stress and fibromyalgia: a review of the evidence suggesting a neuroendocrine link. *Arthrits Res Ther.* 2004;6(3):98-106.

H. Hadhazy VA, Ezzo J, Creamier P, Berman B. Mind-body therapies for the treatment of fibromyalgia. A systematic review. J *Rheum.* 2000 Dec;27(12):2911-8. Review.

Kabat- Zinn, J, Massion, AD, Kristeller, J., Peterson, L.G., Fletcher, K., Linderking, W., Santorelli, SF. Effectiveness of a meditation-based stress reduction program in the treatment of anxiety disorders. *Am J Psychiatry* (1992)149:936-943.

Nielson WR, Jensen MP: Relationship between changes in coping and treatment outcome in patients with fibromyalgia syndrome. *Pain.* 2004 Jun:109(3):232-241.

Sherman JJ, Turk DC, Okifuji A: Prevalance and impact of posttraumatic stress disorder-like symptoms on patients with fibromyalgia syndrome. *Clin J Pain* 2000, 16:127-34.

Thorson, Kristin. *Fibromyalgia Network.* October 2001.

Turk DC, Okifuji A, Starz TW, et al,: Effects of types of symptom onset on psychological distress and disability in fibromyalgia syndrome patients. *Pain* 1996, 68-423-430.

Coping

Backstrom, G., and Rubin, B.R. *When Muscle Pain Won't Go Away.* Dallas, Texas: Taylor Publishing, 1992.

Bishop, G.D., Russell, I.J., Fletcher, E.M., Caro, X., and Wolfe, F. The role of health beliefs in the clinical outcome of fibrositis/fibromyalgia syndrome. (Abstract) University of Texas at San Antonio, 1991.

Gunther, V., et al. Fibromyalgia - the effect of relaxation and hydro galvanic bath therapy on the subjective pain experience. *Clinical Rheumatology*, 13(4):573-8, 1994.

Kaplan, K.H., Goldenberg, D.L., Galvin-Nadeau, M. The impact of a meditation-based stress reduction program in fibromyalgia. *Gen Hosp Psychiatry*, 15(5):284-289, September 1993.

Knipping, Alex, et al. Aspects of coping in fibromyalgia, chronic pain and rheumatoid arthritis. *J Musculoskeletal Pain*, 3(1):102, 1995.

Lewis, K. *Successful Living with Chronic Illness.* Wayne, New Jersey: Avery Publishing, 1985.

Pitzele, S. K. *We are Not Alone: Learning to Live with Chronic Illness.* Minneapolis, Minnesota. Thompson and Company, Inc., 1985.

Register, C. *Living with Chronic Illness: Days of Patience and Passion.* New York: MacMillan, Inc., 1987.

Rotter, J.B. Generalized expectancies for internal versus external control of reinforcement. *Psychological Monographs,* 1960; 80: (1, Whole No. 609), 1960.

White, Kevin P., Nielson, Warren R. Cognitive behavioral treatment of fibromyalgia syndrome: a follow up assessment, *J Rheum,* 22(4):717-721, 1995.

Diet and Nutrition

Abstracts of the Communications Presented at the 10th International Symposium on Transfer Factor, Held in Bologna, Italy. June 23-24, 1995.

Adler GK, Kinsley, BT, Hurwitz S, et al,: Reduced hypothalamic-pituitary and sympathoadrenal responses to hypoglycemia in women with fibromyalgia syndrome. *Am J Med* 1999, 106:534-543.

Ali, Majid. *The Canary and Chronic Fatigue.* Life Span Press, 1994.

Ames, B. MD. Proceedings of National Academy of Sciences 99, 4:2356-61, 2002.

Balch, James R., Balch, Phyllis. *Prescription for Nutritional Healing.* ($16.95)

Baschetti, Riccardo. Chronic fatigue syndrome and Liquorice. *New Zealand Medical Journal* 108: April 26,1995), 156-157.

Behan, P.O., et al. Effects of high doses of essential fatty acids on the post-viral fatigue syndrome. *Acta Neurologica Scaninavica* 82: 3, 211-217, 1990.

Berne, Katrina. *Running on Empty.* Publishers Press, Salt Lake City, 1995. ($14.95)

Bisignano, G, Tomaino A. Lo Cascio R, Crisafi G, Ucella N, Saija A. On the in-vitro antimicrobial activity of oleuropin and hydroxytyrosol. *J Pharm Pharmacol* 1999 Aug; 51(8): 971-4.

Brostoff, Jonathan. *The Complete Guide to Food Allergy and Intolerance.* Crown Publishing, 1989. ($15.00)

Cheney, Paul M.D. *Basic Treatment Plan for Chronic Fatigue Syndrome.* Oct. 2001.

Courmel, Katie. *A Companion Volume to Dr. Jay A. Goldstein's Betrayal By the Brain.* Haworth Medical Press, 1996.

Dalton, Katherina. *Once A Month.* Hunter House, Inc., 1994. ($11.95)

Dalvitt and McPhillips. The Effect of the Human Menstrual Cycle on Nutrient Intake. *Physiol & Behav.* 31 (2):209-12, Aug. 1983.

DeFeudis. Ginkgo biloba Extract (Egb 761) *Pharmacological Activities and Clinical Applications.* Elsevier, Paris, France 1991.

Dufty, William. *Sugar Blues.* Warner Publishing, 1975. ($5.99)

Dyons, et al. Serotonin Precursor Influenced by Type of Carbohydrate Meal in Healthy Adults. *American Journal Clin. Nutr.* 47 (3):433-9, March 1988.

Eisinger J. Ayarni, T., Zakarian H, Plantamura A. Thiamin - Dependent Enzymes Abnormalities in Fibromyalgia. *Journal of Musculoskeletal Pain.* Haworth Medical Press, New York, 3:1 p. 112.

Fedorak Richard N., Madsen, Karen L. Probiotics and Prebiotics in gastrointestinal disorders. *Curr Opin Gastroenterol* 20(2):146-155, 2004.

Ford, Gillian. *Listening to your Hormones.* Prima Publishing, 1996. (916) 632-4400 ($22.95)

Gerwin R., Gervitz R. Chronic Myofoscial Pain: Iron Insufficiency and Coldness in Risk Factors. *Journal of Musculoskeletal Pain.* Haworth Medical Press, New York, 3:1, p. 120, 1995.

Goldberg, B., Trivieri, Jr. *Chronic Fatigue, Fibromyalgia and Lyme Disease.* Second Edition. Celestial Arts, Berkeley, Calif. 2004.

Goldstein, Jay. *Betrayal By the Brain: The Neurological Basisi of Chronic Fatigue Syndrome, Fibromyalgia Syndrome and Related Neural Network Disorders.* Haworth Medical Press, 1996. (800) 342-9678. ($24.95 soft cover) ($39.95 hard cover), plus ($3.00 s&h)

Hugh-Berman, Adriane. *Alternative Medicine: What Works.* Odonian Press, 1996. Box 32375, Tucson, AZ 85751 (520) 296-4056 ($9.00)

Jamaica Dogwood. In: Fleming T.,ed. *PDR for Herbal Medicines,* Montvale, NJ.:Medical Economics Company: 1998: 428-9.

Kelly G. Rhodiola rosea: A possible plant adaptogen. *Alternative Med Rev.* 2001; 6:293-302.

Kleijnen J. and Knipschild P. Ginkgo biloba. *Lancet,* 340:1136-9, 1992.

Kotter, I,. Dick, H., and Schweinsberg, F., Soal, J.G. Selenium Levels in Fibromyalgia. *Journal of Musculoskeletal Pain.* Haworth Medical Press, New York, 3:1, p. 46, 1995.

Kuratsune, H. et al. Acetylcarnitine deficiency in chronic fatigue syndrome. *Clinical Infectious Diseases* 18: Suppl. 1 s62-67. Jan 1994.

Lark, Susan M. *Chronic Fatigue Self-Help Book.* Celestial Arts, 1995. ($16.95)

Lark, Susan M. *PMS Self Help Book.* P.O. Box 7327, Berkeley, CA, 1993. ($16.95)

Lister, RE. An open, pilot study to evaluate the potential benefits of coenzyme Q10 combined with Ginkgo biloba extract in fibromyalgia syndrome. *Int Med Res* 2002. Mar-Apr;30(2):195-9.

Loes, M, MD. *The Aspirin Alternative, The natural way to overcome chronic pain, reduce inflammation and enhance the healing response.* Freedom Press;1999.

Makoul, Sam. Nutrition: Metabolism and Fibromyalgia. *Fibromyalgia Frontiers,* Winter 1996, Vol. 4:1.

Murray, Michael T. *Chronic Fatigue Syndrome.* Prima Publishing, CA, 1994.

Murray, Michael T. *Natural Alternatives to Prozac.* William Morrow & Co., Inc., New York, 1996.

Pfeiffer, Carl C. *Nutrition and Mental Illness.* Healing Arts Press, 1987. ($10.95)

Pierpooli and Regalson. *The Melatonin Miracle.* Simon & Schuster, New York, 1995.

Puri BK. The use of eicosapentaenoic acid in the treatment of chronic fatigue syndrome. Prostaglandins Leukot Essential Fatty Acids. 2004 Apr; 70 (4):399-401.

Rector, Linda G. *Healthy Healing, An Alternative Healing Reference.* Page Publications, 1994. ($27.95)

Researchers track down the relaxin receptor at last. *The Lancet,* Vol 359, Number 9303, Page 323,26 January 2002.

Rogers, S.A. *Tired or Toxic?* Prestige Publishers, 1990.

Romano, T.J. Vitamin A Levels in Patients with Soft Tissue Rheumatism Syndromes. *Journal of Musculosketal Pain,* Haworth Medical Press, New York, 3:1, p. 107.

Russell, I. Jon, Giovengo, S.L. Amino Acids in Cerebrospinal Fluid of Patients with FMS. *Journal of Muskuloskeletal Pain,* Haworth Medical Press, New York, 3:1, p. 9, 1995.

Russell, I. Jon, et. al. Treatment of Fibromyalgia Syndrome with Super Malic: A Randomized, Double-Blinded Placebo Controlled, Crossover Pilot Study, *J. Rheumatology,* 22 (5):953-8, May 1995.

Salmi, H.A. and Sama, S. Effect of silymarin on chemical functional and morphological alterations of the liver. *Scand J Gastroenterol,* 17:517-21, 1982.

Schmidt, Michael A. *Tired of Being Tired: Overcoming Chronic Fatigue and Low Energy.* Frog. Ltd., North Atlantic Books, Berkeley, Calif.

Smith,J.D.,et al. Relief of Fibromyalgia Symptoms Following Discontinuation of Dietary Excitotoxins. *Annals of Pharmacotherapy.* 35(6) (June 2001):702-706.

Somer, Elizabeth. *The Essential Guide to Vitamins and Minerals.* Harper Collins, 1995. ($17.00)

Somer, Elizabeth. *Food and Mood.* Henry Holt, 1996. ($15.95)

Squires, D. Get With the Program. *Health Points* (Vol 7 Issue 4) October 2002, TyH Publications, Fountain Hills, AZ. All rights reserved.

Teitelbaum, J., MD. *From Fatigued to Fantastic.* New York: Penguin Putnam Inc.; 2001.

Teitelbaum, Jacob. *From Fatigued to Fantastic!* Deva Press, Annapolis, MD, 1995.

Thankachen, J. Destress with L-Theanine. *Natural Health*; p.39 Oct/Nov. 2002.

Thorson, Kristin. Does the Food You Eat, Make You Sick? *Fibromyalgia Network,* July 1995.

Tyler, Varro E. *The Honest Herbal & Herbs of Choice.* Pharmaceutical Products Press.

Verillo, Erica F, Gellman, Lauren. *Chronic Fatigue Syndrome: A Treatment Guide.* St. Martin's Griffin, New York. 1997.

Vermeulen, Raud CW, MD, Scholte, Hans, PhD. Exploratory open label, randomized study of Acetyl- and Propionylcarnitine in chronic fatigue syndrome. *Psychosomatic Medicine* 2004 66:276-282.

Vliett, Elizabeth. *Screaming to Be Heard: Hormonal Connections Women Suspect and Doctors Ignore.* M. Evans and Company, Inc., New York, 1996.

Volkmann H, Norregaard J, Jacobsen S, et al. Double-blind placebo controlled cross-over study of intravenous S-adenosyl methionine in patients with fibromyalgia. *Scand J Rheum* 1997; 26:206-11.

Waterhouse, Joyce. Novel Treatment Reduces FMS Symptoms. Controlling Food Sensitivities has Wide Impact, *CFIDS Chronicle,* p. 48, Fall 1996.

Weil, A. *Health and Healing.* Houghton Mifflin, Boston, 1988.

Weil, A. *Natural Health, Natural Medicine.* Houghton Mifflin, Boston, 1990

Alternative Treatments

Goldberg, B., Trivieri, Jr. *Chronic Fatigue, Fibromyalgia and Lyme Disease.* Second Edition. Celestial Arts, Berkeley, Calif. 2004.

Hugh-Berman, Adriane. *Alternative Medicine: What Works.* Odonian Press Tucson, AZ, 1996 $12.75 (800) 788-3123.

Murray, Michael T. *Chronic Fatigue Syndrome.* Prima Publishing, California, 1994.

Murray, Michael T. *Natural Alternatives to Prozac.* William Morrow & Company, Inc. New York, 1996.

Natural Health, April 1996. Boston Common Press. Brookline Village, MA.

Pellegrino, Mark. *The Fibromyalgia Survivor.* Anadem Publishing, Columbus, OH, 1995.

Pioneering Treatments

Aposhian HV., Mobilization of heavy metals by newer, therapeutically useful chelating agents. *Toxicology,* 97(1-3):23-38. 1995. Mar 31.

Almeida TF, Roizenblatt S, Benedito-Silva AA, TufikS: The use of microcurrent electrical therapy and cranial electrotherapy stimulation in pain control., *Clinical Practice of Alternative Medicine* 2(2):99-102, 2001.

Bon-Holaigah, et al. The Relationship Between Neurally Mediated Hypotension and the Chronic Fatigue Syndrome. *JAMA.* 274:961-967, 1995.

Bruno, Richard L. Fainting and Fatigue, Causation or Coincidence? *The CFIDS Chronicle*. pp. 37-39, Spring 1996.

Carpman, Vicki L. Cough Syrup for Pain? Does Unique Treatment Reverse FMS/CFIDS? *The CFIDS Chronicle.*, pp. 46-47, Fall 1996.

Chafety. *Nutrition and Neurotransmitters: The Nutrient Basis of Behavior.* Englewood Cliffs, NJ, 1990.

Crook, William. *The Yeast Connection and the Woman*. Professional Books, Inc., 1995.

Crook, William. *CFIDS and the Yeast Connection.* Professional Books, Inc., 1992.

Donaldson, Stuart, PhD, and Mueller Horst, M.D.. *J Clin Psychol* 2001; 57(7):933-952.

Donaldson C.C.S., Sella, G, Zheng, Y. (2000) Chronic fatigue syndrome, fibromyalgia and neurasthenia. In Zeng, Y. (Ed). *Practice of Biofeedback* (published in China in 2002.)

Donaldson, SS. (1994). The evaluation of trigger points using dynamic EMG techniques. *American Journal of Pain Management* 4(3) : 118-122

Epstein, J.A., Carros, R., Hyman, R.A., Costa, S. Cervical myelopathy caused by developmental stenosis of the spinal cord. *J. Neurosurg,* 51:362-369, 1979.

Estys, Mary Lee, PhD, Perlman, Emily M.S. Neurotherapeutic Treatment of Fibromyalgia Using EEG-Based Stimulation. *Fibromyalgia Frontiers* 2003(vol11, Number 4). Pp.3-13.

Estys, M.L. PhD. The Effect of FNS upon Mild Moderate Brain Traumatic Injury. *The Journal of Head Trauma Rehabilitation,* Vol 16 #3. June 2001.

Gerwin R. A Study of 96 Subjects Examined Both for FMS and Myofascial Pain. *Journal of Musculoskeletal Pain.* Haworth Medical Press, New York, 3:1, p. 121, 1995.

Goldstein, Jay. *Betrayal By the Brain: The Neurological Basis of Chronic Fatigue Syndrome, FM Syndrome and the Related Neural Network Disorders.* Haworth Medical Press, New York, 1996.

Karoliussen, O.H., Kvlheim, L. Effects of Mexiletine on Pain and other Symptoms in Primary Fibromyalgia. *Journal of Musculoskeletal Pain,* 3(1), 26, 1995.

Langfitt, T.W. Cervical spondylosis: the neurological mimic. *W.V. Med J,* 65:97-100, 1969.

Lichtbroun, Alan S., Raicer, Mei-Ming C., and Smith, Ray B. The treatment of fibromyalgia with cranial electrotherapy stimulaton. *Journal of Clinical Rheumatology,* 7(2):72-78, 2001.

Malone, Daniel G. Treatment (RX) of 76 patients with primary fibromyalgia (1^{O} FM) with combined dopaminergic and serotonergic drugs. Poster, ACR Annual Convention, 1996, Orlando, Florida.

Meholic, T.F., Pezzuli, R.T., Applebaum, B.I. Magnetic resonance imaging and cervical spondylotic myelopathy. *Neurosurgery,* 26:217-227, 1990.

Mueller H, Donaldson CC, Nelson D, and Layman M. Treatment of Fibromyalgia Incorporating EEG-driven Stimulation: A Clinical Outcome Study. J *Clinical Psychology* 2001; 57(7),933-952.

Murone, I. The importance of the sagittal diameters of the cervical spinal canal in relation to spondyloses and myelopathy. *J Bone Joint Surg,* 56 B:30-36, 1974.

Rosner, M.J., Banner, S.R., Guin, S., Oper, A.R., Johnson, A.H., Rosner, A.D., Wadlington, V. Response of the cervical spinal cord to decompression for congenital cervical stenosis. Submitted to *Neurosurgery*, 1997. Reference I.D. #2838.

Rowe, P., et al. Is Neurally Mediated Hypotension an Unrecognizable Cause of Chronic Fatigue? *Lancet,* 345:623-24, March 11, 1995.

Rowe, Peter C., Calkins, Hugh. NMH: One Year Later. Johns Hopkins Research Update. *The CFIDS Chronicle,* pp. 49-50, Fall 1996.

Russell, I. Jon, Gilbert,V., Goldstein, Jay. Could low levels of cerebrospinal fluid endothelin explain the vasoconstrictive response seen in pre- and post-treatment brain spect of CFIDS/FMS patients? *Journal of Musculoskeletal Pain,* 3(1), 14, 1995.

Sinclair, David J., et al. Interdisciplinary Treatment for Fibromyalgia: Treatment Outcome and 6 Month Follow-up. 388. Scientific Abstracts. ACR Annual Meeting. October 1996.

Sletvold, M., et al. Information Processing in Primary Fibromyalgia, Major Depression and Healthy Control, *J. Rheumatology* 22 (1):137-42, January 1995.

Sumathi R., Buskaran G., Varalakshmi P. Relationship between glutathione and Dl alpha- lipoic acid against cadmium-induced hepatoxicity. *Jpn J Med Sci Biol,* 49(2):39-48.1996 Apr.

Teitelbaum, Jacob. *From Fatigued to Fantastic!* Deva Press, Annapolis, MD, 1995.

Thorson, Kristin. *Fibromyalgia Network*, October 1995.

Thorson, Kristin. *Fibromyalgia Network*, January 1996.

Thorson, Kristin. *Fibromyalgia Network*, April 1996.

Thorson, Kristin. *Fibromyalgia Network*, January 1997.

Tyers, Steve and Smith, Ray B. A comparison of cranial electrotherapy stimulation alone or with chiropractic therapies in the treatment of fibromyalgia. *The American Chiropractor,* 23(2):39-41, 2001.

REFERENCES

Tyres, Steve and Smith, Ray B. Treatment of Fibromyalgia with cranial electrotherapy stimulation, *The Original Internist,* 8(3):15-17, 2001.

Stejskal, V. Immunological reactions to metal in patients with CFIDS. International symposium on functional medicine. Presentation abstracts. Palm Springs, calif 1994.

Welin, M., Lownertz, M.L., Bragee, B. Is the pain in Fibromyalgia NMDA-receptor Mediated? *Journal of Musculoskeletal Pain,* 3(1), 8, 1995.

Wittrup I, Christiansen M, Jensen B, Markers of Central Nervous System Injury In Two Cohorts of Patients With Fibromyalgia. *J Musculoskeletal Pain* 2001;9:81.

Yudenfreund-Sujka, Shari M. The association of Chronic headaches and fibromyalgia with sexual assault and abuse. *Am. J of Pain Management.* Jan 2003;13(1) 29-32.

REFERENCES

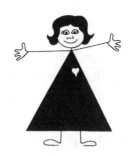

APPENDIX: PHYSICIAN PROTOCOLS

Treatment of Fibromyalgia and Chronic Fatigue Syndrome Using The Oxytocin-Hormonal-Nutrient Protocol

by Jorge D. Flechas, M.D., M.P.H.

Dr. Flechas is a family practitioner in North Carolina who works with patients who have fibromyalgia syndrome (FMS) and patients with chronic fatigue and immune dysfunction syndrome (CFIDS). He has developed a new protocol for treatment of these illnesses using oxytocin (OT), dehydroepiandrosterone (DHEA) and some natural nutrients. He feels both diseases are most likely due to a neuroendocrine/metabolic disorder with chronic hypoxia, which causes abnormalities in the biochemistry of patients.

This summary of information is divided into two sections. Section I contains the technical perspective and Section II the treatment plan. Some readers may wish to review the treatment plan for its applicability to their situation and then become familiar with the technical perspective.

Section I: Medical Perspective

FMS and CFIDS are different diseases but closely related. Patients with these diseases have in common a decrease in corticotrophin releasing hormone (CRH), which controls cortisol output from the adrenals.[1-4] Both groups of patients have shown a decrease in levels of arginine vasopressin (AVP), a hormone that controls the ability of the body to release fluid.[1,2,5] With a lack of this hormone patients feel increasingly thirsty and have frequent urination, about every 20 to 30 minutes. Both of these hormones are produced in an area of the brain called the supraoptic nucleus. Another hormone of importance, called oxytocin (OT), is produced by the same nerve cells. The same neurons that make OT also have the capacity of making CRH and AVP.[6] As of October of 1997, no one in the medical literature had described an OT deficiency. An attempt to define an OT deficiency will be done here.

Oxytocin

OT is a hormone produced in many parts of the body. In the brain, it is produced and released on a daily rhythm with its peak occurring at around noon.[7,8] OT is also produced in the posterior retina, in the pineal gland, thymus, pancreas, testicle, ovary, and adrenal glands. Oxytocin's known functions will be discussed below.

1. OT is known to control the microcirculation of the human body and brain.[9-12] A decrease in OT can cause problems with decreased circulation in the extremities. Therefore, patients often

complain of cold hands and feet, along with a history of recurrent headaches. Oxytocin's ability to vasodilate the blood vessels is due to its capacity to stimulate the body's cells to produce nitric oxide, a powerful vasodilator of microcirculation.[9-11] If vasodilation, such as blushing, does not occur when OT is given intramuscularly, then a serious defect in nitric oxide production is present. This defect of poor circulation is often present among FMS/CFIDS patients.[13-15]

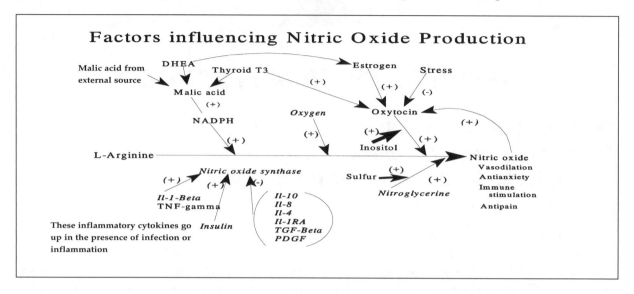

2. OT is released as a mother nurses her baby.[16] Stimulation of the hormone release causes the mother to have an instinct to want to cuddle. As she nurses the child, her desire to cuddle intensifies. This same feeling can be experienced during intimacy–OT has the ability to increase libido.[17,18] Therefore, patients lacking this hormone may often notice that they do not wish to cuddle, to be held, or to be intimate. It has been noticed that stress can restrain the production of OT.[19-21]

3. OT seems to stimulate the ability of the brain to concentrate, contribute to mental alertness, and improve memory. [22] Patients lacking this hormone may find difficulty in concentrating and feel like they are thinking in a fog. This has been noted in FMS.[23-25]

4. OT can occupy multiple hormonal receptor sites in the body. Dr. Flechas theorizes that an empty receptor for OT can potentially cause pain. Administering OT causes the empty OT receptor sites to become full, thereby diminishing or completely obliterating pain. Animal studies reveal that because of this particular characteristic, OT has been an effective tool in weaning addicted animals from narcotics, suggesting that OT has the ability to occupy not only its own receptor sites, but opiate (narcotic) receptor sites as well.[26]

5. OT is produced in the posterior retina of the eye.[27] A decrease in OT level can cause problems with intermittent blurring of vision. When OT is given, it can sharpen the vision. (clinical observation) In patients with reduced levels of OT, one can expect complaints of pain in the posterior eye, sometime so severe that only narcotics provide effective pain relief. Visual disturbances in FMS have been observed.[28,29]

6. OT is also made in the pineal gland of the brain, as is melatonin, a hormone which enhances sleep.[27,30] In animal studies, as the level of OT increases in the brain, the animal is induced into a deeper sleep.[30] (Insomnia is a sleep disorder frequently seen in patients with FMS/CFIDS, and could indicate a deficiency in melatonin.) Note: Recent research indicates that melatonin has the ability to activate the immune system, so the use of this product is usually contraindicated in the presence of autoimmune disease (such as lupus, rheumatoid arthritis).[31]

7. The ovaries make OT.[32,33] In the ovary, OT helps in the fine-tuning of progesterone release.[32] When patients are lacking OT, they may frequently complain of ovarian pain, even though pathology does not support the presence of either cysts or tumors. Ovulation function may be impaired with menstrual irregularity.[28]

8. OT is synthesized in the adrenal glands where it stimulates or inhibits steroid production.[21,34-37] Patients with decreased OT levels often complain of flank pain underneath the posterior ribs. Malfunction in the adrenal steroid production has been seen in FMS.[38,39]

9. OT is created by the thymus gland.[40,41] The thymus gland utilizes OT to help process white blood cells which help control autoimmunity. Normal levels of OT also help stimulate these cells into greater action.[40-46] For example, it is a known fact that women who nurse their children have a much lesser incidence of breast cancer. This hormone may be protective in its ability to prevent breast cancer, through its influences on the immune system.[47]

10. OT is produced by the pancreas.[48] In the pancreas, OT is known to stimulate the production of glucagon, a hormone which helps the intestines to relax.[49,50] Therefore, in treating a patient with decreased levels of this hormone, one would expect to see problems with increased intestinal spasms, secondary to a lack of glucagon production from the pancreas.

11. OT can function as an antianxiety agent in the brain. It can also stimulate social behavior.[51] A lack of this hormone may be expressed as antisocial behavior with some anxiety.

12. OT can function as an antidepressant.[52] In low levels of OT one would expect to see depression, which has been noticed in FMS/CFIDS.[24,53]

13. OT can serve as a regulator of cardiovascular and autonomic nervous system function.[54,55] This explains why patients lacking this hormone have trouble controlling their blood pressure when going from a sitting to upright position, or when standing for a long period of time This is known as neurally mediated hypotension. They often complain of near syncope (light headed) and possible dizziness.[28] OT is found in the sections of the brain where the baroreceptors of the body are controlled.[55] A drop of OT levels in the brain leads to a manifestation of baroreceptor malfunction. Restoration of OT as an oral tablet (Belmar Pharmacy) corrects the symptoms of neurally mediated hypotension. (clinical observation)

14. OT has the capacity to induce the body to mildly retain fluid. This is in part due to its physical and biological similarity to arginine vasopressin.[11,56,57] AVP is a hormone that controls fluid metabolism and memory.[1,2,5] With a lack of OT, patients have increased thirst. They also have increased urinary output due to decreased ability to retain fluid.[28]

As can be seen, the actions and normal functions which have been associated with the use of OT are broad and varied. The following diagram helps to illustrate and contrast the known functions of OT and other symptoms of FMS, which are not commonly known in the regular medical literature.

Dehydroepiandrosterone

In treating FMS/CFIDS patients, a hormone of importance is dehydroepiandrosterone (DHEA). The adrenal glands produce between 30 and 50 mg. of DHEA per day, as compared to 10 mg. of cortisol. Hence, the major steroid released by the adrenals is DHEA. DHEA sulfate is the water-soluble form of the hormone inside the body. DHEA is a waxy substance and is very difficult for the body to transport from the adrenals to the tissues. Therefore, by sulfating the hormone, the body makes it water soluble and easier to transport to the respective tissues that need it. The

Other Symptoms/Syndromes Associated with Fibromyalgia	Functions of Oxytocin
Cognitive difficulties: memory loss, decreased concentration, depression	Increased alertness, concentration, and desire to cuddle
Headaches	Improves and restores memory
Numbness or tingling	Combats depression
Eye complaints	Promotes clear vision
Vestibular complaints: dizziness, vertigo	Stabilizes neurological control of blood pressure
Temporomandibular joint syndrome (TMJ)	Enhances fluid retention
Esophageal dysmotility	Enhances sleep and relaxation
Mitral valve prolapse: heart palpitations, chest pain (non-cardiac)	Enhances microcirculation of hands, feet and head
Lung symptoms	Helps to control pain in muscles and joints
Joint hypermobility	Stimulates or inhibits steroid production in the body
Irritable bowel syndrome	Helps bowels to relax
Painful menstruation	Increases thermogenesis (body warmth)
Interstitial cystitis	Stimulates lactation
Vulvodynia: painful sexual intercourse	Stimulates labor in childbirth
Vestibulitis	Improves sperm function
Female urethral syndrome	Plays an important role in achieving orgasm
Multiple chemical hypersensitivity	Fine tunes progesterone production from ovary
Painful arches of the feet	
Microcirculation disturbances: cold hands and feet	

following paragraphs, one through eleven, explore the physiologic functions of DHEA.

1. DHEA is the primary steroid produced when a baby is in utero.[67,68] At that time, the level of DHEA in the fetus is around 200 mcg./dl. At birth, DHEA levels drop considerably within a period of two to three weeks and will not significantly rise again until the age of 7. The hormone will continue to rise until the age of 25 in males and 32 in females. From these ages on, DHEA levels start dropping, and by age 60 to 70, will be 5 to 10 percent of the hormone level of a normal person 30 years old.[69]

2. DHEA assists in the production of oil in the human skin, as does thyroid and betacarotene. When DHEA is lacking, the skin becomes dry and rough.[70] Patients with low DHEA levels find themselves constantly applying lotion. DHEA also helps to control all hair production in the female, from her head to her toes. A woman experiencing a low level of DHEA will notice a decrease in hair production on the legs, underarms and pubic area and some loss of hair on top of the head. Sometime women will simply notice a need to shave less often. Some patients report that DHEA therapy has helped to increase oil production in their hair. Patients on DHEA hormonal replacement therapy have also noticed that skin and nails begin to get thicker, hair becomes less gray, grows faster, and becomes more dense. Smoother, younger looking skin has been an additional benefit that many patients find attractive while taking DHEA.

3. DHEA helps to maintain skeletal mass. Therefore, patients with a decrease in DHEA will have accelerated problems with loss of bone mass.[71,72]

4. DHEA can stimulate the immune system.[73-78] Therefore, with low DHEA, problems with

APPENDIX

increased infections are noted. In addition, a person with low levels of DHEA requires a longer period of time to recover from a cold and other illnesses, as compared to normal individuals. The steroid also declines with aging.[79]

As mentioned earlier, DHEA is the primary steroid produced by the human adrenal glands.[69] When the body undergoes inflammation from infection or surgical stress, the production of DHEA drops and the adrenal cortisol output increases.[80,81] This process is known in the medical literature as adrenal adaptation syndrome.[80] Chronic inflammation, as seen in lupus, rheumatoid arthritis, tuberculosis, or any long-term infection, is not in the best interest of the body. Overcoming infection when the adrenals are functioning properly is much easier and accomplished in much less time than it is when the immune system is compromised with constant inflammation persisting.

DHEA can override cortisol's immunosuppressive effects on the immune system. One chemical pathway by which DHEA accomplishes this is by reversal of cortisol inhibition of the synthesis and secretion of gamma interferon.[82] Gamma interferon is a hormone produced by white blood cells to help stimulate the immune system to be involved in the protection of the body against infection, as seen in a viral infection.

DHEA is known to inhibit the cellular transformation of Epstein-Barr herpes virus, the virus known to cause mononucleosis.[83,84] When the human body has plenty of DHEA, the immune system is able to control the mononucleosis virus more effectively. When DHEA is low, one would then expect to see reactivation of not only the mononucleosis virus, but possibly other herpetic viruses potentially leading toward a syndrome known as latent herpes virus reactivation phenomena. This would help to explain why patients with CFIDS and FMS may have reoccurrences of herpetic infections such as genital herpes, cold sores, and shingles. Shingles is a reactivation of the chicken pox virus, a known herpes virus.

Patients with AIDS who have low levels of DHEA have been noted in medical studies to die sooner than those with higher levels of DHEA.[85] It appears that an AIDS patient with a higher level of DHEA presents a challenge to the HIV virus.

In laboratory studies, animals given an intentionally lethal dose of a virus predictably died.[85] In these same studies, animals given DHEA a few hours before receiving the "lethal dose" of a virus injection have been shown to survive. This demonstrates DHEA's ability to help the body resist viral infection.

DHEA can increase the size of the spleen germinal centers suggesting stimulation of the B-Lymphocyte dependant areas of the immune system. These cells are responsible for antibody production.[86] DHEA helps in the antibody conversion of IgM to IgG.[75] One of the major antibodies produced by the B-Lymphocyte(s) of the immune system is the IgM antibody. This is a large molecule that needs to be separated to make the IgG antibody. It is felt by some that to separate the IgM molecule into IgG is controlled by DHEA.

Studies performed indicate that DHEA acts as an anti-cancer steroid.[83,87-89] Low levels of DHEA are associated with an increase in breast cancer, bladder, gastric, and prostate cancer.[90-94] A cancer diagnosis could imply that a low level of DHEA probably existed prior to the time of diagnosis.

5. The ability to detoxify chemicals is controlled by the liver. Drugs and other foreign substances in our bodies, such as silicone, antibiotics and other drugs, are referred to as xenobiotics. Metabolism, or detoxification of these xenobiotics, takes place via two different major pathways: Phase I (oxidation) and Phase II (conjugation).

Phase I occurs inside the cell, while Phase II occurs in the liver. It is possible to measure both of these operations to determine whether each is functioning properly. It is not only possible to determine if a patient is suffering from chemical overload, but also to identify which part of the detoxification pathway is damaged. Common problems presenting a chemically sensitive patient are that one or both of the processes are overworked or depleted. This is important so that appropriate nutrient therapy can begin repairing the affected injured pathway.

Testing can also identify whether exposure to chemicals is causing cellular damage and other disease symptoms. Measurements can be taken after a few days at home, then repeated after a few days at work. Using this approach can help to establish which environment is more damaging to the detoxification pathways.

According to experts, most patients suffering from a major illness would exhibit a low level of DHEA if tested. Unfortunately, these untested, chronically ill patients are often the very ones who are investigating detoxification as a potential approach to improve overall health. Experts fear that those initiating a detoxification program with a low DHEA level could potentially place more stress on an already burdened liver. This would in turn prolong the detoxification process and possibly threaten the well-being of the patient.

On the other hand, initiating such a program once the DHEA level is higher could offer the participant less discomfort throughout the detoxification period, as it is known that DHEA has demonstrated the ability to stimulate the Phase II (liver) detoxification process and also assist in Phase I detoxification.[95,96]

Patients receiving DHEA therapy experience less sensitivity to medications. Patients frequently find that they are able to tolerate both increasing the dosage of existing medications and adding additional medications. Clinical observation has suggested that once DHEA therapy is in place, the patient is able to detoxify drugs and other chemicals effectively, as the body approaches a normal detoxification process.

6. DHEA has unique properties that are responsible for the ways it interacts with itself. DHEA has no feedback on itself.[97] There is no documented evidence of DHEA production being inhibited with hormonal replacement therapy of DHEA.[98] It is known that the self-production of thyroid greatly decreases when patients are given oral thyroid hormone. This same principle holds true for the administration of cortisol; the adrenal gland slows production of cortisol when a patient receives cortisol preparations.

DHEA also has unique functions when interacting with other hormones. The active hormone produced by the thyroid is a hormone called thyroid T3. Although DHEA has no direct effect on the T3 levels of the body, recently it has been shown that DHEA works to potentiate the active free T3 function, making it more effective in its work at the cellular level.[99]

In diabetes, it has been noted that DHEA helps to enhance insulin binding to its receptors on the cell membrane and also to its action on cells.[100,101]

It is felt that DHEA is the main hormone which helps to control the female libido.[102] Most female sex steroid hormones are dependent on DHEA for their existence.[102] Therefore, DHEA controls the production of estrogens and androgens (male hormones). This can potentially influence fertility, libido, and improve PMS. (Clinical observation)

7. Inside each cell of the body are approximately 800 mitochondria which help produce energy for the cells. This energy can be used by cells for normal cellular function or be used to help heat

the body. The process of heating the human body is called thermogenesis. It has been shown that when DHEA is given, thermogenesis increases.[103] Patients receiving oral DHEA therapy report feeling warmer.

Inside the mitochondria, DNA is present and helps to produce some of the enzymes inside the mitochondria. DHEA is known to stimulate the DNA production of these enzymes.[104,105] DHEA has been shown to increase basal oxygen consumption.[99] The hormone, when added to thyroid T3, has been shown to be helpful in activation of the malic enzyme gene transcription inside the mitochondria.[104] Overall, DHEA and thyroid T3 interact synergistically to stimulate the body to have more energy via the cellular mitochondria.

8. In human studies DHEA has been used in the treatment of cirrhosis,[106-108] psoriasis (as a topical solution),[109-112] lupus,[113] hereditary angioneurotic edema,[114] arteriosclerotic heart disease,[115] AIDS,[84] porphyria,[116] and has been shown to increase natural killer cells cytotoxicity.[117] DHEA has now been used in the treatments of disease such as multiple sclerosis,[118,119] post-menopausal depression,[120] and gout.[120] Clinically, it has been successfully used to treat a patient with porphyria. The patient could not tolerate five minutes of sunshine. When exposed to the sun, her skin would develop blisters and cause her to have severe itching. Within one month of hormonal replacement therapy with oral DHEA, she was able to be in the Florida sunshine for greater than eight hours per day with no reaction to the sun.

In the presence of DHEA, natural killer cells of the immune system are able to kill cancer cells and yeast cells more effectively. Clinically, it has been noted that yeast infections come under better control with less recurrences in the presence of taking DHEA. The overall number of natural killer cells is increased in the presence of DHEA.[117]

9. DHEA has been shown to be an anti-aging hormone. Clinical observations show that patients who have high levels of this hormone suffer less from the ravages of aging as compared to those who have lesser amounts of this hormone.[96]

10. DHEA has recently been shown to stimulate the production of serotonin, a chemical used by the brain to inhibit depression.[121] Hence, low levels of DHEA can manifest as depression. In FMS, plasma serotonin levels have been found to be low.[122-124]

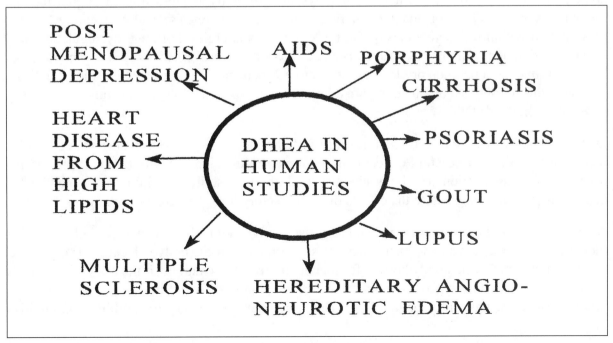

APPENDIX

221

11. In recent medical literature, Dr. I. Jon Russell, a prominent FMS researcher, and others have shown that patients with FMS have much lower levels of DHEA sulfate as compared to normal patients.[38,39]

The relationship between Oxytocin and DHEA

OT travels to its receptor sites in certain cell membranes of the body, binds, and activates a chemical messenger called cyclic AMP (cAMP).[32] This cAMP creates a signal which moves through the cell membrane directly into the cell, then activates the inositol triphosphate system. Research literature supports that this inositol phosphate system is DHEA dependent and necessary for optimum OT function.[125] When this system is activated, the cells of the body are free to do the jobs they are designed to perform. OT acts much like a fine tuner, enhancing the functions which the body is already performing on its own.

Inositol

Inositol is a substance found in the liver, kidneys, skeletal and heart muscle, and is part of the vitamin B complex. Its highest levels are found in the brain.[126,127] In nature it is found in brown rice, vegetables and fruit. The activity of cells throughout the body is governed by an intricate network of signaling systems which translate outside information into internal signals, or second messengers. Inositol acts as a signal enhancer to transduct many cellular processes, such as secretion, metabolism, cell growth, and neurotransmission of light.[128-132] Inositol in a cell helps to increase cellular calcium. This helps the cell perform functions such as contract, produce a hormone, etc. Secondary messengers, or signal transductors, are important because it is thought that an imbalance of these messengers may be at least partially responsible for normal cells converting into cancerous ones. This system is also responsible for the ability of a cell to produce nitric oxide.[133]

At this point it is important to recognize that other natural chemicals have been found to enhance the human body's response to OT and DHEA. These are choline, malic acid, magnesium, creatine and thyroid T3.

Choline

This nutrient is involved in protein, fat, and normal carbohydrate metabolism. Its highest concentration in nature is found in the soybean. Although phosphatidyl choline (PC) is a natural component of every single membrane, it plays an especially notable role in supporting the membranes responsible for making energy, detoxifying chemicals, and preventing cancer. Dysfunction within the membranes of the body produces allergies, hormone dysregulation, and disease. A deficiency in this essential nutrient can slow the improvement or recovery phase of an illness, produce gradual memory loss, and encourage chemical over-sensitivity. Studies indicate the use of this nutrient in combination with others has been successful in slowing down some early cases of Alzheimer's Disease.

Diets are usually lacking in sufficient quantities of choline, as well as other nutrients needed for metabolism of PC. Successful PC treatment requires careful balancing with these other nutrients necessary for assimilation into body chemistry. Experts describe this nutrient's potential for healing as phenomenal because the effects of a satisfactory level are so far-reaching.

As the body detoxifies chemicals, even more phosphatidyl choline is needed, especially since our modern world exposes us to so many chemicals. If one part of the body is lacking sufficient PC to perform its job, it will simply borrow from another area. For example, if the body's liver needs more and elects to borrow from the brain, the brain becomes deficient in this substance and can produce mood swings and poor memory. The components necessary for building PC are also necessary for forming acetylcholine, which is the main neurotransmitter of the brain and a potent stimulator of nitric oxide production.[134,135] Correcting a PC deficiency often produces marked improvement in short-term memory, as well as in overall health.

According to nutritional experts, a dosage which supplies approximately 3 gm. of phosphatidyl choline is preferred. This dosage is sufficient to increase the choline levels in the brain by 50%; 9 gm. can actually double the brain's choline level. However, manufacturers are constantly changing formulations and diluting the product to become more cost effective, so finding the appropriate dosage can be a challenge.

Malic Acid

Malic acid is a valuable adjunct to this therapy because it plays an essential role in sugar metabolism and in the formation of ATP, the energy currency for physical activity and other important body functions. The energy we use to perform physical and mental tasks as well as to maintain normal function of the organs in our body comes from food product combustion after digestion. Energy comes from these combusted, digested food products combined with oxygen. This energy is stored as ATP for future use. ATP production requires magnesium, oxygen, phosphates, and oxygen. Conditions such as hypoxia (reduced oxygen supply) can lower ATP production. Further, conditions such as lower than optimal levels of magnesium, phosphate, and substrates will literally "shut down" the complete utilization of sugar for the manufacture of ATP.

As a result, the body will then switch to a very inefficient system of generating ATP. This involves the breaking down of proteins in muscles and other tissues. This is harmful to the body in the long run, resulting in damage to the affected parts. Physical symptoms usually associated with this breakdown are pain, decreased function, and fatigue. ATP levels have been found low in FMS.[136,137]

When OT levels are low, the cells of the body go into a state of hypoxia. This happens because OT via nitric oxide acts as a vasodilator to the capillaries. A lack of OT can potentially cause blood vessels to spasm, creating vicious cycles of more spasms which worsens the condition. It also further decreases the oxygen supply and food substances needed for ATP production. Malic acid is unique in its ability to increase the utilization of substances needed for ATP synthesis, and also has oxygen-sparing effects because it is able to generate ATP effectively by using sugar as fuel, even under low-oxygen conditions. This increase of ATP production under hypoxic conditions actually reverses blood vessel spasms and increases the amount of oxygen and food substances available to muscles and other tissues. Malic acid has also found uses in the treatment of liver disease because of its ability to eliminate ammonia, a substance very toxic to the brain. There are no known contraindications for the use of malic acid.[138]

Magnesium

In addition to malic acid, the other major player is magnesium, the fourth most abundant mineral in the body, and the second most abundant in muscles and organs. Magnesium is required for normal activity of 300 enzymes, including those involved in energy transfer from food to ATP and for transfer of energy from ATP to physical and mental activity. ATP forms a complex with magnesium, in order to stabilize the ATP molecule. An inadequate supply of magnesium can inhibit this process of energy production and the stability of its major energy component, ATP.[138] Magnesium insufficiency has presently been documented in both FMS/CFIDS.[138-140]

Creatine

Both FMS/CFIDS patients have low levels of creatine phosphate.[141-143] In the body creatine is used as a chemical to store energy. It can also serve as a major fuel for normal brain metabolism and as a stimulant for muscle building.[144-146]

Thyroid T3

The thyroid produces two major hormones, T4 and T3. Thyroid T4 will be absorbed in certain cells of the body where it is converted into T3. Many cells, such as liver, heart, skeletal muscles, and kidney cells, do not have the ability to convert T4 into T3 and must absorb T3 directly from the plasma. Thyroid T3 does its work in the DNA of the nucleus and of the mitochondria. The conversion of T4 to T3 will decrease under certain conditions. Some factors are aging, infection, inflammation, selenium deficiency, massive weight loss, fasting, and drugs.[147-153] When the thyroid T4 blood level is normal and the free T3 blood level is low, this is called Euthyroid Sick Syndrome.[154] FMS has been associated with hypothyroidism (low thyroid).[155-157]

How Are DHEA, T3, Malic Acid, Magnesium, Choline, Inositol, and Oxytocin Related?

The production of oxytocin and nitric oxide are dependant upon those substances below them in the following pyramid.

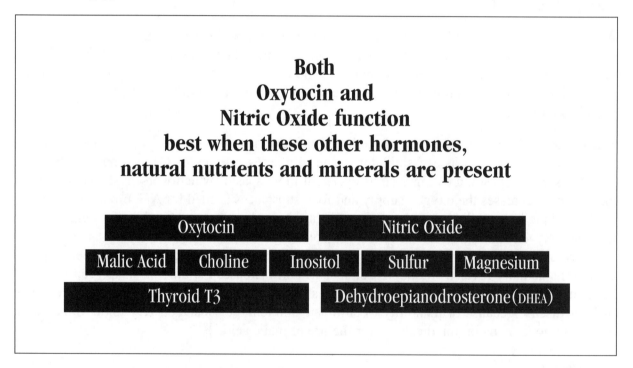

Both Oxytocin and Nitric Oxide function best when these other hormones, natural nutrients and minerals are present

Oxytocin			Nitric Oxide	
Malic Acid	Choline	Inositol	Sulfur	Magnesium
Thyroid T3		Dehydroepianodrosterone (DHEA)		

Section II: Treatment Plan

Understanding that the true success of any approach to treatment lies in the ability to reach patients outside the parameters of a single medical practice, a protocol has been developed for other treating physicians, using the aforementioned preparations. Double-blind, placebo-controlled testing of these hormones and nutrients has not been performed because of lack of funding. The clinician may wish to try them sequentially in individual patients.

First Office Visit

During this visit the diagnosis is made of a patient's medical problem. Lab work is done to get a baseline on the patient. Thyroid T3 and DHEA sulfate blood levels are measured on all FMS/CFIDS patients. The recommendations of DHEA researchers is that the blood levels of both male and female patients should be around 200 mcg. per dl. or greater. If the DHEA sulfate level is lower in a patient, then he or she is started on hormonal replacement therapy with DHEA. If the patient does not respond to the OT test dose with facial flushing and redness of the ears, then he or she is placed on DHEA in the A.M. for three months. If the DHEA-S04 value is below 200 mcg./dl., a good starting point is to begin treatment with DHEA 25 mg. p.o. (by mouth), every morning. DHEA converts to DHEA-S04 in the liver and is a stable hormone; a steady state exists between DHEA and DHEA-SO4. Therefore, treatment with DHEA-SO4 would not be of value. Please see below for dosage based on blood levels.

Recent work on neurosteroids from the brain has shown that DHEA in some patients may be excitatory to the brain. Hence, if one experiences problems with insomnia with DHEA, then the hormone should be taken in the morning. DHEA stimulates the DNA of the cells to produce the enzymes of the inositol triphosphate system. This allows the cells to be more reactive to OT stimulation when it occurs. This increase in reactivity of cells to OT may take up to three months to become fully operational. An easy way to probe this reactivity is by giving a patient a test dose of OT 10 units IM in the office along with .25 cc. of xylocaine without epinephrine. OT injectable is a liquid. It has a pH of around 2 to 4 and can cause significant burning pain when given, hence the use of the xylocaine. If within the first 2 to 3 minutes the patient feels his or her face becoming warmer and the ears warm, the patient would then seem to have adequate amounts of DHEA. The cells should respond to the use of oral OT tablets. It is still recommended that a DHEA sulfate level be drawn to get a baseline level on the patient. This will give a starting point for this particular patient's treatment.

During the first office visit a RBC magnesium level is drawn. If the RBC magnesium level is low, the patient should be started on Mag 200, two tablets twice daily. MAG 200 is a magnesium product that was developed to give the least amount of bowel irritation with excellent absorption.

Also measured at the first visit is the creatine blood level. If found low, replacement therapy is begun. Once the patient is responding to the therapy as listed in this paper, he or she can then be started on creatine monohydrate one teaspoon four times per day for one week, then two teaspoons every morning. Creatine can be mixed with juice, water, or applesauce. It is best given in the morning. If it is taken at night, it can keep an individual awake. Some patients with sensitive stomachs may have difficulty in taking creatine monohydrate and may need a lower starting dose.

If no blushing occurs at the time of giving the initial dose of oxytocin, patients are then requested to start on choline, inositol, and paba (five tablets per morning). Choline and inositol help load the enzymes that are being made by DHEA in order to help the inositol triphosphate system to respond to OT. Choline (1500 mg.) and inositol (1500 mg.) may also be found in the local health food stores.

At this point we need to focus on a new finding. As noted above, OT can stimulate the body to vasodilate its capillaries to give a person better circulation. Two recent medical papers have now shown that OT vasodilates the body's small blood vessels via the mechanism of stimulating production of nitric oxide. Nitric oxide is a very potent gas produced at the capillary level of the tissues. One of its major jobs is to improve tissue oxygenation. A few patients are having trouble making this gas, even in the presence of the hormones and nutrients thus far discussed.

During the last few months, we have learned to improve our therapy. We do this by giving sublingual nitroglycerin 1/2 tablet of .3 mg. every four hours. (Nitrostat .3 mg. sl q4hrs) This therapy can increase the blood supply to the brain, heart and tissues. A sign the therapy is working is when the patient develops a headache. This headache is due to increased blood supply to the brain. The headache will last one to fifteen minutes and then disappear. When the headache is gone, the individual will also notice a greater relief from their fibromyalgia pain. The pain relief will last about four to six hours before another sublingual tablet is required. The nitroglycerin works best in the presence of OT. If nitroglycerin is given by itself, a poor response may occur. The first pill should always be given in a doctor's office in case hypotension should develop. Therapy with nitroglycerin should always be started on those patients with weak or no blushing when given OT.

Since FMS patients have so much pain, they are placed on Super Malic, a malic acid and magnesium preparation that has undergone the rigors of a double-blind placebo-controlled trial and proven itself to be effective to reduce FMS pain. Three to six tablets twice per day is the recommended amount.[158] Currently in the USA there are many malic acid and magnesium preparations being sold. None of these have stood the rigors of medical testing to prove that they work. This is why only Super Malic can be recommended without reservation. The magnesium in Super Malic can encourage loose bowel movements, so it may be advisable to begin with one tablet three times a day, and eventually work up to a daily dose of three to four tablets three times a day, unless liquid stools develop. Increasing the dosage by one tablet per day every four to five days may be the best approach to use in the initial stages of treatment, when trying to establish an individualized dose response.

There seems to be a metabolic disturbance of the ability of the body to handle glucose in patients with FMS.[158] Because of this, patients are started on Super Malic to help correct the metabolism disorder in conjunction with DHEA.

Second Office Visit

After the patient has been on DHEA, magnesium, and Super Malic for three months and the inositol choline treatment, a challenge dose of intramuscular OT 10 U with lidocaine 1% 0.25 cc should be administered, unless the patient is sensitive to lidocaine or similar preparations. Within five minutes the patient should start to feel very warm and relaxed, and within twenty minutes notice a reduction of pain. Once the physician is satisfied that the patient has responded to OT, the patient can then start an oral dose of 10 U each morning. An upper limit of 40 U daily has been established for this therapy. Oral OT tablets were developed at Belmar Pharmacy from Lakewood, Colorado, and have been shown to be biologically active (unpublished data). Oral oxytocin tablets should be taken in the morning.

Observations at the office have also indicated that patients who smoke have not responded as well to the OT therapy. This is presumably because the chemicals in cigarette smoke may block OT receptors.

At the second office visit, repeat blood work should be done to monitor hormone and mineral blood levels for those patients that are receiving replacement therapy.

During the initial or subsequent office visits, many patients report a problem with a decreased desire for intimacy. This is a very private and understandably sensitive issue. However, we feel a responsibility to address the problem because so many women injured by FMS/CFIDS are affected; yet embarrassment and fear of further rejection prevent most from discussing it with treating physicians. It is important to realize that there are true physical reasons for this lack of desire, and that most women injured by FMS/CFIDS share this problem. Although medical opinions may differ as to the actual causes, the end results are essentially the same. No longer desiring to be intimate with a partner represents yet another insult from the ILLNESS, because it affects the well partner deeply, and it can affect the security of the marriage directly or indirectly.

Chronic illness imposes a real mix of limitations, experienced by both the injured and the well partner. It is as though personal identity and sense of purpose take up new residence in the background, as THE DISEASE and all that entails takes over. In addition, most families affected by FMS/CFIDS illness also suffer financial embarrassment, due either to mounting medical bills or to the sick partner's inability to work, or both. Adding the sick partner's chronically low or non-existent libido to this picture of intimacy for both partners is a challenge at best. However, striving to accomplish this can be absolutely devastating when perhaps the single most powerful ingredient for establishing and maintaining closeness has simply been removed.

For this reason, finding a treatment program with the potential to restore a healthy desire for intimacy, while at the same time reducing pain and increasing mobility, has seemed like an answered prayer to many chronically ill women.

Treatment Summary

Overall, FMS/CFIDS patients who are involved in this particular regimen seem pleased. However, as with any therapy involving medications, side effects do exist and should be researched before treatment is initiated. Although the information provided in this paper is accurate, it should by no means be considered complete.

Reported benefits of this therapy include a reduction of both pain and fatigue. Although still in the early stages, the above outlined interactive OT-Hormonal-Nutrient Treatment Protocol provides an exciting new alternative to the traditional methods of FMS/CFIDS treatment. Generally, mainstream medicine is geared toward treating symptoms. Because of time constraints, physicians may be more interested in reducing the severity of symptoms than identifying the cause. As identified earlier in the text, traditional methodology is now being challenged, as more and more FMS/CFIDS affected patients regain control over their lives and make a commitment to take an active role in their own recovery. As with anything else, it is important to conduct your own research, and decide on your own what seems to be the most reasonable approach for your personal treatment.

Side Effects

The following side effects have been associated in the medical literature with DHEA, Inositol, OT, Malic Acid, Magnesium:

DHEA/Side Effects

An increase in DHEA has been known to cause increased hair growth on the head, legs, underarms and the pubic area. (This is not normally considered to be a problem, because a decreased level of DHEA has usually created a reduction of hair growth in these areas.) This increase in hair growth can be witnessed by increased itching of the scalp and skin. The itching is actually secondary to the hair growth.

In addition, an increase of facial hair has been noted on rare occasions, but is not a frequently noted problem.

Because DHEA can also stimulate oil glands to increase oil production, an increase in acne may be seen.[159]

These side effects as listed are the natural effects of this hormone, so anytime an excess of DHEA is present, an increase in these areas can be expected.[68,70,98]

An increase in muscle mass and a slight increase in the fat mass around the abdomen has also been observed. (Clinical observation) If DHEA is taken at night, it can cause insomnia. This can be due to the fact that it is a neuroexcitatory hormone of the brain.[160-165]

Although DHEA is capable of increasing thermogenesis, patients receiving this hormone who normally complain of being hot all the time have reported feeling comfortably cooler. This would suggest that DHEA might play a role in helping to control the thermal settings of the brain which determine whether a patient is too hot or too cold.

DHEA/Undesirable Combination/Side Effects

The combination of thyroid hormone supplementation, DHEA, and injectable estrogen given to the same patient at the same time was noted to produce an overactive libido, to the extent the labia became painfully engorged. This extremely painful physical condition persisted for a period of 14 to 21 days. (clinical observation)

Oxytocin/Side Effects

OT therapy helps to stimulate the micro-circulation, thereby increasing body temperature which can make some patients feel uncomfortably warm.[10,54,166] Still, complaints of cold hands and feet are usually diminished, as the patient experiences increased circulation to these areas. Correct dose regulation can alleviate tissues that seem too warm.

OT therapy increases circulation to the head and can produce headaches, but they usually disappear within a short time after starting treatment.

Patients with congestive heart failure or decreased renal function are not good candidates for OT therapy because of its propensity to cause fluid retention.

OT should not be given to a pregnant patient as it may cause some fluid retention, or even miscarriage.

If a patient does not have enough DHEA or inositol on board at the time OT therapy is initiated, the addition of OT can actually cause agitation rather than produce its normal calming effect. This would suggest that this patient is not ready to begin OT therapy and would probably benefit from taking supplemental DHEA and inositol for a few months, before trying OT again.

On the other hand, too much OT could theoretically cause patients to experience a psychiatric problem known as obsessive compulsive disorder. This is based on data from one study only.[167]

In addition, an increase in the manic phase of patients diagnosed with manic-depressive illness is seen as a disorder of inositol.[125,127] This increase in the manic phase comes under quick control as soon as either the hormones or inositol are withdrawn.

Some patients have noted an increase in the size of breast tissue, sometimes necessitating a corresponding change in bra cup size. Increased breast and nipple tenderness have been reported by patients, while others report reduced breast tenderness before their monthly cycle. Patients have also reported greater sensation and sexual excitation when the breast is caressed.

Malic Acid/Magnesium/Side Effects

Gastric irritation can occur in the presence of malic acid.[158,168] Taking the nutrient with at least one eight ounce glass of water seems to minimize this reaction, although some still find it necessary to experiment until an appropriate personalized dosage of malic acid is reached.

Magnesium is contained in Super Malic and may cause problems with frequent loose bowel movements.[138,169] Many patients with constipation find this side effect of their therapy to be helpful. If liquid stools develop, reducing the Super Malic until two or three soft bowel movements per day are achieved seems to work well.

As previously described, this combination of preparations has been known to produce effects ranging from decreased fatigue and pain to clearer vision and improved thinking. Many symptoms are eliminated, such as being lightheaded, irritable bowel syndrome, cramps, cold hands and feet, foggy concentration, and muscle pain. Other improvements include better circulation, better temperature regulation, more energy, reduced skin sensitivity, and less agitation.

Please consider the above outlined plan for informational purposes only; patients are encouraged to use this as a starting point to further their own research for therapies which may bring them better health. If one is interested in this particular approach to treatment, this text with the above mentioned protocol can easily be taken to your own physician, who can initiate the program and monitor your progress.

As these and other treatment modalities surface, hope looms on the horizon for both women and men suffering from FMS/CFIDS related illnesses. The future holds even more promise!

Source of Medication

Belmar Pharmacy, Lakewood, Co., compounds a highly bioavailable form of DHEA as well as oxytocin. Both these hormones are available by prescription. Super Malic (Optimox Cooperation) is available without medical claims as a source of both malic acid and magnesium, and can be purchased at your local pharmacy or health food store as an over the counter product. It can also be purchased through Belmar, along with inositol/choline and Mag 200. The medication is shipped directly to the patient after a prescription has been faxed to the pharmacy from the doctor's office.

Orders should be faxed to: 303-763-9712

> Belmar Pharmacy
> 12860 W. Cedar Dr. #210
> Lakewood, Colorado 88228
> Telephone: 800-525-9473

Reprints of a publication featuring an open clinical trial with Super Malic can be obtained free of charge to your physician upon request from:

> Optimox Corporation
> P.O. Box 3378
> Torrance, California 90510-3378
> Telephone: 800-223-1601

Medication Orders (should look like this)

1. DHEA 50 mg. 1 qam #100 for DHEA levels less than 100mcg./dl.; 25 mg. of DHEA for levels between 100-200 mcg./dl.

2. Super Malic 3-6 bid #180.

3. Thyroid T3 60 or 90 mcg. 1 qam #100 (This pill is sustained release.)

4. Choline-Inositol-Paba 5 qam #250.

5. Mag 200 2 bid #120.

6. Oxytocin 10 unit tab 1-3 tab qam #100.

7. Creatine monohydrate 2 tsp. qam in juice #300 gms.; creatine should only be started after oxytocin has been initiated.

8. Nitrostat .3mg. sl q4-6hr #100; first dose should always be given in a doctor's office; try giving 1/2 tablet first.

Once the prescription is faxed to Belmar, have your patient call their 800 number to make financial arrangements to have the medications sent to them.

For more information about DHEA and Oxytocin therapy contact: Dr. Jorge D. Flechas, 724 5th Avenue West, Hendersonville, NC 28739; (828) 693-3015.

Your phone call will be returned as a collect call as time allows.

Special thanks is given to Sarah Templeton for her donated time and talent in originally typing this manuscript.

REFERENCES

1. Crofford, L.J., Pillemer, S.R., Kalogeras, K.T., Cash, J.M., Michelson, D., King, M.A., et al. Perturbations of Hypothalamic-Pituitary-Adrenal Axis Function in Patients with Fibromyalgia. *American College of Rheumatology*, 1993; 36:C195.
2. Crofford, L.J., Pillemer, S.R., Kalogeras, K.T., Cash, J.M., Michelson, D., Kling, M.A., et al. Hypothalamic-Pituitary-Adrenal Axis Pertubations in Patients with Fibromyalgia. *Arthritis & Rheum*, 1994; 37:1583-1592.
3. Demitrack, M.A., Dale, J.K., Straus, S.E., Laue, L., Listwak, S.J., Kruesi, J.P., et al. Evidence for Impaired Activation of the Hypothalamic-Pituitary-Adrenal Axis in Patients with Chronic Fatigue Syndrome. *Journal of Clinical Endocrinology and Metabolism*, 1991; 73:1224-1234.
4. Demitrack, M.A., Crofford, L.J. Hypothalamic-Pituitary-Adrenal Axis Dysregulation in Fibromyalgia and Chronic Fatigue Syndrome: An Overview and Hypothesis. *Journal of Musculoskeletal Pain*, 1995; 3:67-73.
5. Bakheit, A., Behan, P.O., Watson, W.S., Morton, J.J. Abnormal Arginine-Vasopressin Secretion and Water Metabolism in Patients with Postviral Fatigue Syndrome. *Acta Neurol Scand*, 1993; 87:234-238.
6. Crowley, W.R., Armstrong, W. Neurochemical Regulation of Oxytocin Secretion in Lactation. *Endocrine Reviews*, 1992; 13:33-65.
7. Amico, J.A., Robinson, A.G. The Radioimmunoassay of Oxytocin: New Developments. In: Amico, J.A,. Robinson, A.G., editors. *Oxytocin - Clinical and Laboratory Studies*. A.E. Amsterdam: Elsevier Science Publishers, B.V.. 1985:3-15.
8. Amico, J.A., Tenicela, R., Johnston, J., Robinson, A.G. A Time-Dependent Peak of Oxytocin Exists in Cerebrospinal Fluid but Not in Plasma of Humans. *Journal of Clinical Endocrinology and Metabolism*, 1983; 57:947-951.
9. Argiolas, A., Melis, M.R. Oxytocin-Induced Penile Erection: Role of Nitric Oxide. In: Ivell, R., Russell, J.A., editors. *OXYTOCIN: Cellular and Molecular Approaches in Medicine and Research*. New York: Plenum Press, 1995:247-254.
10. Suzuki, Y., Satoh, S.I., Kimura, M., Oyama, H., Asano, T., Shibuya, M., et al. Effects of Vasopressin and Oxytocin on Canine Cerebral Circulation in vivo. *J Neurosurg*, 1992; 77:424-431.
11. Oyama, H., Suzuki, Y., Satoh, S.I., Kajita, Y., Takayasu, M., Shibuya, M., et al. Role of Nitric Oxide in the Cerebral Vasodilatory Responses to Vasopressin and Oxytocin in Dogs. *Journal of Cerebral Blood Flow and Metabolism*, 1993; 13:285-290.
12. Katusic, Z.S., Shepherd, J.T., VanHoutte, P.M. Oxytocin Causes Endothelium-Dependent Relaxations of Canine Basilar Arteries by Activating V1-Vasopressinergic Receptors. *The Journal of Pharmacology and Experimental Therapeutics, 1985;* 236:166-170.
13. Mountz, J.M., Bradley, L.A., Modell, J.G. Fibromyalgia in women. Abnormalities of regional cerebral blood flow in the thalamus and the caudate are associated with low pain threshold levels. *Arthritis Rheum*, 1995; 38:926-938.
14. Henriksson, K.G. Aspects of the Pathogenesis of Chronic Muscular Pain. *Journal of Musculoskeletal Pain*, 1995; 3:35-41.
15. Hau, P.P., Scudds, R.A., Harth, M. An Evaluation of Mechanically Induced Neurogenic Flare by Infrared Thermography in Fibromyalgia. *Journal of Musculoskeletal Pain*, 1996; 4:3-20.
16. Moos, F,. Freund-Mercier, M.J., Guerne, Y., Stoeckel, M.E., Richard P. Release of oxytocin and vasopressin in Magnocellular Nuclei in Vitro: Specific Facilitatory Effect of Oxytocin on its Own Release. *Journal of Endocrinology*, 1983; 63-72.
17. Carmichael, M.S., Humbert, R., Dixen, J., Palmisano, G., Greenleaf, W., Davidson, J.M. Plasma Oxytocin Increases in the Human Sexual Response. *Journal of Clinical Endocrinology and Metabolism*, 1987; 64:27-31.
18. Pedersen, C.A., Caldwell, J.D., Jirikowski, G.F. Oxytocin and Reproductive Behaviors. In: Yoshida, S., Share, L., editors. *Recent Progress in Posterior Pituitary Hormones*. Amsterdam: Elsevier Science Publishers, B.V., 1988:141-149.

APPENDIX

19. Nussey, S.S., Page, S.R., Ang, V.T.Y., Jenkins, J.S. The Response of Plasma Oxytocin to Surgical Stress. *Clinical Endrocinology*, 1988; 28:277-282.

20. Altemus, M., Deuster, P.A., Galliven, E., Carter, C.S., Gold, P.W. Suppression of Hypothalmic-Pituitary-Adrenal Axis Responses to Stress in Lactating Women. *J of Clinical Endocrinology and Metabolism*, 1995; 2954-2959.

21. Gibbs, D.M. Vasopressin and Oxytocin: Hypothalamic Modulators of the Stress Response: A Review. *Psychoneuroendocrinology,* 1986; 11:131-139.

22. Burbach, P.H., Bohus, B., Gabor, L.K., Van Nispen, J.W., Greven, H.M., De Wied, D. Oxytocin Is A Precursor of Potent Behaviourally Active Neuropeptides. *European Journal of Pharmacology*, 1983; 94:125-131.

23. Clauw, D.J., Morris, S., Starbuck, V. Impairment in Cognitive Function in Individuals with Fibromyalgia. *Arthritis Rheum*, 1994; 37:s347

24. Kaplan, R.F., Meadows, M.E., Vincent, L.C. Memory impairment and depression in patients with Lyme encephalopathy. Comparison with fibromyalgia and nonpsychotically depressed patients. *Neurology*, 1992; 42:1263-1267.

25. Slotkoff, A.T., Clauw, D.J. Fibromylgia: When Thinking is Impaired. *The Journal of Musculoskeletal Medicine*, 1996; 32-36.

26. Yoshida, S., Share, L. Oxytocin and Experimental Drug Addiction: Receptor-Related Effects. In: Kovacs, G.L,. editor. *Recent Progress in Posterior Pituitary Hormones,* 1988. Amsterdam: Elsevier Science Publishers, B.V., 1988:127-132.

27. Gauquelin, G., Gharib, C., Krasnov, I.B., Geelen, G., Allevard, A.M., Brun, J., et al. Hypopyseal Hormones in the Retina, Pineal and Harderian Glands of the Rat. Modifications Induced by Environmental Factors. In: Yoshida S, Share L, editors. *Recent Progress in Posterior Pituitary Hormones*. Amsterdam: Elsevier Science Publishers, B.V, 1988:293-301.

28. Clauw, D.J. Fibromyalgia: More than just a Musculoskeletal Disease. *American Family Physician*, 1995; 52:843-851.

29. Rosenhall, U., Johansson, G., Orndahl, G. Eye Mobility Dysfunction in Chronic Primary Fibromyalgia with Dysesthesia. *Scand J Rehab Med*, 1987; 19:139-145.

30. Voloschin, L.M., Tramezzani, J.H. Milk Ejection Reflection Linked to Slow Wave Sleep in Nursing Rats. *Endocrinology*, 1979; 105:1202-1207.

31. Reiter, R.J., Robinson, J. Atypical Reactions. In: Reiter, R.J., Robinson, J, editors. *Melatonin: Your Body's Natural Wonder Drug*. New York: Bantam Books, 1995; 206-207.

32. Mayerhofer, A., Sterzik, K., Link, H., Wiemann, M., Gratzl, M. Effect of Oxytocin on Free Intracellular CA2+ Levels and Progesterone Release by Human Granulosa-Lutein Cells. *Journal of Clinical Endocrinology and Metabolism*, 1993; 77:1209-1214.

33. Behrens, O., Maschek, H., Kupsch, E., Fuchs, A.R. Oxytocin Receptors in Human Ovaries during the Menstrual Cycle. In: Ivell, R., Russell, J.A., editors. *OXYTOCIN: Cellular and Molecular Approaches in Medicine and Research*. New York: Plenum Press, 1995:485-486.

34. Legros, J.J., Chiodera, P., Geenen, V. Inhibitory Action of Exogenous Oxytocin on Plasma Coritsol in Normal Human Subjects; Evidence of Action at the Adrenal Level. *Neuroendocrinology*, 1988; 48:204-206.

35. Ang, V.T.Y., Jenkins, J.S. Neurohypophyseal Hormones in the Adrenal Medulla. *Journal of Clinical Endocrinology and Metabolism,* 1984; 58:688-691.

36. Hinson, J.P., Vinson, G.P., Porter, I.D., Whitehouse, B.J, Dept.of Biochemistry MC, Charterhouse Square, et al. Oxytocin and Arginine Vasopressin Stimulate Steroid Secretion by the Isolated Perfused Rat Adrenal Gland. *Neuropeptides,* 1987; 10:1-7.

37. Taylor, A.H., Whitley, G.S., Nussey, S.S. The Interaction of Arginine Vasopressin and Oxytocin with Bovine Adrenal Medulla. *Journal of Endocrinology,* 1987; 121:133-139.

38. Russell, I.J., Vipraio, G.A., Abraham, G.E. Serum Dehydroepiandrosterone Sulfate (DHEA) in Fibromyalgia Syndrome (FS) Rheumatoid Arthritis (RA), Osteoarthritis (OA) and Healthy Normal Controls (HC). *Arthritis & Rheumatism*, 1993; 36:S223.

39. Nilsson, E., de la Torre, B., Hedman, M. Blood DHEA-S levels in polymyalgia rheumatica/giant cell arteritis and primary fibromyalgia. *Clinical & Experimental Rheumatology,* 1994; 12:415-417.

40. Johnson, H., Torres, B. Regulation of Lymphokine Production by Arginine Vasopressin and Oxytocin: Modulation of Lymphocyte Function by Neurohypophyseal Hormones. *Journal of Immunology*, 1985; 135:773s-775s.

41. Johnson, H., Torres, B., Farrar, W. Vasopressin Replacement of Interleukin 2 Requirement in Gamma Interferon Production: Lymphokine Activity of a Neuroendocrine Hormone. *Journal of Immunology*, 1982; 139:983-986.

42. Geenen, V., Robert, F., Fatemi, M., Defresne, M.P., Boniver, J., Legros, J.J., et al. Vasopressin and Oxytocin: Thymic Signals and Receptors in T Cell Ontogeny. In: Yoshida, S., Share, L., editors. *Recent Progress in Posterior Pituitary Hormones*. Amsterdam: Elsevier Science Publishers, B.V., 1988:303-310.

43. Elands, J., Resink, A., De Kloet, E. R. Neurohypophyseal Hormone Receptors in the Rat Thymus, Spleen, and Lymphocytes. *Endocrinology,* 1990; 126:2703-2711.

44. Elands, J., Resink, A., De Kloet, E. R. Oxytocin Receptors in the Rat Thymic Gland. *European Journal of Pharmacology*, 1988; 151:345-346.

45. Geenen, V., Defresne, M.P., Robert, F., Legros, J.J,. Franchimont, P., Boniver, J. The Neurohormonal Thymic Microenvironment: Immunocytochemical Evidence that Thymic Nurse Cells Are Neurendocrine Cells. *Neuroendocrinology,* 1988; 47:365-368.

46. Caldwell, J.D., Walker, C., Noonan, L., Peterson, G., Pedersen, C.A., Mason, G. Thymic Oxytocin Receptors During Development and After Steroid Treatments in Adults. *Annals of the New York Academy Of Science,* 1995; 429-432.

47. Bussolati, G., Cassoni, P., Negro, F., Stella, A., Sapino, A. Effect of Oxytocin on Breast Carcinoma Cell Growth. In: Ivell, R., Russell, J.A. *CIN: Cellular and Molecular Approaches in Medicine and Research*. New York: Plenum Press, 1995:553-554.

48. Page, S.R., Ang, V.T.Y., Jackson, R., Nussey, S.S. The Effect of Oxytocin on the Plasma Glucagon Response to Insulin-Induced Hypoglycemia in Man. *Diabetes & Metabolism*, 1990; 16:252.

49. Milenov, K., Kasakov, L. Effect of Synthetic Oxytocin on the Motor and Bioelectrical Activity of the Stomach and Small Intestines. *Acta Physiological Bulg,* 1979; 34:31-40.

50. Milenov, K. Effect of estradiol, progesterone and oxytocin on smooth muscle activity. In: Bulbring, E., Shuba, M.F., editors. *Physiology of Smooth Muscle*. New York: Raven Press, 1976:395-402.

51. McCarthy, M.M. Estrogen Modulation of Oxytocin and Its Relation to Behavior. In: Ivell, R., Russell, J.A., editors. *OXYTOCIN: Cellular and Molecular Approaches in Medicine and Research*. New York: Plenum Press, 1995:235-246.

APPENDIX

52. Arletti, R., Bertolini, A. Oxytocin Acts as an Antidepressant in Two Animal Models of Depression. *Life Sciences,* 4195; 1725-1729.

53. Buchwald, D., Garrity, D. Comparison of patients with chronic fatigue syndrome: A comprehensive approach to its definition and study. *Arch Intern Med,* 1994; 154:2049-2053.

54. Argiolas, A., Gessa, G.L. Central Functions of Oxytocin. *Neuroscience & Biobehavioral Reviews,* 1991; 15:217-231.

55. Jenkins, J.S., Nussey, S.S. The Role of Oxytocin: Present Concepts. *Clinical Endocrinology,* 1991; 34:515-525.

56. Sukhof, R.R., Walker, L.C., Rance, N.E., Price, D.L., Young, III. Vasopressin and Oxytocin Gene Expression in the Human Hypothalamus. *J Comparative Neurology,* 1993; 337:306

57. Fabian, M., Forsling, M.L., Jones, J.J., Pryor, J.S. The Clearance and Antidiuretic Potency of Neurohypophyseal Hormones in Man and Their Plasma Binding and Stability. *J Physiol,* 1969; 204:653-668.

58. Pellegrino, M.J., Van Fossen, D., Gordon, C., Ryan, J.M., Waylonis, G.W. Prevalence of Mitral Valve Prolapse in Primary Fibromyalgia: A Pilot Investigation. *Arch Phys Med Rehabil,* 1989; 70:541-543.

59. Triadafilopoulos, G., Simms, R.W., Goldenberg, D.L. Bowel Dysfunction in Fibromyalgia Syndrome. *Digestive Diseases and Sciences,* 1991; 36:59-64.

60. Wilke, W.S. FIBROMYALGIA: Recognizing and addressing the multiple interrelated factors. *Postgraduate Medicine,* 1996; 100:153-170.

61. Hiltz, R.E., Gupta, P.K., Maher, K.A., Blank, C.A., Benjamin, S.B., Katz, P., et al. Low Threshold of Visceral Nociception and Significant Objective Upper Gastrointestinal Pathology in Patients with Fibromyalgia Syndrome. *Arthritis & Rheumatism,* 1993; 36:93.

62. Whitehead, W.E., Holtkotter, B., Enck, P., Hoelzl, R., Holmes, K.D., Anthony, J., et al. Tolerance for Rectosigmoid Distention in Irritable Bowel Syndrome. *Gastroenterology,* 1990; 98:1187-1192.

63. Granges, G., Littlejohn, G. Pressure Pain Threshold in Pain-Free Subjects, in Patients with Chronic Regional Pain Syndromes, and in Patients with Fibromyalgia Syndrome. *Arthritis and Rheumatism,* 1993; 36:642-646.

64. Lurie, M., Caidahl, K., Johansson, G., Bake B. Respiratory function in Chronic Primary Fibromyalgia. *Scand J Rehab Med,* 1990; 22:151-155.

65. Wallace, D.J. Genitourinary Manifestations of Fibrositis: An Increased Association with the Female Urethral Syndrome. *The Journal of Rheumatology,* 1990; 17:238-239.

66. Simm, R.W., Goldenberg, D.L. Symptoms Mimicking Neurologic Disorders in Fibromyalgia. *The Journal of Rheumatology,* 1988; 15:1271-1273.

67. Rainey, W.E., Bird, I.M., Mason, J.I., Carr, B.R. Angiotensin II Receptors on Human Fetal Adrenel Cells. *American Journal of Obstetrics and Gynecology,* 1988; 122:2012-2018.

68. Parker, L.N. Adrenarche and Puberty. In: Parker, L.N., editor. *Adrenal Androgens in Clinical Medicine.* San Diego: Academic Press, Inc., 1989:98-117.

69. Hornsby, P.J. Biosynthesis of DHEAS by the Human Adrenal Cortex and Its Age-Related Decline. In: Bellino, F.L., Daynes, R.A., Hornsby, P.J., Lavrin, D.H., Nestler, J.E., editors. *Dehydroepiandrosterone (DHEA) And Aging.* New York: Annals of the New York Academy of Sciences, 1995:29-46.

70. Parker, L.N. Skin Disease. In: Parker, L.N., editor. *Adrenal Androgens in Clinical Medicine.* San Diego: Academic Press, Inc. 1989:339-351.

71. Spector, T.D., Thompson, P.W., Perry, A., Grunnos, A.C. The Relationship Between Sex Steroids and Bone Mineral Content in Women Soon After Menopause. *Clin Endoc,* 1991; 34:37-41.

72. Szathmari, M. DHEA Hormone and Osteoporosis Prevention. *Osteoporosis Int,* 1994; 4:84-88.

73. Garg, M., Bondada, S. Reversal of age associated decline in immune response in PNU immune vaccine by supplementation with the steroid hormone DHEA. *Infect Immun,* 1993; 61:2238-2241.

74. Araneo, B.A,. Dowell, T., Diegel, M., Daynes, R.A. Dehydrotestosterone Exerts a Depressive Influence on the Production of Interleukin-4 and y-Interferon, But Not IL-2 by Activated Murine T Cells. *Blood,* 1991; 78:688-699.

75. Daynes, R.A., Araneo, B.A. Natural Regulators of T-Cell Lymphokine Production In Vivo. *Journal of Immunotherapy,* 1992; 12:174-179.

76. Ridson, G., Cope, J., Bennett, M. Mechanisms of Chemoprevention by Dietary Dehydroisoandrosterone. *American Journal of Pathology,* 1990; 136:759-769.

77. Ridson, G., Kumar, V., Bennett, M. Differential Effects of Dehydroepiandrosterone (DHEA) on Murine Lymphopoiesis and Myelopoiesis. *Exp Hematol,* 1991; 19:128-131.

78. Daynes, R.A., Dudley, D.J., Araneo, B.A. Regulation of Murine Lymphokine Production In Vitro. *Eur J Immunol,* 1990; 20:793-802.

79. Neifeld, J.P., Lippman, M.E., Tormey, D.C. Steroid Hormone Receptors in Normal Human Lymphocytes. *Journal of Biological Chemistry,* 1977; 252:2972-2977.

80. Parker, L.N., Levin, E.R., Lifrak, E.T. Evidence for Adrenocortical Adaptation to Severe Illness. *Journal of Clinical Endocrinology and Metabolism,* 1985; 947-952.

81. Gordon, G.B., Bush, T.L., Helzlsouer, K.J., Miller, S.R, Comstock, G.W. Relationship of Serum Levels of Dehydroepiandrosterone and Dehydroepiandrosterone Sulfate to the Risk of Developing Postmenopausal Breast Cancer. *Cancer Research,* 1990; 50:3859-3862.

82. Daynes, R.A., Araneo, B.A., Dowel, T.A. Regulation of Murine Lymphokine Production In Vivo. III The Lymphoid Microenvironment Exerts Regulatory Influences Over T Helper Function. *J Exp Med,* 1991; 171:979-996.

83. Gordon, G.B., Shantz, L.M., Talalay, P. Modulation of Growth, Differentiation and Carcinogenesis by Dehydroepiandrosterone. *Advances in Enzyme Regulation,* 1987; 26:355-383.

84. Henderson, E., Yang, J.Y., Schwartz, A. Dehydroepiandrosterone (DHEA) and Synthetic DHEA Analogs Are Modest Inhibitors of HIV-1 IIIB-Replication. *Aids Research and Human Retroviruses,* 1992; 8:625-631.

85. Jacobson, M.A., Fusaro, R.E., Galmarini, M., Lang, W. Decreased Serum Dehydroepiandrosterone Is Associated with an Increased Progression of Human Immunodeficiency Virus in Men with CD4 Cell Counts of 200-499. *Journal of Infectious Diseases,* 1991; 64:864-868.

APPENDIX

86. Loria, R.M., Inge, T.H., Cook, S.S., Szakai, A.K., Regelson, W. Up-Regulation of the Immune Response and Resistance to Virus Infection with Dehydroepiandrosterone (DHEA). In: Lardy, H., Stratman, F., editors. *Hormones, Thermogenesis, and Obesity.* New York: Elsevier Science Publisher, B.V., 1989:427-437.

87. Schwartz, A.G., Whitcomb, J.M., Nyce, J.W., Lewbart, M.L., Pashko, L.L. Dehydroepiandrosterone and Structural Analogs: A New Class of Cancer Chemopreventive Agents. *Advances in Cancer Research,* 1988; 51:390-421.

88. Schwartz, A.G., Pashko, L.L., Whitcomb, J.M. Inhibition of Tumor Development by Dehydroepiandrosterone and Related Steroids. *Toxicologic Pathology,* 1986; 14:362.

89. Schwartz, A.G., Hard, G.C., Pashko, L.L., Abou-Gharbia, M., Swern, D. Dehydroepiandrosterone: An Anti-Obesity and Anti-Carcinogenic Agent. *Nutrition and Cancer,* 1981; 3:46-53.

90. Helzlsouer, K.J., Gordon, G.B., Alberg, A.J., Bush, T.L., Comstock, G.W. Relationship of Prediagnostic Serum Levels of Dehydroepiandrosterone and Dehydroepiandrosterone Sulfate to the Risk of Developing Premenopausal Breast Cancer. *Cancer Research,* 1992; 52:1-4.

91. Zumoff, B., Levin, J., Rosenfeld, R.S., Markham, M,. Strain, G.W., Fukushina, D.K. Abnormal 24-Hr. Mean Plasma Concentrations of Dehydroisoandrosterone and Dehydroisoandrosterone Sulfate in Women with Primary Operable Breast Cancer. *Cancer Research,* 1981; 41:3360-3363.

92. Stahl, F., Schnorr, D., Pilz, C., Dorner G. Dehydroepiandrosterone (DHEA) Levels in Patients with Prostatic Cancer, Heart Diseases and Surgery Stress. *Exp Clin Endocrinol,* 1992; 99:68-70.

93. Gordon, G.B., Helzlsover, K.J., Alberg. Serum levels of dehydroepiandrosterone and DHEA Sulfate and the risk of developing gastric cancer. *Cancer Epidemiol Biomakers Prev,* 1993; 2:33-35.

94. Gordon, G.B., Helzlsover, K.J., Comstock, G.W. Serum levels of DHEA and its sulfate, and the risk of developing bladder cancer. *Cancer Research,* 1991; 51:1366-1369.

95. Prough, R.A., Lei, X.D., Xiao, G.H., Wu, H.Q., Geoghegan, T.E., Webb, S.J. Regulation of Cytochromes P450 by DHEA and Its Anticarcinogenic Action. In: Bellino, F.L., Daynes, R.A., Hornsby, P.J., Lavrin, D.H., Nestler, J.E., editors. Dehydroepiandrosterone And Aging. *Annals of the New York Academy of Sciences,* 1995:187-199.

96. Milewich, L., Catalina, F., Bennett, M. Pieotropic Effects of Dietary DHEA. In: Bellino, FL, Daynes, R.A., Hornsby, P.J., Lavrin, D.H., Nestler, J.E., editors. Dehydroepiandrosterone And Aging. *Annals of the New York Academy of Sciences,* 1995:149-170.

97. Parker, L.N. Control of Adrenal Androgen Secretion. In: Parker, L.N., editor. *Adrenal Androgens in Clinical Medicine.* San Diego: Academic Press, Inc., 1989:30-57.

98. Parker, L.N., Odell, W.D. Control of Adrenal Androgen Secretion. *Endocrine Reviews,* 1980; 1:393-411.

99. McIntosh, M.K., Berdanier, C.D. Influence of Dehydroepiandrosterone (DHEA) on the Thyroid Hormone Status of BHE/cdb Rats. *J Nutr Biochem,* 1992; 3:194-199.

100. Schroick, E.D., Buffington, C.K., Hubert, G.D., Kurtz, B.R., Kitabchi, A.E., Buster, J.E., et al. Divergent Correlations of Circulating Dehydroepiandrosterone Sulfate and Testosterone with Insulin Levels and Insulin Receptor Binding. *Journal of Clinical Endocrinology and Metabolism,* 1988; 66:1329-1331.

101. Haning, Jr., R.V., Flood, C.A., Hackett, R.J., Loughlin, J.S., McClure, N., Longcope, C. Replacement of Dehydroepiandrosterone (DHEA) Enhances T-Lymphocyte Insulin Binding in Postmenopausal Women. *Fertil Steril,* 1995; 63:1027-1031.

102. Davis, S.R., Burger, H.G. Androgens and the Postmenopausal Woman. *J of Clinical Endocrinology and Metabolism,* 1996; 81:2759-2763.

103. Lardy, H., Su, C.Y., Kneer, N., Wielgus, S. Dehydroepiandrosterone Induces Enzymes that Permit Thermogenesis and Decrease Metabolic Efficiency. In: Lardy, H., Stratman, F., editors. *Hormones Thermogenesis and Obesity.* New York: Elsevier Science Publisher, 1989:415-426.

104. Song, M.K.H., Grieco, D., Rall, J.E., Nikodem, V.M. Thyroid Hormone Mediated Transcription Activation of the Rat Liver Malic Enzyme Gene by Dehydroepiandrosterone. *J Biol Chem,* 1989; 264:18985.

105. Marrarer, M,. Prough, R.A., Frenkel, R.A., Milewich, L. Dehydroepiandrosterone Feeding and Protein Phosphorylation, Phosphates, and Lipogenic Enzymes in Mouse Liver. *Proc Soc Exp Biol Med,* 1990; 193(2):110-117.

106. Sonka, J. *Acta Univ,* 1976; 71:146-171.

107. Sonka, J., Stravkova, M. *Aggressologie 5,* 1970; 5:421-426.

108. Lanthier, A., Pantalioni, P. *J Steroid Biochem,* 1987; 28:697-701.

109. Dennenbaum, R., Hoffman, G., Oertel, G.W. *Horm Metab,* 1972; 4:383-385.

110. Hoffman, G., Modsches, B., Dohler, U. *Rach Derm Forsch,* 1972; 243:18-30.

111. Holzman, H., Krapp, R., Morsches, B. *Aerptliche Forsch,* 1971; 25:345-353.

112. Holzman, H., Morsches, B., Knapp, R., Hoffman, G. *Arch Derm Forsch,* 1973; 247:23-28.

113. Lang, R.E., Heil, W.E., Ganten, D., Hermann, K., Unger, T., Rascher, W. Oxytocin Unlike Vasopressin Is a Stress Hormone in the Rat. *Neuroendocrinology,* 1983; 37:314-316.

114. Koo, E., Feher, K.G., Feher, T., Fust, G. *Klin Woehenschr,* 1983; 61:701-717.

115. Felt, V., Starka, l. Metabolic Effects of Dehydroepiandrosterone and Atromid in Patients with Hyperlipaemia. *Corvasa,* 1966; 8:40-48.

116. Honer, W.G.T., Lightman, C. No Effect of Naloxone on Plasma Oxytocin in Normal Men. *Psychoneuroendocrinology,* 1986; 11:245-248.

117. Casson, P.R., Andersen, R.N., Herrod, H.G., Stentz, F.B., Straughn, A.B., Abraham, G.E., et al. Oral Dehydroepiandrosterone in Physiologic Doses Modulates Immune Function in Postmenopausal Women. *American Journal of Obstetrics and Gynecology,* 1994; 169:1536-1539.

118. Calabrese, V.P., Isaacs, E.R., Regelson, W. Dehydroepiandrosterone in Multiple Sclerosis: Positive Effects on the Fatigue Syndrome in a Non-Randomized Study. In: Kalimi, M., Regelson, W., editors. *Biologic Role of Dehydroepiandrosterone (DHEA).* New York: Walter de Gruyter, 1990:95-100.

119. Roberts, E., Fauble, T. Oral Dehydroepiandrosterone in Multiple Sclerosis: Results of a Phase One, Open Study. In: Kalimi, M., Regelson, W., editors. *Biologic Role of Dehydroepiandrosterone (DHEA).* New York: Walter de Gruyter, 1990:81-93.

APPENDIX

120. Regelson, W., Kalimi, M., Loria, R.M. DHEA: Some Thoughts as to its Biologic and Clinical Action. In: Kalimi, M., Regelson, W., editors. *Biologic Role of Dehydroepiandrosterone*. New York: Walter de Gruyter, 1990:405-445.

121. Wolkowitz, O.M., Reus, V.I., Roberts, E., Manfredi, F., Chan, T., Ormiston, S., et al. Antidepressant and Cognition-Enhancing Effect of DHEA in Major Depression. In: Bellino, F.L., Daynes., R.A., Hornsby, P.J., Lavrin, D.H., Nestler, J.E., editors. Dehydroepiandrosterone And Aging. New York: *Annals of the New York Academy of Science,* 1995:337-339.

122. Russell, I.J., Michalek, J.E., Vipraio, G.A., Fletcher, E.M., Javors, M.A., Bowden, C.A. Serum Serotonin and Platelet 3H-Impramine Binding Receptor Density in Patients with Fibromyalgia/Fibrositis Syndrome. *J Rheum,* 1991.

123. Russell, I.J., Michalek, J.E., Vipraio, G.A. Serotonin [5HT] in Serum and Platelets [PLT] from Fibromyalgia Patients [FM] and Normal Controls. *Journal of Musculoskeletal Pain,* 1995; 3:144

124. Russell, I.J. Neurohormonal: Abnormal Laboratory Findings Related to Pain and Fatigue in Fibromyalgia. *Journal of Musculoskeletal Pain,* 1995; 3:59-65.

125. Fujii, E., Oku, M. Effects of Steroid Hormones on Change in [Ca2+] and on PI Response Following Oxytocin Stimulation in Cultured Human Myometrial Cells. *Acta Obst Gynaec Jpn,* 1995; 47:94-100.

126. Margolis, R.U., Press, R., Altszuler, N., Stewart, M.A. Inositol Production by the Brain in Normal and Alloxan-Diabetic Dogs. *Brain Research,* 1971; 28:535-539.

127. Berridge, M.J. Inositol Trisphosphate, Calcium Lithium and Cell Signaling. *JAMA,* 1989; 262:1834-1842.

128. Fein, A., Payne, R., Corson, D.W., Berridge, M.J., Irvine, R.F. Photoreceptor Excitation and Adaption by Inositol 1,4,5-Trisphosphate. *Nature,* 1984; 311:157-160.

129. Sakakibara, M., Alkon, D., Neary, J.T., Heldman, E. Inositol Trisphosphate Regulation of Photoreceptor. *MemJ Biophysial Society,* 1986; 50:797-803.

130. Ehrlich, B.E., Watras, J. Inositol 1,4,5 Trisphosphate Activates a Channel from Smooth Muscle Sarcoplasmic Reticulum. *Nature,* 1988; 336:583-586.

131. Irvine, R.F., Moor, R.M., Pollock, W.K., Smith, P.M., Wreggett, K.A. Inositol Phosphates: Proliferation, Metabolism and Function. *Phil Trans Soc Lond,* 1988; B320:281-298.

132. Berridge, M.J., Irvine, R.F. Inositol Trisphosphate: A Novel Second Messenger in Cellular Transduction. *Nature,* 1984; 312:315-321.

133. Busse, R., Mulsch, A., Fleming, I., Hecker, M. Mechanisms of Nitric Oxide Release from the Vascular Endothelium. *Circulation,* 1993; 87-V:18-25.

134. Goadsby, P.J., Kaube, H., Hoskin, K.L. Nitric Oxide synthesis couples cerebral blood flow and metabolism. *Brain Research,* 1992; 595:167-170.

135. Chowienczyk, P.J., Cockcroft, J.R., Ritter, J.M. Blood flow responses to intra-arterial acetylcholine in man: effects of basal flow and conduit vessel length. *Clinical Science,* 1994; 87:45-51.

136. Russell, I.J., Vipraio, G.A., Abraham, G.E. Red Cell Nucleotide [RCN] Abnormalities in Fibromyalgia Syndrome. *Arthritis and Rheumatism,* 1993; 36:S223.

137. Russell, I.J. Biochemical Abnormalities in Fibromyalgia Syndrome. *The Journal of Musculoskeletal Pain,* 1994; 2:101-115.

138. Abraham, G.E., Flechas, J.D. Management of Fibromyalgia: Rationale for the Use of Magnesium and Malic Acid. *Journal of Nutritional Medicine,* 1992; 3:49-59.

139. Clauw, D.J., Ward, K., Katz, P., Sunder, R. Muscle Intracellular Magnesium Levels Correlate with Pain Tolerance in Fibromyalgia (FM). *Arthritis and Rheumatism,* 1994; 37:R29.

140. Clauw, D., Blank, C., Hewett-Meulman, J., Katz, P. Low Tissue Levels of Magnesium in Fibromyalgia. *Arthritis and Rheumatism,* 1993; 61.

141. Bengtsson, A., Henriksson, K.G., Larsson, J. Reduced High-Energy Phosphate Levels in The Painful Muscles of Patients with Primary Fibromyalgia. *Arthritis and Rheumatism,* 1986; 29:817-821.

142. Wortmann, R.L. Searching For The Cause of Fibromyalgia: Is There A Defect In Energy Metabolism? *Arthritis and Rheumatism,* 1994; 37:790-793.

143. McCully, K.K., Natelson, B.H., Iotti, S. J.S.J. Reduced Oxidative Muscle Metabolism in Chronic Fatigue Syndrome. *Muscle & Nerve,* 1996; May:621-625.

144. Bessman, S.P., Savabi, F. The Role of the Phosphocreatine Energy Shuttle in Exercise and Muscle Hypertrophy. In: Taylor, A.W., Golnick, P.D., Green, H.J., Ianuzzo, C.D., Noble, E.G., Metivier, G.S., editors. *Biochemistry of Exercise.* Champaign: Human Kinetics Publishers, 1990:167-178.

145. Spriet, L.L., Soderlund, K., Bergstrom, M., Hultman, E. Anaerobic Energy Release in Skeletal Muscle During Electrical Stimulation in Men. *American Physiological Society,* 1987; 611-615.

146. Wallimann, T., Wyss, M., Brdiczka, D., Nicolay, K. Intracellular Compartmentation, Structure and Function of Creatine Kinase Isoenzymes in Tissues with High and Fluctuating Energy Demands: The 'Phosphocreatine Circuit' for Cellular Energy Homeostasis. *Biochem J,* 1992; 281:21-40.

147. Boelen, A., Platvoet-ter, Shiphorst, M.C., Wiersinga, W.M. Soluble Cytokine Receptors and the Low 3,5,3' Triiodothyronine Syndrome in Patients with Nonthyroidal Disease. *J Clinical Endocrinology,* 1995; 80:971-976.

148. Szabolcs, I., Weber, M., Kovacs, Z., Irsy, G., Goth, M., Halzsz, T., et al. The Possible Reason For Serum 3,3'5' - (Reverse) Triiodothyronine Increase In Old People. *Acta,* 1982; 39:11-17.

149. Surks, M.L., Sievert, R. Drugs and Thyroid Function. *New England J Med,* 1995; 333:1688-1693.

150. Vagenakis, A.G. Division of Peripheral Thyroxine Metabolism From Activating To Inactivating Pathways During Complete Fasting. *J Clin Endocrine Metab,* 1975; 41:191-194.

151. Elliott, D.L. Sustained Depression of Resting Metabolic Rate After Massive Weight Loss. *Am J Clin Nutr,* 1989; 49 (1):93-96.

152. Komorowski, J. Increased Interleukin-2 Level in Patients with Primary Hypothyroidism. *Clinical Immunology & Immunopathology,* 1992; 63:200-202.

153. Arthur, J.R., Nicol, F., Beckett, G.J. Selenium Deficiency, Thyroid Hormone Metabolism, and Thyroid Hormone Deiodinases. *Am J Clin Nutr Suppl,* 1993; 57:236S-239S.

154. Wartofsky, L., Burman, K.D. Alterations in Thyroid Function in Patients with Systematic Illness: the "Euthyroid Sick Syndrome." *Endocrine Reviews,* 1982; 3:164-217.

234

155. Wilke, W.S., Sheeler, L.R., Makarowlki, W.S. Hypothyroidism Presenting Symptoms of Fibrositis. *Journal of Rheumatology*, 1987; 8:626-631.

156. Meeck, G., Riedel, W. Thyroid Function in Patients with the Fibromyalgia Syndrome. *Journal of Rheumatology*, 1992; 19:1120-1122.

157. Jurell, K.C., Zanetos, M.A., Orsinelli, A., Tallo, D., Waylonis, G.W. Fibromyalgia: A Study of Thyroid Function and Symptoms. *Journal of Musculoskeletal Pain*, 1996; 4:49-59.

158. Russell, I.J., Michalek, J.E., Flechas, J.D., Abraham, G.E. Treatment of Fibromyalgia Syndrome with Super Malic: A Randomized, Double Blind, Placebo Controlled, Crossover Pilot Study. *Journal of Rheumatology*, 1995; 22:5:953-958.

159. Qde, Raeve, L., De Schepper, J., Smitz, J. Prepubertal Acne: A Cutaneous Marker of Androgen Excess? *J of the American Academy of Dermatology,* 1995; 32:181-184.

160. Baulieu, E.E., Robel, P. Neurosteroids: A New Brain Function? *J Steroid Biochem Molec Biol,* 1990; 37:395-403.

161. Baulieu, E.E. Steroid Hormones in the Brain: Several Mechanisms. Fuxe, K., Gustafsson, J.A., Wetlerberg, L., eds. *Steroid Hormone Regulation of the Brain*. Oxford Pergamon, 1975; 3-14.1975; 3-14.

162. Robel, P., Baulieu, E.E. Neurosteroids Biosynthesis and Function. *Trends Endocrinol Metab,* 1994; 5:1-9.

163. McEwen, B.S. Steroid Hormones Are Multifunctional Messengers to the Brain. *Trends Endocrinol Metab,* 1991; 62-67.

164. Robel, P., Kawa, Y., Corpechot, C., Zhong-Yi, H., Jung-Testas, I., Kabbadj, K., et al. Neurosteroids: Biosynthesis and Function of Pregnenolone and Dehydroepiandrosterone in the Brain. In: Motta, M., editor. *Brain Endocrinology,* Second Edition. New York: Raven Press, Ltd., 1991:105-131.

165. Freiss, E., Trachsel, L., Guldner, J., Schier, T., Steiger, A., Holsboe, F. DHEA Administration Increases Rapid Eye Movement Sleep and EEG Power in the Sigma Frequency Range. *American Physiological Society,* 1995; E107-E13.

166. Altura, B.M., Altura, B.T. Vascular Smooth Muscle and Neurohypopyseal Hormones Oxytocin. *Federation Proceedings,* 1977; 36:1853-1860.

167. Leckman, J.F., Goodman, W.K., North, W.G., Chappell, P.B., Price, L.H., Pauls, D.L., et al. Elevated Cerebrospinal Fluid Levels of Oxytocin in Obsessive Compulsive Disorder. *Arch Gen Psychiatry,* 1994; 51:782-792.

168. Flechas, J.D. Clinical Effect of Super Malic (SM), a Malic Acid/Magnesium Oral Supplement, on Fibromyalgia Patients: Long Term Follow-up. *Journal of Musculoskeletal Pain,* 1995; 3:54.

169. Matz, R. Magnesium: Deficiencies and Therapeutic Uses. *Hospital Practice,* 1993; 79-92.

Medically reviewed and edited by Jorges D. Flechas, M.D., M.P.H.

Address: **Dr. Jorges D. Flechas**
724 5th Avenue West
Hendersonville, NC 28739
Phone (828) 693-3015 • Fax (828) 693-4471

APPENDIX

My Approach to Fibromyalgia

by Michael McNett, M.D.

When approaching a patient with fibromyalgia, my first responsibility is to make sure that they actually have FMS. I commonly see patients misdiagnosed with fibromyalgia who actually have diffuse myofascial pain syndrome, polymyalgia rheumatica, or a variety of other diseases. The history, physical, and initial lab tests often help to establish whether the patient actually has another condition or whether another illness (hypothyroidism, rheumatoid arthritis, etc.) is contributing to their problem.

Once the diagnosis is confirmed, our clinic offers a multidisciplinary approach; this has been shown in numerous studies to be the best form of treatment. Our program includes the following components:

- ▲ **Provides optimal medication management for pain, fatigue, sleep disorder, associated symptoms, and underlying causes.**

- ▲ **Includes a structural/postural analysis and follow up treatment.**

- ▲ **We provide myofascial trigger point therapy, osteopathic manipulation, self-care training(which includes appropriate stretching and strengthening exercises tailored to each individual which can be done at home) and trigger point (TP) injections when appropriate.**

- ▲ **Prolotherapy treatment is available.**

- ▲ **Nutritional counseling for candida and other dietary concerns, such as reactive hypoglycemia.**

- ▲ **Counseling for grief work, stress management, interpersonal relationships, psychological reactions such as depression and anxiety, and keeping healthy attitudes about the illness.**

In this article, I will detail how I provide optimal management of a patient's medications.

Medication management is very complex and must be structured to each individual – I could write an entire book about this subject alone. In general, medical management has three aspects:

1. Treating symptoms.

2. Controlling other conditions that are commonly associated with fibromyalgia such as: depression, irritable bowel syndrome, migraine headaches, sleep disorder, pain, etc.

3. Treating possible underlying problems that may be causing the fibromyalgia. Of course, the medications should be chosen to minimize interactions with the patient's other medications, should cause as few side effects as possible, and, ideally, would be inexpensive. I usually start at low levels and gradually increase the dose, since fibromyalgia patients are so sensitive to side effects.

Medications to treat fibromyalgia symptoms come from several general classes. First are the antidepressants. Many fibromyalgia patients are reluctant to take these because they feel it indicates that they have a mental problem, and they're sick and tired of being told "it's all in your head." In fact, that has nothing to do with why we use antidepressants in fibromyalgia. Some antidepressants are sedating and not only put a person to sleep but actually improve the quality of their sleep by increasing the amount of time they spend in deep, non-dreaming sleep. Other antidepressants (especially those that raise the concentration of the neurotransmitter norepinephrine) can cause the spinal cord to act as a "pain filter," keeping pain signals from reaching the brain where they would be experienced. Some antidepressants can also increase energy, counteracting the fatigue of fibromyalgia. And, since fibromyalgia patients commonly get depressed due to the pain and horrible life impact of the disease, antidepressants can prevent a difficult situation from becoming worse—as if fibromyalgia isn't bad enough without depression adding to it!

Sleep agents are important in fibromyalgia, since poor sleep not only turns a person's night into a nightmare, but it also contributes to fatigue during the day, undermines job performance, hurts relationships by making the person irritable – I could go on and on. Sedating antidepressants are the first line here, since they're not addictive, improve sleep quality, are inexpensive and well-tolerated. I don't like tricyclic antidepressants like amitriptyline (Elavil), nortriptyline (Pamelor) or cyclobenzaprine (Flexeril) because they cause a nasty increase in brain fog in the majority of patients treated with them – something fibromyalgia patients struggle with anyway. I also don't like benzodiazepines (the Valium/Klonopin class) because they're potentially addictive, don't increase deep sleep, and interfere with the stress response (the "HPA axis").

In general, I haven't had much success with muscle relaxants. They don't relax trigger points, and they tend to be too sedating for most of my patients to tolerate. Sometimes they can be useful to help with sleep.

I also rarely prescribe arthritis medication. The recent controversy over heart problems with COX-II inhibitors (Vioxx, et. al.) has cast doubts on their use. The other major class is a group of aspirin-related compounds known as nonsteroidal anti-inflammatory agents (NSAIDs). First of all, they don't work very well for most fibromyalgia patients. Secondly, they interfere with platelets in the blood, which prevents clotting. Thirdly, they cause ulcers. (And the last thing you need with a bleeding ulcer is a drug interfering with clotting!) Every three years we kill as many people in the US with NSAIDs as died in the entire Vietnam War. Certainly, these medications should only be used in people who get a major benefit from them, and most fibro patients don't.

Anticonvulsants (drugs used to treat epilepsy) can be very helpful for fibromyalgia pain. An easy way to understand how they work is to think of them as making nerves less irritable. This is how they prevent seizures. Since they also make pain nerves less irritable, they can help fibromyalgia pain, as well. Since many of these medications work in different ways, a patient may have to try several before deciding on the best one for them.

Pain medications are important in fibromyalgia. Studies have shown that fibromyalgia patients truly are suffering:

- ▲ **They have high levels of pain-causing chemicals in their spinal cord**
- ▲ **Microelectrode studies have documented hyperactivity of pain processing nerves in the spinal cord**
- ▲ **PET and functional MRI scans have shown that the pain areas of the brain are extremely active in fibromyalgia patients**

As a result, I consider it cruel not to provide pain relief. Acetaminophen (Tylenol) can be used if it works, but many patients need something stronger. Tramadol (Ultram) is a virtually non-addictive opiate (narcotic) medication that I have used with great success in my patients; if necessary, it can be made more effective by taking dextramethorphan (a common cough suppressant) along with it. If absolutely necessary—and only as a last resort—I'll use stronger opiates such as codeine, hydrocodone, oxycodone, methadone, or morphine. For me to prescribe these, the patient must be taking the other, non-addictive medications listed previously and must be participating in the multidisciplinary aspects of our program.

The fatigue of fibromyalgia can be intense and even crippling. It can cost a person their job or prevent them from doing simple housework. If it's severe, stimulants can be used, though they're controversial. The nutritional supplements malic acid and ginseng are mildly beneficial. Caffeine and over-the-counter decongestants help some people, though they often have side effects. Some antidepressants and anticonvulsants have stimulant properties and are generally well-tolerated. Modafenil (Provigil) is a stronger stimulant which tends not to cause the hypertension and irregular heartbeats that can occur with amphetamines, which I generally avoid.

Treating other medical conditions associated with fibromyalgia is important to a patient's life, as well. These conditions include migraines, myofascial pain syndrome, sleep apnea, depression, anxiety (including panic disorder), irritable bowel, irritable bladder, vulvovaginitis, restless legs, and sicca syndrome (dry eyes and mouth). While a full discussion of these treatments is beyond the scope of this paper, suffice it to say that there are a number of medications available to treat each of these conditions, and patients should not settle for being told that there's nothing that can be done for them.

Treating underlying causes is difficult, since we know so little about what causes fibromyalgia. Still, some treatments show promise at improving overall fibromyalgia symptoms. It is my belief that, by studying how these treatments may be producing their benefit, they could lead us to a breakthrough in understanding what causes fibromyalgia. It should be noted that some of these conditions are viewed as alternative medicine by many doctors. I have reviewed them in detail and fully believe that there is good scientific evidence for them and that they will be accepted by the medical community once rigorous scientific studies had documented their benefit. Our clinic is in the process of setting up a research foundation to perform these studies. Because fibromyalgia is a condition which may have a number of underlying causes, one or more of these therapies may need to be used in a specific individual. Since these treatments and/or conditions are detailed elsewhere in this book, I'll simply list them here:

▲ **Treating candida hypersensitivity syndrome**

▲ **Treating hidden hypothyroidism**

▲ **The use of pramipexole (Mirapex)**

▲ **Treating adrenal depletion syndrome**

▲ **The use of sodium oxybate (Xyrem)**

▲ **Guaifenesin treatment**

▲ **Testing for a growth hormone deficiency and use of the appropriate treatment**

▲ **Appropriate diagnosis and referral for neurological problems such as Chiari Syndrome or cervical cord compression**

▲ **Treating chronic subclinical infections**

▲ **Determining food allergies (including IgG)**

In summary, there is a tremendous amount that can be done to help fibromyalgia patients. Proper use of medications as well as the other aspects of our multidisciplinary program has provided a substantial benefit in the large majority of our patients—many of whom had been told by their other doctors that there was no more help for them. We even have a significant number of people who are in complete remission. Fibromyalgia patients are suffering, and there's a lot that can be done to improve them.

Never give up hope.

Medically reviewed and edited by Michael McNett, M.D.

Address: **Dr. Michael McNett**
Fibromyalgia Treatment Centers of America
4332 N. Elston
Chicago, Illinois 60641
Phone: 773-604-5321 • Fax 773-604-5231
www.ftcoa.com

Protocol for Fibromyalgia Treatment

By Thomas J. Romano, M.D., Ph.D., FACP, FACR

Dr. Romano is a compassionate and dedicated rheumatologist living and practicing in Martins Ferry, Ohio. He has treated many FMS patients, authored a number of research articles on the topic and is very interested in the treatment of fibromyalgia. He serves on the Board of Advisors and Board of Directors of the American Academy of Pain Management and is on the editorial board of the Journal of Musculoskeletal Pain. He has served as president of the AAPM Board of Directors and is chairman of its examination committee.

My approach to the fibromyalgia (FMS) patient is very similar to that of Travell and Simons with regard to patients with myofascial pain. That is, perpetuating factors need to be identified and eliminated/ameliorated in order for the patients to benefit from medical intervention. Typically, I look for nutritional inadequacies, metabolic and endocrine inadequacies, psychological factors, postural problems, concomitant inflammatory diseases such as lupus or rheumatoid arthritis, etc. and should one or several of these problems exist, all efforts would be made to correct the situation in order for the FMS treatment to be successful. For example, some patients with FMS have vitamin deficiencies typically of one or more of the B vitamins or vitamin C or they have an excessive amount of vitamin A. Some FMS patients have growth hormone, thyroid hormone or have other types of hormone imbalances. Of course, a history and physical examination should be done and appropriate testing be performed. Naturally, not every FMS patient can be tested for every conceivable perpetuating factor, but some elements of the history can tip off a clinician and point to a reasonable course of investigation. For example, a patient taking diuretics on a chronic basis might develop hypomagnesemia, hypokalemia and/or other electrolyte imbalances. A patient who complains of being cold might have low serum ferritin or a low level of thyroid hormone. When women preferentially gain a lot of weight in their mid section as well as having cold intolerance, decreased energy and deceased stamina, one should think of adult growth hormone deficiency. While thought to be rare, I have found it to be quite common in my patients who often have levels of insulin dependent growth factor one (a byproduct of growth hormone) far below what they should be. Once this is corrected, the patients tend to do a lot better with regards to many of the FMS symptoms. A thorough history and physical examination are critical and can alert the clinician to possible perpetuating factors. In a patient whose FMS seems to be resistant to medical intervention, getting vitamin levels is a reasonable strategy. I have observed that many patients with vitamin imbalances respond better to medical treatment after their vitamin imbalances are corrected.

Once perpetuating factors have been dealt with, I aim at correcting the stage four non-REM delta wave sleep disorder that seems to be characteristic of the vast majority of, if not all, FMS patients. Medications such as tricyclic drugs, serotonin reuptake inhibitors, mild tranquilizers, can all be used effectively in helping to alleviate the sleep disorder. I tend to question the patient about "jerking" at bedtime. This can alert the clinician that the patient may have nocturnal myoclonus and that the patient's abnormal movements may actually be interfering with stage four sleep. If the patient gives such a history or if the patient's spouse notices that the patient "jerks" or "twitches" at night, then a trial of Klonopin 0.5mg. po qhs will be a reasonable way of suppressing these abnormal movements, thus allowing the patient to sleep more normally. I frequently use medications for pain. I tend to use the nonacetylated salicylates such as Trilisate or Disalcid at a dose of up to 3 grams per day. These are anti-inflammatory medications with analgesic properties. They are selective prostaglandin inhibitors, so they do not predispose the patient to peptic ulcer disease, renal plasma flow problems (which could cause difficulty with fluid retention) and they do not thin the blood or cause easy bruising. Therefore they are the safest of all anti-inflammatories and seem to be fairly effective if used in conjunction with other medications for the treatment of patients with FMS. Newer pain medications such as Tramadol (Ultram) can also be useful if given in doses of approximately 50 mg. every four to six hours as needed for pain. If a patient needs a strong anti-inflammatory, the selective COX 2 inhibitors may be a good choice. They are safer than traditional NSAIDs. One can use celecoxib (Celebrex) 100 to 200 mg. per day, or Valdecoxib (Bextra) 10 to 20 mg. per day if necessary. I encourage the use of aerobic exercise where appropriate. Some patients are so deconditioned that they cannot do aerobics on land but need to start with an aquacise of water aerobics program and then graduate to more vigorous activity, but this should be done gradually and slowly so as not to cause relapses. One must, of course, understand that weather changes, increased activity, emotional stress, etc., can all make symptoms of FMS worse, so these must be taken into account in designing any type of exercise program. Furthermore, patients with myofascial bands, trigger points and muscle spasm may be unable to exercise on certain days or perform certain activities, so the patient must be thoroughly examined for these and these should be dealt with accordingly. I tend to use tender point and/or trigger point injections in my practice as the situation dictates. I don't think there is any ironclad rule one way or the other regarding the use of these injections, but I let the patient's condition dictate the type of therapy. For example, some FMS patients have no trigger points and their muscles do not appear to be very tight most of the time. These patients probable would not benefit from soft tissue injections. However, there are many fibromyalgia patients that have concomitant myofascial pain syndromes with trigger points, myofascial bands and spasm. Injection of such trigger points can be very useful in alleviating specific niduses of musculoskeletal pain.

I instruct my patients to obtain a book called *Pain Erasure* by Bonnie Prudden, Ballantine Books, New York, 1980. This book is a very useful manual in that it teaches patients why muscles get tight, how massage and myotherapy (i.e., ischemic compression) can be helpful and can serve as a good handbook for deep tissue massage. Oftentimes a member of the household, such as the patient's spouse or friend, can perform this treatment with good temporary relief of pain. I also use a lotion called Aurum lotion. It has been shown to be of help in patients with FMS and applying this lotion and massaging it into painful tight muscles three to four times a day has helped to ease pain in many of my patients. However, there are some patients that require the use of professional massage therapists to help ease muscle pain. I certainly would encourage this. However, I rarely ask the patients to see a massage therapist with no follow-up at home. Rather, I encourage the patient to use a massage therapist as a resource in getting rid of the most recalcitrant areas of muscle spasm and tightness, whereas most of the areas of tight muscle can be treated at home with regular massage and stretching.

I encourage FMS patients to ask questions, especially about new modalities, nutritional supplements, etc. However, I stress to the patient that one particular medication or mode of therapy is often insufficient in controlling most of the symptoms. Rather, a combination of avoidance of perpetuating/aggravating factors, the enhancement of stage four sleep, the use of anti-inflammatories/analgesic medication and/or the use of muscle relaxants, the "hands-on" treatment, such as myotherapy/ischemic compression and massage therapy, as well as the judicious use of injections, need to be done in a concerted and coordinated manner for the patient to achieve the proper result. It is important to understand that anxiety, self-doubt and depression can also mitigate against the successful outcome in patients with FMS. When necessary, referral of an FMS patient with such symptoms to a counselor and possibly even to a psychiatrist would be a reasonable thing to do and can be very therapeutic. It is important to explain to the patient that even though he or she may need to see a mental health professional, the FMS is not a psychological problem; rather, they may need specific psychological/psychiatric intervention in order to handle the stresses that this chronic condition imposes upon them and their loved ones.

The key to FMS treatment, in my opinion, is coordination of different modalities of care, individualization of treatment, education, support, and constant reassessment of the treatment modalities in order for the patient to get optimal care. This, of course, includes the identification and elimination/amelioration of perpetuating factors and the use of counseling where appropriate.

As with just about every other medical condition, FMS patients vary in many ways including the degree of severity of their illness. Many patients with FMS can work having to modify their behavior in terms of changing work hours, changing work conditions, making the work place more suitable ergonomically, taking rest periods if possible at work, etc. However despite the best efforts of patients and health care professionals, some patients with FMS are so severely affected that they are unable to work on a regular and sustained basis at any occupation in our society. Such patients should receive disability benefits since they are truly unable to work. It is important to note that many of the usual measures of impairment/disability, such as functional capacity assessments and even the AMA's book on the evaluation of permanent impairment have rate limitations in the assessment of FMS patients since FMS patients have an inability to perform repetitive muscular tasks, often have severe cognitive difficulties and have symptoms that wax and wane depending on many factors as noted above. Forcing or pressuring a patient to work in a situation that is unhealthy for them will only perpetuate their symptoms. Thus when the clinician takes a careful history, does a thorough physical examination and is guided by the appropriate lab tests, he has a much better chance of helping the patient with FMS to improve to the point where they can start enjoying life more and even continue working at their chosen career or job. However the physician should also be forthright in his opinion regarding the patient's disability/impairment status. Only in this way can the health care professional fulfill his obligations to both the patient and society.

Medically reviewed and edited by Thomas J. Romano, M.D., Ph.D., FACP, FACR

Address: **Dr. Thomas J. Romano**
205 North 5th Street
Martins Ferry, Ohio 43935
Phone: (740) 633-2449 • Fax (740) 633-2016

APPENDIX

Effective Treatment Approaches for CFS, Fibromyalgia and Myofascial Pain-

by Jacob Teitelbaum M.D.

For years, many of us have dreamt of the day when we would see the headline "EFFECTIVE TREATMENT FOR CHRONIC FATIGUE SYNDROME, FIBROMYALGIA (CFS/FMS), AND MYOFASCIAL PAIN SYNDROME (MPS) DEVELOPED!" We are very excited to report that that day has arrived!

The lead article in a recent edition of the Journal of Chronic Fatigue Syndrome is titled "Effective Treatment of Chronic Fatigue Syndrome and Fibromyalgia -- the Results of a Randomized, Double-Blind, Placebo-Controlled Study!" After decades of hard work by hundreds of researchers in the field, we have progressed to the point where effective treatment is now available for these illnesses! In our study, over 90 percent of patients improved with treatment.

In the average patient, after two years of treatment, the average improvement in quality of life was 90 percent. Pain decreased by over 50 percent on average. Many patients no longer even qualified for the diagnosis of CFS or fibromyalgia after treatment! Interestingly, many of the same principles for treating fibromyalgia also apply to myofascial pain syndrome

That the vast majority of patients improved significantly in the active group while there was minimal improvement in the placebo group proves two very important things. The first is that these are very treatable diseases. The second is that anyone who now says that these illnesses are not real or are all in your head are clearly both wrong and unscientific. The full text of the studies can be seen at: www.vitality101.com

A new day is dawning in how CFS/fibromyalgia/MPS will be treated. In support of our work, an editorial in the April, 2002 journal of a major multidisciplinary medical society for pain management in United States noted "the comprehensive and aggressive metabolic approach to treatment detailed in the Teitelbaum study are all highly successful approaches and make fibromyalgia a very treatment responsive disorder. The study by Dr. Teitelbaum et al. and years of clinical experience make this approach an excellent and powerfully effective part of the standard of practice for treatment of people who suffer from fibromyalgia and myofascial pain syndrome."

It is important to recognize that these syndromes can be caused and aggravated by a large number of different triggers. When all these different contributing factors are looked for, and treated effectively, patients improved significantly and often get well!

What is causing these illnesses?

As we noted above, CFS/FMS/MPS is not a single illness. Our study has shown that it is a mix of many different processes that can be triggered by many causes. Some of you had your illness caused by any of a number of infections. In this situation, you can often give the time that your illness began almost to the day. This is also the case in those of you who had an injury (sometimes very mild) that was enough to disrupt your sleep and trigger this process. In others the illness had a more gradual onset. This may have been associated with hormonal deficiencies (e.g. low thyroid, estrogen, testosterone, cortisone, etc.) despite normal blood tests. In others, it may be associated with chronic stress, antibiotic use with secondary yeast overgrowth, and/or nutritional deficiencies. Indeed, we have found well over 100 common causes of, and factors that contribute to, these syndromes.

APPENDIX

What these processes have in common is that most of them can suppress a major control center in your brain called the hypothalamus. This center controls sleep, your hormonal system, temperature, and blood flow / blood pressure. When you don't sleep deeply, your immune system also stops working properly and you'll be in pain. When we realized this, the myriad symptoms seen in CFS/fibromyalgia suddenly made sense. It also gave us a way to effectively treat you!

Four main categories of problems need to be treated.

A half-century of work by Dr. Janet Travell, the White House physician for Presidents Kennedy and Johnson and author of the *Trigger Point Manual* showed that the same problems caused by hypothalamic suppression resulted in muscles getting stuck in the shortened position. Chronic muscle shortening then causes myofascial and fibromyalgia pain. As she laid the groundwork for effective treatments these processes, our research team dedicated our published study to her memory. These are the four key areas that need to be treated for Chronic Fatigue syndrome, fibromyalgia and muscle pain to resolve:

1. **Disordered sleep.** Most patients with these illnesses find that they are unable to get 7-8 hours of deep sleep a night without taking medications. In part, this occurs because hypothalamic function is critical to deep sleep. Unfortunately, many of the most common sleep medications actually aggravate the sleep problems by **decreasing** the amount of time spent in deep sleep. **For patients to get well, it is critical that they take enough of the correct sleep medications to get 8 to 9 hours sleep at night**! These medications include Ambien, Desyrel, Klonopin, Xanax, Soma and, if you don't have Restless Leg Syndrome, Flexeril and/or Elavil. In addition, natural remedies can help sleep. An excellent one (which I developed -Revitalizing Sleep Formula by Enzymatic Therapy - 100 percent of my royalty for all products I develop is donated to charity) includes theanine, Jamaican Dogwood, wild lettuce, valerian, passionflower, and hops. Other natural sleep aids include Krebs Calcium-Magnesium Chelates (1-5 at bedtime), 5-HTP (100-300mg), Kava (125-375mg-do not use if you have liver disease), and melatonin (3/10-1mg). Some patients find that over-the-counter antihistamines such as doxylamine (Unisom for sleep) or Benadryl can also help. In the first six months of treatment, it is not uncommon to sometimes need to take even six to eight different products **simultaneously** to get 8 hours of sleep at night. After 6-18 months of feeling well, most people can come off of most sleep (and other) medications. I'm starting to believe that, to offer a margin for safety during periods of stress, it may be wise to stay on 1/2 to 1 tablet of a sleep medication for the rest of your life. Your doctor may initially be uncomfortable with this. Nonetheless, our experience with over 2000 patients and 2 research studies have found this approach to be safe and critical to people getting well. When one recognizes that CFS/FMS is a hypothalamic sleep disorder - not poor sleep hygiene - this approach makes sense. Otherwise, it is as if your doctor would immediately try to stop blood pressure or diabetes medicines every time the patient was doing better!

2. **Hormonal deficiencies.** The hypothalamus is the main control center for most of the glands in your body. Most of the normal ranges for our blood tests were not developed in the context of hypothalamic suppression or these syndromes. Because of this (and for a number of other reasons) it is usually necessary, albeit controversial, to treat with thyroid, adrenal (very low dose cortef; DHEA), and ovarian and testicular hormones—despite normal blood tests! These hormones have been found to be reasonably safe when used in low doses. Growth hormone has also been shown to be helpful in fibromyalgia. We don't use it because, unfortunately, it can cost over $15,000 a year and is given by injection. Fortunately, there may be a cheaper way to raise your low growth hormone. Most growth hormone is made during deep sleep. This may be another reason why **getting 8 to 9 hours of deep-sleep a night can be critical!**

3. **Unusual infections.** Many studies have shown immune system dysfunction in FMS/CFS. Although there are many causes of this, I suspect that poor sleep is a major contributor. The immune dysfunction can result in many unusual infections. These include viral infections (e.g. - HHV-6, CMV, and EBV), parasites and other bowel infections, infections sensitive to long-term treatment with the antibiotics Cipro and Doxycycline (e.g. mycoplasma, chlamydia, Lyme's, etc) and fungal infections. Although the latter is controversial, both our study and another recent placebo-controlled study found treating with an antifungal to be very helpful with the symptoms seen in these syndromes.

4. **Nutritional supplementation.** Because the western diet has been highly processed, nutritional deficiencies are a common problem. In addition, bowel infections can cause poor absorption, and the illness itself can cause increased nutritional needs. The most important nutrients include: a) vitamins - especially the B vitamins (most at 25-50 mg/day), vitamin B12 (50-3000mcg/day), antioxidants (e.g. - vitamin C and E). b) Minerals - especially magnesium, zinc, and selenium and c) amino acids (proteins). To replace the 25 - 35 tablets that people needed to take, I developed a good tasting product that contains 50 key nutrients in 1 capsule and 1 scoop of a good tasting powder taken daily. It is called "Energy Revitalization System" by Enzymatic Therapy, and is available at health food stores or on my web site.

There are many other treatments available as well. Although space does not allow for a full discussion of these in this article, I discuss them at length in my book *From Fatigued to Fantastic!* and at my www.Vitality101.com (click on the "Treatment Protocol" link on the bottom left for detailed instructions on treatments for each of these problems).

So can I make my pain go away?

Fibromyalgia and Myofascial Pain and associated nerve entrapments are now very responsive to treatment! In many cases, they usually will improve dramatically and often even go away if you simply get the eight hours of sleep a night I discuss above, take the vitamin powder, take thyroid hormone, and treat the underlying yeast infections. Other patients require the more thorough evaluation and treatment. Localized myofascial pain also requires an evaluation for structural causes.

Aspirin family medications (including ibuprofen) are not very effective for most Fibromyalgia and Myofascial Pain patients. I avoid Tylenol because it can markedly deplete a critical antioxidant (glutathione). The medications I find to be most helpful for myofascial pain include Celebrex (celecoxib) and Skelaxin (which are not sedating) and Neurontin, Baclofen, Zanaflex, and Ultram which can be sedating. Lidocaine patches and creams creating a mixture of medications can also be highly effective for local areas of pain without significant side effects. There are many other medications and other effective ways to treat pain as well. These can be used to help keep you comfortable while we go after the pain's underlying causes.

How do I go about getting well?

My best-selling book *From Fatigued to Fantastic* has been dramatically updated. It will supply you and your physician with all the information that you need to get treated effectively. It also contains the full text of our double blind, placebo-controlled study which proves that effective pain treatment is now available.

Because determining which treatments are needed by any given individual and then teaching them how to use them can be very difficult and time consuming (even for doctors that are very skilled in treating these syndromes - a new patient visit in my office usually takes at least four hours of my "one-on-one" time), I've created a sophisticated computer program on my Web site (*www.endfatigue.com*) that is like a **computerized CFS/Fibromyalgia specialist! It can analyze your history and lab tests to tailor a treatment protocol to your case using both natural and prescription therapies.** The good thing about it being a computer program is that it has both the time and ability to guide almost everyone with these syndromes back to health!

In addition, our website also contains:

1. Copies of both of our research studies demonstrating effective treatment for these illnesses. The first one, published in 1995, was an open (not placebo-controlled) study in which over 90 percent of patients improved. The second is the placebo-controlled study I've discussed above. Feel free to make copies of this study for your physicians, friends, and for anybody in the news media you think might be interested.

2. A referral list of over 700 health care professionals (with an area for patient comments) who asked to be listed. If you have (or are) a good health care provider who uses a significant part of our protocol, please encourage them to go on our site and add their name to our list. Because we do not know many of the health care professionals who asked to be on our list, please add your comments about the ones you are familiar with. This will help to let people know who are the "diamonds" versus the "lumps of coal". I would recommend you begin with the separate list of practitioners who have done my 2 day workshops for health care professionals (both physicians and non-physicians).

3. A question, answer, and comments area.

4. A section or you can vote for which of over 200 treatments helped or didn't help. You can also see how others voted, and their comments.

5. A shop where you can order supplements or books

6. Articles of interest, and more.

The purpose of our web site is to supply, in one place, all of the resources that you need in order to get well.

How can I get treated if I don't have much money?

Although some of the treatments for these syndromes can be very expensive, it is often possible to do the treatment protocol in an affordable manner. The key tests that are needed include the blood count (CBC), ESR, general chemistry, free T4 level (thyroid test), vitamin B12, iron, and DHEA-S level. Although many other tests can be very helpful, one can often rely on symptoms alone to make the other treatment decisions. The following medications and supplements can be found fairly inexpensively, and will often be helpful. The vitamin powder can be adequate for basic nutritional support. Flexeril and Elavil, although more likely than some other medications to cause side effects, are inexpensive. Desyrel and Klonopin, in generic form, are also reasonably priced. These four can be very helpful for sleep, and your doctor is likely to be comfortable prescribing the first three of these. Thyroid, cortef, DHEA, and estrogen, can also be found for a fairly low price. For infections, nystatin and tetracycline are also inexpensive. Most drug companies offer medications for free to those who cannot afford them. Although many of the other treatments can often be very helpful, these inexpensive ones may be enough to help you get well.

In last 25 years, my associates and I have had a wonderful time in our quest to make the possibility of effective treatment available for everyone with CFS, & FMS related problems. Finding effective treatment, doing the research to prove its effectiveness, writing a book that teaches people how to get well (and their doctors how to treat them), and creating the web site educational program that can help you tailor a treatment program for your specific situation has fulfilled this goal!

At this time, you now have all the tools you need to get well! We wish you all God's blessings and our best wishes in reclaiming vibrant health!

With appreciation for all you've been through,

Jacob E Teitelbaum MD

Dr. Teitelb⋯ ⋯ internist and director of the Annapolis Research Center for Effective ⋯ uffered with and overcome these illnesses in 1975, he spent the next 28 years ⋯ t effective therapies. He sees CFS/Fibromyalgia/Chronic pain patients from ⋯ olis, Maryland (410-266-6958). He lectures internationally. He is also the ⋯ Fatigued to Fantastic!" and the just released "Three Steps to Happiness! ⋯ e found at: *www.vitality101.com*

⋯ *FIDS/Fibromyalgia*

⋯ *gued To Fantastic" by Jacob Teitelbaum, M.D.*
⋯ *be ordered from 800-333-5287 or our Web site at*

⋯ n treatments used in treating CFIDS/FMS. I would use this list as a record of your treatments and have it with you for follow-up/phone visits. Put a line through the number in front of any treatment you stop and note the reason stopped and date. Put the date started in front of the other treatments. Although it can take 6 weeks to see a treatment's benefits, most of the medications' side effects will usually occur within the first few days of starting a treatment. Except for treatment #1 through 21 which can all be started in the first 1 to 3 days, add in 1 new treatment each 1 to 3 days. If a side effect occurs, stop the last 2 or 3 treatments for a few days and see if it goes away. If the side effect is worrisome, call your family doctor (or go to the E.R.) immediately. If needed, all treatments (except if you've been on #27, 35, 41, 92 through 99 or 122 and 126 for over 2 months - then taper these off) can be stopped until the situation is clarified. Do not get pregnant on treatment or drive if sedated. It is normal for a woman's periods to be irregular during the first 3 to 4 months of treatment. On average, it takes 3 months to start feeling better. You can begin to slowly taper off most treatments when you feel well for 6 months. Stop things one at a time (e.g., one pill every 1 to 2 weeks) so you can see if you still need it. If needed, any or all of these can be used forever (usually not necessary). Some prescriptions can be obtained at a much lower cost from Consumers Discount Drug Company (323-461-3606). We priced 100 Sporanox tablets (100mg) - they would cost $793.55 at a local food chain pharmacy vs. $189.95 at Consumers Discount Drug. Do not take any treatments below that you are allergic to or that have caused prohibitive side effects. Prescription items have "Rx" after their names. If a recommended (i.e., checked off) treatment has a * by the number, it is more likely to be important to take. If you choose to simplify your program, you can begin with just the *'d items that are checked off.

We have listed natural/over-the-counter alternatives for most prescription therapies that can be substituted for and/or added to the prescription ones. We recommend products made by

Enzymatic Therapies or Phyto Pharmica as these have proven potency and purity. Dr. Teitelbaum does not accept money from any company whose products he recommends. He has directed all his royalties for products he makes be donated to charity. Only the items that are checked off are the ones recommended for you.

Nutritional Treatments

___ 1.* **Energy Revitalization System** - 1/2 - 1 scoop of powder a day (as feels best) blended with juice, water or yogurt with 1 capsule of Daily Energy B-Complex (also available separately). If diarrhea occurs, start with a lower dose and work your way up to the best dose that feels best or divide the daily dose into smaller doses and take 2-3 times a day. These products are made by Enzymatic Therapies and are available from our Web site at *www.endfatigue.com* and most health food stores. You can substitute 3, 4, 7, 9, 12B, 13, 20, 105 and 107 below. These would, however, only replace a small part of the over 25 tablets worth of supplements in one scoop of the powder.

___ 2.* **Complete GEST Enzymes** - 2 capsules with each meal to help digest your food properly - by Enzymatic Therapies.

___ 3. **Betaine HCL (Hydrochloric Acid)** - 650mg capsules. Take 3-7 capsules during each meal. Use less or stop if heartburn occurs. Do not use if you have ulcers.

___ 4. **Magnesium Glycinate 75mg/Malic Acid 300mg** - 2 tablets 3 x a day for 8 months, then 2 tablets a day (less if diarrhea is a problem. Start with 1 to 2 a day and slowly work up as able without getting uncomfortable diarrhea. You can take up to 10 a day for constipation. Taking it with food may lessen diarrhea. If pain or fatigue recur on lowering the dose, increase it. Taken at bedtime, it helps sleep.

___ 5. **Calcium** - 500 to 1000 mg daily with 400 units of vitamin D (a chewable calcium or Calcium Chelate is recommended). If you get a non-chewable tablet, see if it dissolves in 2 to 3 inches of vinegar over 1 hour (swirl a few times). If not, it won't dissolve in your stomach, and you need to get a different brand. (Do not drink the vinegar). You can also avoid this problem by using capsules or liquid filled gelcaps. Taken at bedtime, it may help sleep.

___ 6. **Lipoic Acid** - 200mg a day (protects the liver) **whenever you're on Sporanox or Diflucan (#60).** If you have active Hepatitis or Cirrhosis, consider 300 to 2000mg a day depending on it's severity.

___ 7. **Vitamin B12** - ____mcg under your tongue daily.

___ 8.* **Vitamin B-12** - 1 I.M. injection (1cc = 3000 mcg) 3 to 7 times weekly for 15 doses, then as needed (e.g., 1 to 12 times a month). This needs to be made by a compounding (holistic) pharmacy (e.g., Cape Drugs 800-248-5978).

___ 9.* **NAC (N-Acetyl - L - Cysteine)** - 500-650mg a day for 3 months. Makes Glutathione.

___ 10.* **Chromagen FA (Rx, iron)** - one tablet a day. Do not take within 6 hours of thyroid hormone preparations or Cipro (antibiotic), as this can prevent their absorption. Take on an empty stomach (i.e., take between 2 and 6PM on an empty stomach). It is OK to miss up to 3 doses a week. Stop in 4 to 6 months or when your Ferritin blood test is over 40. It may turn your stool black. Flora Dix iron is much easier on the stomach if this is a problem.

___ 11.　**Flaxseed/Borage Oil** - 1050mg - 3 capsules 2 times a day (or 1/2 - 1 tablespoon a day) for 9 months. Use Flaxseed oil **without** Borage oil if manic/depressive. Dry eyes, mouth, hair and excessive hard ear wax suggest a need for this. Use Enzymatic Therapies, PhytoPharmica or Barleans brands.

___ 12.　**Vitamin C** - 500-1000mg 2 times a day.

___ 12A.　**Grape Seed Extract** - 50-100mg a day for 6 months.

___ 13.　**Vitamin E** - 400 units a day (natural).

___ 13B.　**Imuplus** - 1 packet 2 times a day.

　　　　OR ImmunoPro 1 scoop a day (for more information see *www.GenomicWhey.com*)

___ 14.　**Zinc Picolinate or Sulphate** - 25mg 2 times a day for 6 weeks and then stop.

___ 14A　**Chromium (GTF or Picolinate)** - 200-250mcg a day for 6 months (helps hypoglycemia).

___ 14B.　**Potassium - Micro K Extentabs 10 MEQ (Rx)** - _____ 1 capsule 1-2 times a day for 8 weeks.

Mitochondrial Energy Treatments

Use these for 4-9 months. Then drop the dose to the lowest dose that maintains the effect (or stop it if no benefit).

___ 15.　**Acetyl-L-Carnitine** - 500 mg 1 capsule twice a day for 3 months. Then 250 to 500 mg/day or stop it. Although important in CFS/FMS, it is even more important to take this if you also have Mitral Valve Prolapse and/or elevated blood triglycerides. Take less or L-Carnitine can be substituted if the cost is prohibitive. This helps with weight loss.

___ 16.　**Coenzyme Q10** - 200 mg - 1 x a day. Especially important if taking cholesterol lowering prescriptions (e.g., Mevacor). Take it with a meal that has fat, oil supplements or in an oil based form to improve absorption. Vitaline makes the best form.

___ 17.　**L-Lysine** - 1000 mg - 1-3 x a day for 3 months, then 1000 mg a day. Take also if you have oral cold sores or genital Herpes to suppress them. Helps make Carnitine.

___ 18.　**L-Arginine** - 2000mg 1 to 3 times a day (do not take if it flares Herpes or take Valtrex with it). May raise growth hormone.

___ 19.　**Magnesium/Potassium Aspartate** - two 500mg capsules- 2 x a day (need to use a "fully reacted" brand) for 3 to 4 months.

___ 20.　**Daily Energy B-complex** - 1 capsule in the morning or mid day (by Enzymatic Therapies).

___ 21.   **NADH (Enada brand)** - 5 mg- 2 tablets each morning. Take it on an empty stomach first thing in the morning (leave it by your bedside in the bottle or foil wrap with a glass of water) at least 1 hour before eating, drinking coffee/juice or taking any medication or supplements (except thyroid, which you can take with the NADH). It takes 2 months to see if it works. 15 to 20mg a day may be more effective and is safe. **Don't take vitamin C, Malic Acid, Lipoic Acid, vitamins or other acids within 2 to 3 hours of NADH, as acid destroys NADH.**

Sleeping Aids For Fibromyalgia

You can try these in the order listed or as you prefer based on your history. ****ADJUST DOSE AS NEEDED TO GET 7-9 HOURS OF SOLID SLEEP WITHOUT WAKING OR HANGOVER.** No going to the bathroom if you wake up unless you still have to go 5 minutes later. Mixing low doses of several treatments is more likely to help you sleep without a hangover than a high dose of 1 medication. You can take up to the maximum dose of all checked off treatments simultaneously. Do not drive if you have next day sedation (adjust your treatment to avoid this). If you're not sleeping 7-8 hours a night without waking on the checked off treatments, do not wait until your next appointment to let us know or contact your physician! Ambien, Klonopin, Xanax and Soma are considered potentially addictive. If you have next day sedation, try taking the medications (except the Ambien) a few hours before bedtime. The antidepressants (e.g., Prozac/Paxil) can improve sleep a lot after 6 weeks. * 126 & 127 can also help sleep. **TAKING YOUR MAGNESIUM AND/OR CALCIUM AT NIGHT ALSO CAN HELP SLEEP. YOU CAN TRY THE NATURAL PRODUCTS IN COMBINATION FIRST TO SEE IF THEY GIVE YOU 8 HOURS OF SLEEP A NIGHT. ADD THEM IN THIS ORDER #24, 28, 33, 26, 32, 36B, 44A.** Use 36C if pain keeps you up and #29 is also helpful and is non-prescrition.

___ 22.*   **Ambien (Rx, zolpidem)** - 10 mg- 1/2 to 1-1/2 at bedtime. If you tend to wake during the night, leave an extra 1/2 to 1 tablet at bedside and you can take it as needed to help you sleep through the night.

___ 23.*   **Desyrel (Rx, trazodone)** - 50 mg - 1/2 to 6 at bedtime. Although sedating, it can be used (50-250mg at a time) for anxiety. Do not take over 450mg a day (or 150mg a day if on other antidepressants).

___ 24.   **Revitalizing Sleep Formula (by Enzymatic Therapies & PhytoPharmica)** - Valerian 200mg, Passion Flower 90mg, L-Theanine 50mg, Hops 30mg, Piscidia 12mg and Wild Lettuce 28mg. Take 2-4 capsules each night 30 to 90 minutes before bedtime. Can also be used during the day for anxiety. Do not take more than 4 capsules a day. If Valerian energizes you (occurs in 5-10% of people) use the other components.

___ 25.   **Krebs Calcium magnesium Chelate. 1-5 tabs at bedtime (less if diarrhea from magnesium) from PhytoPharmica.**

___ 26.   **Delta Wave Sleep Inducing CD/Tape. This helps with no side effects.** Play to fall asleep and if you wake during the night. They can be played throughout the night if desired (order from 800-333-5287 for our Web site at *www.endfatigue.com*). You can use either of the CD's.

___ 27.*   **Klonopin (Rx, clonazepam)** - 1/2 mg - begin slowly and work your way up as sedation allows. Take 1 tablet at bedtime increasing up to 6 tablets at bedtime as

needed. Can be **very** effective for sleep, pain and Restless Leg Syndrome.
Klonopin may be addictive.

___ 28. **Melatonin** - 1/2 mg - 1mg at bedtime (available at health food stores). If you feel wide awake at bedtime, try 5mg at 3 to 5 hours before bedtime. Don't use a higher dose unless you find it more effective (.5mg is usually as effective as 5mg and may be safer).

___ 29. **Doxylamine (Unisom For Sleep)** - 25 mg at night (an antihistamine).

___ 30. **Soma (Rx, carisprodol)** - 1/2 to 1 at bedtime. This is very good if pain is severe. Soma may be addictive.

___ 31. **Flexeril (Rx, cyclobenzaprine)** - 10 mg- 1/2 to 2 at bedtime. Muscle relaxant - can cause dry mouth.

___31A. **Sonata (Rx)** 10mg - Take 1-2 capsules during the night if you wake after 3 AM. Effects only last 3-4 hours.

___ 32. **Kava Kava** - 30% extract - 250mg capsules - 1 to 3 capsules at night (if a rash develops add a B-complex 50mg at night - and stop/decrease the dose/frequency of use. If the rash persists, see your family doctor). Do not use if you have liver inflammation. May rarely cause liver inflammation.

___ 33. **5 HTP (5 Hydroxytryptophan)** - 200 to 400mg at night. Naturally stimulates Serotonin. Don't take over 250mg a day if you are on Prozac, Paxil, Zoloft, Desyrel or Celexa. Can help with pain and weight loss at 300mg a day for at least 3 months.

___ 34A. **Remeron (Rx, mirtazapine)** - 15mg - 1 to 3 tablets at bedtime (especially helpful if you feel like you're "hibernating" during the day).

___ 34B. **Elavil (Rx, amitriptyline)** - 10 mg- 1/2 to 5 tablets at bedtime. May cause weight gain or dry mouth. Good for nerve pain and vulvadynia.

____ 34C. **Doxepin (Rx, Sinequan)** - 5-10mg, 1-3 capsules at bedtime or Doxepin liquid 10mg/cc. If lower dose is needed you can start with 1-3 drops at night. A powerful antihistamine.

___ 35. **Xanax (Rx, alprazolam)** - 1/2 mg - 1/2 to 4 tablets at bedtime. This is short-acting and gives a good 3 to 5 hours sleep with less hangover in the morning. Xanax may be addictive.

___ 36A. **Sinemet 10/100 (Rx)** - 1 at 6 to 9PM each evening for Restless Leg Syndrome. Can substitute Mirapex.

___ 36C. **Cuddle-Ewe Mattress Pad** - Use if pain interferes with sleep (800-328-9493, ext. 000 - company may offer a 90-day money back guarantee).

Hormonal Treatments

Thyroid supplementation - several studies show that thyroid therapies can be very helpful in CFIDS/FMS - even if your blood tests are normal. This treatment is, however, very controversial

- even though it's usually very safe. All treatments (even aspirin) can cause problems in some people though. The main risks of thyroid treatment are:

1.   Triggering caffeine-like anxiety or palpitations. If this happens cut back the dose and increase by 1/2 to 1 tablet each 6 to 8 weeks (as is comfortable) or slower. Sometimes taking vitamin B1 (thiamine) 100 to 200mg a day will also help. If you have severe, persistent racing heart, call your family doctor and/or go to the emergency room.

2.   Like exercise (i.e., climbing steps), if one is on the edge of having a heart attack or severe "racing heart" (atrial fibrillation), thyroid hormone can trigger it. In the long run though, I suspect thyroid may decrease the risk of heart disease. If you have chest pain, go to the emergency room and/or call your family doctor. It will likely be chest muscle pain (not dangerous) but better safe than sorry. To put it in perspective, I've never seen this happen despite treating many hundreds of patients with thyroid. Increasing your thyroid dose to levels above the upper limit of the normal range may accelerate Osteoporosis (which is already common in CFIDS/FMS). Because of this, you need to check your thyroid (Free T4 - not TSH) levels after 4 to 8 weeks on your optimum dose of thyroid hormone. All this having been said, we find treatments with thyroid hormone to be safer than Aspirin and Motrin. If you have risk factors or Angina, do an exercise stress test to make sure your heart is healthy before beginning thyroid treatment. These risk factors include: 1. Diabetes, 2. Elevated cholesterol, 3. Hypertension, 4. Smoking, 5. Personal or family history of Angina, 6. Gout, 7. Age over 50 years old.

There are several forms of thyroid hormone, and one kind will often work when the other does not. **Do not take thyroid within 6 hours of iron or calcium supplements or you won't absorb the thyroid.** It can take 3 to 24 months to see the thyroid's **full** benefit.

___ 37.   **Synthroid (Rx)** - (L-Thyroxine) 50mcg - (100mcg=.1mg)

___ 38.*   **Armour Thyroid (Rx)** - 30mg (1/2 grain = 30mg) (natural thyroid glandular). If #41 (Cortef) is checked, begin the Cortef and/or adrenal support 1-7 days before starting the thyroid.

For each of these 3 forms (#37-39), take 1/2 tablet each **morning** on an empty stomach for 1 week and then 1 tablet each morning. Increase by 1/2 to 1 tablet each 2 to 6 weeks (till you're on 3 tablets or the dose that feels best). Check a repeat Free T4 blood level when you're on 3 tablets a day (or your optimum dose) for 4 weeks. If okay, you can continue to raise the dose by 1/2 to 1 tablet each morning each 6 to 9 weeks to a maximum of 5 a day and then recheck the Free T4 4 weeks later. Adjust it to the dose that feels the best (lower the dose if shaky or if your pulse is regularly over 88/minute). Do not go over 5 tablets a day without discussing it with your doctor. When on your optimum dose, you can often get a single tablet at that strength. Interestingly, thyroid hormone (about the same as Armour called "Bio-throid") can be mailed to the U.S. without a prescription from *www.antiaging-systems.com*. **Only use thyroid under a doctor's supervision.** If your energy wanes too early in the day, you can also take part of your thyroid dose between 11AM and 3PM.

OR

_____   **Iodine** - 1500 mcg a day for 2 months (if you have daytime body temperatures under 98.3 degrees). May flare Hashimoto's Thyroiditis.

_____   **Thyroid Glandulars** - _____mg capsules in the morning and at noon. Thyroid L-Tyrosine by Enzymatic Therapies or Tyrosine Complex by PhytoPharmica. Take 1-2 capsules up to 3 times a day.

_____   **Dessicated Thyroid** - 130mg from *www.nutri-meds.com* - it is over-the-counter. 1/2-2 tablets each morning (caution - contains active thyroid hormone).

___ 39.   **Thyrolar (Rx)** - 1/2 (this equals T4 25mcg plus T3 6.25mcg)

___ 40.*   **Cytomel (Pure active T3) (Rx)** - 5 and 25mcg tablets. In Fibromyalgia, resistance to normal thyroid doses may occur and patients often need very high levels of T3 Thyroid to improve. Dr. John Lowe's research group feels that the average dose needed in FMS is 75-125mcg each morning - much higher than your body's normal production. Because we are often going above normal levels with T3, the risks/side effects noted above increase. Because of this, if you have risk factors, it is more important to consider an exercise stress test to make sure your heart is healthy (i.e., no underlying Angina) before beginning this protocol. Also, consider a Dexa (Osteoporosis) Scan each 6 to 18 months while on treatment. There may be initial bone loss the first year, then increased bone density. Bone density may decrease at 6 months and then increase after that. This having been said, in our experience this treatment has been quite safe and, in some FMS patients, dramatically effective. Begin with 5mcg each morning and continue to increase by 5mcg each 3 days until you're at 75mcg a day and then increase by 5mcg a day each 2 to 6 weeks until (whichever comes first):

1. You reach 125mcg each morning (or 60mcg if you're over 50 years old unless approved by your physician).

2. You feel healthy.

3. You get shakiness, worsening significant palpitations (occasional "flip flops" are common), anxiety, racing heart, sweating or other uncomfortable side effects. If this happens, lower the dose a bit for 2-4 weeks and then try raising again till you note significant improvement WITHOUT uncomfortable side effects or you tried to raise it 3 times and still became shaky/hyper.

Blood tests for thyroid hormone or TSH are not reliable or useful on this regimen. If you feel no better even on the maximum dose, taper off (decrease by 5mcg each 3 days until you're at 15mcg a day. Take 15mcg a day for 3 weeks and then drop to 5mcg a day for 3 weeks - then stop).

After being on treatment for 3 to 6 months, some patients can lower the T3 dose or stop it. Feel free to try dropping the dose. If you feel better initially and then worse (beginning more than 4 weeks after starting a new dose), you probably need to lower the dose. If you lose too much weight, try to eat more (and discuss this with your physician).

APPENDIX

Adrenal Hormones, Glandulars & Support

Helps your body deal with stress and maintains blood pressure.

___ 41.* **Cortef (Rx)** - 5 mg tablets - 1/2 to 2 1/2 tablet(s) at breakfast, 1/2 to 1 1/2 tablets at lunch and 0 to 1/2 tablets at 4 PM. Use the lowest dose that feels the best. Most patients find that 1 to 1 1/2 tablets in the morning and 1/2 to 1 tablet at noon is optimal. Take it with food if it causes an acid stomach. Do not take over 4 tablets a day without discussing the risks with your physician. Take Calcium (see #5) if on Cortef. If taken too late in the day, Cortef can keep you up at night. You can double the dose for up to 1 to 3 weeks (to maximum 7 tablets a day), during periods of severe stress (e.g., infections - see or call your doctor for the infection and let him/her know you're raising the dose). If routinely taking over 4 tablets a day, wear a "Med-Alert bracelet" that says "on chronic Cortisol treatment." After 9 months, you can try to wean off the Cortef (decrease by 1/2 tablet a day each 2 weeks) if you feel OK (or no worse) without it.

OR

41A &/or G are best. Can also add 41 B,C , D, E or F

___ 41A. **Adrenal Stress- Free** - An excellent Adrenal glandular and the best natural remedy for stress and adrenal fatigue. From Enzymatic Therapies or PhytoPharmica. Take 1-2 capsules each morning (or 1-2 in the morning and 1 at noon). Take less or take with food if it upsets your stomach.

___ 41B. **Adreset** - Contains Ginseng, cordyceps & Rhodiola Root for adrenal support. Take 1 twice a day.

___ 41C. **Vitamin B5 (Pantothenic Acid)** - 1000mg 1-2 times a day (take 1st dose in the morning) of a sustained release form.

___ 41D **Panax Ginseng** - 100-200mg twice a day can help your adrenals to heal.

___ 41E. **Drenatrophin (Adrenal Glandular from Standard Process)** - Take 1-2 tablets in the morning. May add one at noon. Use the lowest dose that gives you the optimum effect.

___ 41F. **Drenamin (Adrenal Support)** - Take 3-6 tablets in the morning and 3 at lunch for 3-7 days. Then lower the dose (e.g., 3 a day) to what feels best.

___ 41G. **Isocort (Adrenal Glandular)** - Contains 2 1/2 mg Cortisol (Cortef) per pellet (see #41 above for directions). Order from 800-743-2256.

___ 42.* **DHEA** - _____ mg each morning or twice daily (lower the dose if acne or darkening of facial hair occurs). Keep your DHEA-Sulphate levels between 140-180mcg/dL for females and 300-500mcg/dL for males. If you have breast cancer, do not use without your physician's OK. See information sheet for dosing.

___ 43. **Florinef (Rx)** - (fludrocortisone) - 0.1 mg- 1 each morning. Begin with 1/4 tablet and increase by 1/4 tablet each 3 to 7 days. Increase more slowly if headache occurs. Increase your water, salt and potassium (e.g., 12 oz V-8 juice and one banana a day) intake. See the NMH information sheet and check a potassium level and blood pressure each 6 weeks for 4 months and then each 3 to 4 months.

OR 43B plus #95 A (Acceleration Capsules)

___ 43B.   Increase your salt (to about 4 to 8gms a day) and water (approximately 1 gallon a day) intake a lot. If your mouth and lips are dry (and you're not on Elavil) you're dehydrated - drink more water (or herbal tea or lemonade sweetened with Stevia - see #54B), **not** sodas or coffee. Celtic Sea Salt is an excellent form to use (800-867-7258).

Other Hormones

___ 44.   **Oxytocin (Rx)** - 10 units each morning; ____ by mouth or nose spray: ____ by I.M. injection - as is helpful. The injections may sting. If so, you can add Lidocaine 2/10 to 5/10cc (**without** Epinephrine) to the Oxytocin. Try the tablets, nose spray & injections and use the one you prefer.

___ 45.*   **Natural Estrogen (Rx)** - ____ take Estrace (estradiol) 1mg, 1 to 2 times a day, OR ____ put a Climara .05 to .1mg patch on each Sunday, OR take a Biestrogen 2 1/2 mg 1 to 2 times a day. If you have not had a hysterectomy, you must be on progesterone with the estrogen to prevent uterine cancer. If you are on the patch and it seems to stop working the last 1 to 2 days of the week, you can change the patch every 5 days. Use the Estrogen ____ every day; ____ day 1 through 25 of your cycle (day 1 of your period is day 1 of your cycle). It is normal for your periods to be irregular for 3 to 4 months. If your symptoms (including migraines and anxiety) worsen for the week you are off the Estrogen, we can add a Climara .025mg patch for that week. If they worsen a few hours before you take the Estrogen by mouth, divide the dose up through the day (e.g., 1/2 tablet - 4 times a day vs. 2 tablets each morning). If you order your Estrogen/Progesterone capsules from Cape Apothecary, Tom will be glad to work with you in adjusting the dose (800-248-5978 or 410-757-3522).

OR   **Natural Non-Prescription Estrogen/Progesterone** (from 800-743-2256); ____ Phyto B - 8 pellets a day (= 2 1/2 mg Triest + 50mg progesterone); ____ Osta B3 - 8 pellets a day (= 2mg Estradiol + 50mg Progesterone) OR; ____ Osta Derm Cream 1/2 teaspoon a day (= 2mg Triest + 66mg Progesterone).

OR   Can also take Lignans (e.g., 5-10gm of Flax Seed) a day and/or Soy Isoflavons 100mg/day (e.g., 1 cup soymilk or 1/2 cup tofu or 3 capsules of Soy Extract by Enzymatic Therapies - each have 40mg isoflavons) plus exercise (weight bearing) plus #1, 5 and vitamin K 300mcg a day plus ipriflavones.

OR   Menopause AM/PM - From Enzymatic Therapies/PhytoPharmica.

AND/OR

____   **Remifenin (Black Cohosh)** - 2 tablets 2 times a day for 2 months and then you can lower to 1 tablet twice a day (for hot flashes). Can take 6 weeks to work.

___ 46.   **Ortho-novum 1/35 (Rx)** - Begin the Sunday after this period. It's effectiveness as birth control begins after you've been on it the first week. If you miss a pill, add alternate contraception that cycle. It's effectiveness as birth control is decreased while on Doxycycline or Amoxicillin/Augmentin family antibiotics. If you feel poorly the week off the pill, you can take it every day till you get your period (or 5 months - whichever comes first). Then stop the pill for 5-7 days and then repeat this cycle.

___ 47.* **Natural Progesterone (Rx)** - (Prometrium - available in most pharmacies) - 100 mg daily if over 48 years old **OR** 200 mg a day for the 16th to 25th day of your cycle if under 48 years old. Take it at night. Available without prescription from 800-743-2256. As Progerol Cream (66mg/1/2 teaspoon) or _____ Progon B 12 1/2mg per pellet.

___ 47A. **Fosamax (Rx)** - 70mg each Sunday. For Osteoporosis. Do not lay down for 1 hour after taking.

___ 47B. **Relaxin (Vitalaxin 20)** - 20mcg tablets. Take 1 to 2 tablets 1 to 2 times a day. Often takes 3 months to see the benefit (from 612-946-1550). May have morning sickness and/or _____ during the first month of use. Start with 1 tablet at night _____ - if OK take 1 tablet twice a day for 5 days _____.

___ 48A.* **Testosterone (Rx)** - Males 100mg (1/2cc) shot every 7 days or 25 to 50mg (order 100mg/gm of cream) 2 to 3 times a day (less if acne occurs). Rub the cream into an area of thin skin on the abdomen, inner thigh or inner arms. The cream is available by prescription from 877-340-5922 (ask for Ron).

___ 48B. **Testosterone (Rx)** - Females 2mg tablets or cream, 1 to 2 times a day - make 4mg/gm of cream (less if acne or darkening of facial hair occurs). Rub the cream into an area of thin skin on the abdomen, inner thigh or inner arms. The cream is available by prescription from 877-340-5922 (ask for Ron).

___ 49*. **Somatomed** - Helps make growth hormone - take 2 tablets on an empty stomach (at least 2 hours after eating), 1 hour before bedtime on weeknights (don't take Saturday and Sunday night). After 3 months, stay off of it for 2 to 4 weeks.

___ 49A. **Mestinon (Pyridostignanine) 60mg** - Take 1/2 tablet in the morning and again 60 minutes before exercise (enhances exercise induced growth hormone release 8 fold)

Antiviral Agents - (See the article "Treating Respiratory Infections Without Antibiotics" in my book, Volume 2, Issue 2 of my newsletter or on our web site at *www.endfatigue.com*. For HHV-6, CMV & EBV Infections, see Vol. 4, Issue 1 of our newsletter.

___ 50. **Transfer Factor 540 for Epstein Barr, Transfer Factor 560 for HHV-6** - 1-3 capsules each morning on an empty stomach.

___ 50A. **Famvir (Rx)** - 750mg 3 times a day.

___ 51. **Lithium (Rx)** - 300mg ____ times a day. If tremor, take 2 teaspoons of Expeller Pressed Safflower Oil from a health food store (uncooked - e.g., as salad dressing) daily or lower the dose. Check a Lithium level 1 month after beginning medication. Then check a Lithium and thyroid blood test (Free T4) each 6 to 12 months.

___ 51A. **Symmetrel (Rx, Amantadine)** - 100mg 2 times a day.

___ 52. **Monolaurin** - 300 mg capsules. Take 9 capsules once a day on an empty stomach for 1 week, followed by 6 capsules once a day for 20 days. Take Lysine 1500 mg twice a day while on Monolaurin.

___ 53. **Olive Leaf** - 500mg - 3 to 4 capsules 3 times a day for 10 to 14 days for respiratory infections or 3 to 4 capsules, 3 times a day for 6-24 weeks for chronic infections (e.g., HHV-6, Epstein Barr, etc).

___ 53A. **Kutapressin (Rx)** - 2cc daily or 3 times a week for 14 weeks by subcutaneous injection. If not better use 4cc daily or 3 times a week for 14 more weeks. (Costs approximately $160 for 20cc.)

Anti-Yeast Treatments

___ 54.* **Avoid sweets** - this includes sucrose, glucose, fructose, corn syrup, or any other sweets until the doctor says that it is okay to include them in your diet again. Avoid fruit juices, which are naturally sweet. Having 1-2 fruits a day (the whole fruit as opposed to the juice) is okay. Stevia is a great sugar substitute.

___ 54B. **Stevia** is a wonderful herbal sweetener. A great tasting one is available from 800-478-3842. Use all you want.

___ 55. **Acidophilus or Milk Bacteria** - 2-4 billion units (1 unit = 1 bacteria) a day. Do not take within 6 hours of taking an antibiotic (e.g., take it midday, if you take the antibiotic morning and night). Use the Enzymatic Therapy/PhytoPharmica Acidophilus or Probiotic Pearls form (contains 2 billion units - even though box says only 1 billion) as in many other brands the bacteria are not viable.

___ 56. **Cellulase** - Enzyme which digests yeast. E.g., SMI Formula - 1 level tablespoon (mixed in water) for 2 containers - then as needed.

___ 56A. **Caprylic Acid** - 680mg - 1 to 2 capsules 3 times a day with meals for 3 to 4 months and then as needed (1800 to 3600mg a day). May cause acid tasting reflux.

___ 56B. **Citricidal** - 4 drops or 100mg 1-3 times a day.

___ 56C. **Ammonium Chloride** - 322mg - 1-3 capsules a day from Allergy Research. Take 3 tablets a day.

___ 56D. **Pau D'Arco**

___ 57. **Garlic** - 1 clove 1 to 3 times a day with meals (crushed in olive oil with salt tastes great on bread).

___ 58. **Mycelex Oral Lozenges (Rx, for Thrush and/or "in the mouth" sores)** - Suck on 1 lozenge, 5 times a day for 1 to 4 days (as needed). After sucking on it awhile (e.g., 10 minutes), put pieces of the lozenge up against sore(s) until you are tired of it being there.

___ 59.* **Nystatin (Rx)** - 500,000 units - 2 tablets 2 x a day. Begin with 1 a day and increase by 1 tablet a day until you are up to the total dose. Your symptoms may initially flare as the yeast die off. If this occurs, decrease the dose and then increase the Nystatin more slowly or stop for awhile until symptoms decrease. The Nystatin is usually taken for 5 to 8 months. If nausea occurs take 2 twice a day and/or switch to the Nystatin powder in capsules or mixed in water (available from Cape Drug at 800-248-5978). Repeat Nystatin for 4 to 6 weeks anytime you take an antibiotic or have recurrent bowel symptoms.

___ 60.* **Diflucan (Rx)** - 200mg a day. Or, if not covered by insurance - Nizoral 200mg a day. **IMPORTANT - begin taking the Diflucan 4 weeks after starting the Nystatin.**

OR

___ **Sporanox (Rx)** - (itraconazole) - 100 mg, take 2 each day (simultaneously) with food.

OR #55, 56, 56A, 56B, 56C, 56D and 61

Begin taking the **Diflucan or Sporanox** 4 weeks after beginning the Nystatin. If the symptoms have improved and then worsen when you stop the antifungal, refill the prescription for another 6 weeks. (Note: A 6-week supply costs over $500!) If your symptoms flared when you began the Nystatin, begin with 1/4 to 1/2 the above dose for the 1st week. **Do not take Seldane, Hismanyl, Propulcid, cholesterol lowering agents related to Mevacor or antacids (e.g., Tagamet) while on Sporanox!** Diflucan 200mg a day may be substituted for Sporanox if you are on antacids. **Do not take Seldane, Hismanyl, Propulcid or Mevacor family medications with Diflucan!** Take Lipoic Acid (#6) any time you take Sporanox or Diflucan. Also, taking Betaine HCL (stomach acid to help digestion - available at most health food stores) at the same time as the Sporanox, can dramatically increase Sporanox's absorbtion and effectiveness. Lipoic Acid may decrease the risk of liver inflammation from the Diflucan or Sporanox. If you need to stay on these medications more than 3 months, check liver blood tests (ALT, AST) every 3 months. If you feel well and symptoms (especially bowel symptoms) recur over time, consider retreating yourself with Nystatin and/or Caprylic Acid and Oregano Oil and/or Sporanox (or Diflucan) for 1 month as needed. If you have a low income and no prescription insurance the Diflucan company may supply it for free. Call 800-869-9979 for information (let them know you have immune suppression and fungal overgrowth).

___ 61. **Oregano Oil (enteric coated)** - Candida Formula from Enzymatic Therapies. 2 capsules on an empty stomach 1-2 times a day for 3 to 4 months, then as needed for yeast overgrowth.

Immune Stimulants

___ 62. **Echinacea** - 300 to 325 mg - 3 x a day (also take while on Famvir). Stay off the Echinacea for 1 week each month (or it will stop working). It may also improve adrenal function.

___ 63. **Thymic Protein - (AKA- Proboost and Bio Pro A)** - Dissolve the contents of 1 packet under your tongue - any that is swallowed is destroyed! _____ times a day for _____ weeks, then 1 a day for _____ weeks. Also take it 3 times a day at first sign of any infection until the infection resolves (it is approximately $2.00 a packet). Order from our office 800-333-5287.

___ 64. **ImmPower** - 500mg capsules - Take 2 capsules 3 times a day for 3 weeks. Then take 1 twice a day. This natural product **triples** some important components (natural killer cells) of your immune system. It is expensive.

___ 65. **Selenium** - 200mcg a day (in addition to the Selenium 200mcg in your multi-vitamin) for 6 months. You may get toxic if you take over 200mcg a day for over 6 months.

___ 66. **Saventaro Cat's Claw - use this form.** 1 capsule 3 times a day for 10 days, then once a day. Available from our office (800-333-5287) or Phyto Pharmica (800-553-2370). Also helps indigestion.

___ 67. **IP- 6** - Take 5 to 8 grams a day. Take for 1 to 2 months and then 1 gram twice a day. May block absorption of minerals if taken within 2 hours of each other.

For Brain Fog

___ 68. **Ginkgo Biloba (standardized to 24%)** - 60mg _____ 1 twice a day for brain fog; _____ 2 twice a day for depression or sexual dysfunction from antidepressants (takes 6 weeks to work).

___ 68A. Remember (Enzymatic Therapies) or Mental Acuity (PhytoPharmica) - 2 capsules a day. 2 Capsules contains 120mg Ginkgo Biloba, 300mg Bacopa and 600mg Lipoic Acid.

___ 69. **Vinpocetine 10mg plus Ginkgo 60mg** - 1 capsule 2-3 times a day.

___ 70. **Piracetam (Rx)** - 1200mg twice a day for 2 weeks, then take 2400mg twice a day for 2 weeks. Then adjust to optimum dose (up to 4800mg a day). Can be ordered from England. Take with Hydergine (#71) (Web site - antiaging systems.com).

___ 71. **Hydergine (Rx)** - 4 to 6mg each morning.

___ 72. **DMAE** - up to 400mg a day.

For Migraines

Magnesium (see #4) is also very important.

___ 73. **Vitamin B2 (riboflavin)** - 400mg a day to prevent migraines.

___ 74. **Feverfew** - 250mg 1 to 3 times a day to prevent migraines.

___ 74A. **Petadolex (butterbur)** - 50mg one 3 times a day for 1 month and then 1 twice a day. Can take 2 every 3 hours up to 6 capsules for acute migraines. Use only Enzymatic Therapy or PhytoPharmica brands - others often have impurities and do not contain the amount of Butterbur the label claims.

*Treatment For Parasites

If your stool test shows parasites, recheck the stool test 3 to 4 weeks after finishing the treatment below. **Can use the natural remedies #82 and #82A with either #84 or #85.**

___ 75.* **Flagyl (Rx, metronidazole)** - 750mg 3 x a day for 10 days. Followed by Yodoxin for many parasites. For Clostridium Difficile take 250mg, 4 times a day or 500mg, 3 times a day. It may cause nausea/vomiting (uncomfortable but usually not worrisome). Do not drink alcohol while on this medication as it will make you vomit. The SR (sustained release) form is easier on the stomach (as is the Brand name form). If you get numbness/tingling in your fingers (or it worsens if you usually have it) stop the Flagyl.

___ 76. **Yodoxin (Rx, iodoquinol)** - 650 mg- 3 x a day for 20 days after Flagyl is completed.

___ 77. **Tinidazole (Rx)** - 2000mg - ____ Once daily for 3 consecutive days with food (for Entamoeba Histolytica) **OR** ____ 3 doses - each 2 weeks apart (for Giardia or Dientamoeba Fragilis); Available at Clark's Prescriptions 800-480-3432.

___ 78. **Humatin (Rx, Paromomycin)** - 500mg 3 times a day for 10 days (for Cryptosporidium). For Blastocystis add Yodoxin.

___ 79. **Zithromax (Rx)** - 250mg 1 a day on an empty stomach for 10 days, along with Bactrim 1 tablet twice a day for 10 days (alternate treatment for Cryptosporidium). Add Artemesia (#84).

___ 80. **Bactrim DS (Rx)** - 1 twice a day plus Yodoxin 650mg 3 times a day with food for 10 days. Do not take Folic acid supplements (e.g., B Complex or multivitamins) for these 10 days (for Blastocystis).

___ 81. **Amphotericin B (Rx)** - 100mg twice a day plus Tinidazole 500mg twice a day plus Furoxone (Furazolidone) 1 tablet twice a day. Take these 3 together with food for 5 to 7 days (Amphotericin B and Tinidazole are available from Clark's Pharmacy 800-480-3432) (treatment for refractory Blastocystis).

___ 82. **Parastat (Holarrhena Antidysenterica)** - 500mg - you can take up to 8 capsules a day. From Premier Research Labs (800-325-7734).

___ 82A. **Lactoferrin** - 350mg, 1 to 3 capsules at bedtime.

___ 83. **Multi-pure Water Filter** - Most other filters except reverse osmosis are ineffective. Available from Bren Jacobson, 410-224-4877).

___ 84. **Artemesia Annua (an herbal antiparasitic)** - 500 mg- 2 tablets 3 x a day for 20 days.

___ 85. **Tricyclin (an herbal antiparasitic)** - 2 tablets 3 x a day after meals for 6-8 weeks (concentrated Artemesia).

___ 86. **Colostrum (mother's milk)** - 3 capsules 3 x a day for 6-9 months. Then stop or use the lowest dose needed for symptoms. If nausea or indigestion occurs, lower the dose to a comfortable level for 1-2 weeks till it passes. Take on an empty stomach. May increase "Growth Hormone Effect" by raising IGF-1 - it takes 5 months to see this effect.

___ 87. **Quinacrine** - 100mg a day for 5 days. May be useful for empiric therapy of suspected but not identified parasites.

___ 88. **Albendazole** - 400mg a day for 5 days. May be useful for empiric therapy of suspected but not identified parasites.

Treatment for Bacterial, Mycoplasma, Chlamydia, Bladder Infections With E-Coli or Other Infections

These infections usually take months to years to eradicate. It is common to flare your symptoms (from the infection "die off") the first 2-6 weeks of treatment. Take the antibiotics for 6 months and, if better, then repeat 6 week cycles till your symptoms stay gone. Antidepressants, Neurontin, and/or Codeine may block the antibiotic's effectiveness. Be sure to take Nystatin 2 tablets twice a day and Acidophilus while on the antibiotics. If you have occasional low grade fever (i.e., if over 98.6 (F), check your oral temperature occasionally to see if the antibiotic reduces or eliminates the fever. If so, stay on that antibiotic. See Dr. Nicholson's Web site (*www.immed.org*) for more information. **CAN ATTEMPT IMMUNE STIMULATION WITH #62-67 PLUS OLIVE LEAF (#53) (INSTEAD OF OR WITH ANTIBIOTICS).**

___ 89A.   Cipro (Rx) - (ciprofloxacin) - 750mg - twice a day for 6 months. Do not take magnesium products (e.g., Fibrocare, some antacids, Pro Energy, From Fatigued To Fantastic (Formula) within 6 hours of Cipro or you won't absorb the Cipro).

OR

___ 89B.*   **Doxycycline (Rx)** - (a tetracycline) - 100 mg - 3 x a day for 6 months. If symptoms recur when the Doxycycline is completed, keep repeating 6 week courses until the symptoms stay resolved. Take Nystatin (at least 2 twice a day) while on the antibiotic. Your birth control pill may not work while on Doxycycline. Do not take any Doxycycline tablets older than it's expiration date (very dangerous).

OR

___ 89C.   **Zithromax (Rx, azithromycin)** - 600mg tablets - 1 tablet a day (take with food if it bothers your stomach). Don't take magnesium containing products within 6 hours of the Zithromax.

___ 89D.   **Biaxin (Rx)** - 500mg, 2 times a day.

___ 89E.   **D-Mannose** - 1/2 teaspoon (1 gram) stirred in water every 2 to 3 hours while awake for 2 to 5 days for acute bladder infections (may use 1-2 times a day long term for chronic infections) caused by E.Coli (this causes approximately 90% of bladder infections). If not much better in 24 hours, get a urine culture and consider an antibiotic. D-Mannose is available from BioTech (800-345-1199), our office or our Web site Vitamin Shop.

___ 89F.   **Sinusitis Nose Spray** - By prescription from Cape Drug (800-248-5978). Contains Sporanox, Xylitol, Bactroban, Beclamethasone and Nystatin. Use 1-2 sprays each nostril twice a day for 6-12 weeks. If it irritates the nose, use nasal saline spray just before using the prescription.

Nonspecific Treatments

(#92 through 99 may help treat NMH and decrease pain as well as helping energy).

___ 90.   **N.A.E.T.** - Allergy Desensitization (see *www.naet.com* for more information). In Annapolis see Laurie Teitelbaum at 410-266-6958.

___ 90B.   **Myers Cocktail** - I.V. nutritional therapies (very helpful). ___ I.V. Bradford Protocol. In Annapolis - call Rhonda Kidd at 410-571-6337 or Kim Weiss at 410-280-1655.

___ 91.   **Antioxynol (grapeseed extract)** - 50mg - _____ capsules _____ times a day.

___ 92.   **Dexedrine (Rx)** - (dextroamphetamine) - 5mg - 1 to 2 tablets in the morning; plus 1/2 to 1 1/2 tablets at noon; or **Concerta** 18mg take1-2 each morning and/or _____ **Provigil (Rx)** 200mg - up to 1 in the morning and 1 at noon, as needed for energy. Dexedrine is an amphetamine family stimulant similar to Ritalin and may be addictive. Take less if you have caffeine-like shakiness. Most patients use 1 tablet of Dexedrine in the morning and 1/2 at noon. If appetite and/or weight loss is a problem you can add **Periactin (Rx)** 4mg (antihistamine & anti-serotonin) up to 5 tablets a day.

OR #95A below

___ 92A.   **Midodrine (Rx, Proamatine)** - 5mg 1-2 tablets. Take 1/2 -1 hour before 'exercise/activity' up to 3 times a day (for NMH).

___ 92B.   **Mestinon (Rx, Pyridostigmine)** - 60mg - Take 1/2 to 1 tablet up to 1 hour before 'exercise/activity' up to 6 times a day. Restores normal Growth Hormone secretion that occurs with exercise.

___ 93.   **Zoloft (Rx)** - (sertraline) - _____mg - _____ tablet(s) each morning or evening.

___ 94.   **Paxil (Rx)** - (paroxetine) - 20 mg - _____ tablet(s) each morning.

___ 95.   **Prozac (Rx)** - (fluoxetine) - 20 mg - _____ capsule(s) each morning. Begin with 10mg a day the first week if the full dose makes you hyper.

___ 95A.   **Acceleration or Escalation** - By Enzymatic Therapies/PhytoPharmica. Take 1 capsule 1-3 times a day. A powerful stimulant. It contain Cola Nut, Ephedrine and green tea. Do not use if you have heart problems or high blood pressure. Do not combine with any other stimulants, decongestants or diet pills. Adding Willow Bark or 1 Baby Aspirin a day to this makes it a powerful tool for losing weight. It may disrupt sleep if taken after 1 PM. Read the product label and follow the directions.

___ 96.   **Effexor (Rx)** - (venlafaxine) - 37 1/2 mg _____ tablets - _____ times a day.

___ 97.   **Serzone (Rx)** - (nefazodone) - 100 mg - 2 x a day for 1 week, then 150 mg 2 x a day.

___ 98.   **Celexa (Rx)** - 20mg ____ tablet(s) a day OR #109.

___ 99.   **Wellbutrin (Rx)** - (bupropion) - _____ mg - _____ x a day.

___ 100.   **Deprenyl (Rx, Selegiline)** - 10mg ___ times a day (first dose in the morning).

___ 101.   **Aspirin** - 81mg a day.

___ 102.   **Oxygen 10 Liters/minute** - Via a partial re-breather mask (set at F102 35-40%). One hour a day. The oxygen mask must expand and contract during breathing.

___ 102A.   **Cold Water Therapy**

___ 103.   **Heparin (Rx, blood thinner)** - _____units (_____cc) subcutaneously twice a day for 3 months. Then switch to Heparin in lozenge form 5000 units and suck on one twice a day. Avoid any traumatic injuries. There are 10,000units/cc. If you have preloaded syringes (____units/cc) use 1 syringe 2 times a day. This is a blood thinner - call immediately if you have any bleeding problems. Check the Platelet Count and PTT blood tests (#147) each 3 days for 9 days then every 2 weeks while on Heparin injections. Inject it into the fat (not muscle) in your abdomen. Use a different spot each time (you may get a bruise where the injection is given). Can cause a (potentially fatal) bleeding problem or drop in platelet count.

AND/OR   **Nattokinase (natural powerful blood thinner)** - 138mg. Take 1 tablet at night or twice a day (from Allergy Research).

AND/OR   **Protease Enzymes** (e.g. Trauma or Wobenzyme) plus Vascular enzymes.

___ 103B.   **Naltrexone (Rx) (Low Dose)** - 3-4 1/2 mg at bed time (stop in one month if not helping) - from Cape Drugs (800-248-5978). This is an immune stimulant and may enhance the effectiveness or Morphine. Only if taken at extraordinarily low doses (e.g., 1-2 micrograms) See www.lowdosenaltrexone.org.

___ 104.   **Coumadin (Rx, blood thinner)** - _____mg each morning. Reacts with many medications. Be sure to check with your doctor before adding or deleting any medicines (even Aspirin) while on Coumadin. Check P.T./INR blood tests as noted in #148. Begin 3 days before stopping Heparin - see Coumadin/Heparin instruction sheet for how to dose.

___ 105.   **MSM (sulfur = methyl sulfonyl methane)** - 2000-6000mg - 2 times a day for 2-3 months, then as needed for allergies, wound healing, and arthritis. Take vitamin C 500mg with each dose to improve absorption. This is O.K. to take even if you are Sulfa allergic.

___ 105A.   **Food Allergy Elimination Diet**

___ 106.   **Humibid (Rx, guaifenisin)** - 600mg _____ tablets _____ times a day (see instruction sheet). No aspirin or herbals can be taken while on Guaifenisin. GuaiLife - a shorter acting form may be more effective.

___ 106B.   **For pesticide detoxification** (usually takes 3-10 months to start working and symptoms may initially flare). Add 50gm choline and 25gm vitamin C to 500cc (-1 pint) of flavored water. Take 10cc (2 teaspoons) 3 x a day for 1 month then 5cc (1 teaspoon) 2 times a day. Choline can cause a fishy smell at a higher dose. If this a problem, lower the dose. Reference *Journal of Chronic Fatigue Syndrome 6* (2) 2000, p 11-21.

___ 106C.   For severe dry eyes - Use #1, #11 and Testosterone cream applied to eyelids.

___ 107.   **L-Serine** - 250mg - 2 to 6 capsules a day (from 800-366-6056).

___ 108.   **Iberogast (digestive system herbal)** - Take 20 drops 3 times a day in warm water with meals. Very helpful for indigestion (takes 4 to 8 weeks to work). From Phyto Pharmica.

___ 108B   **Interferon (Rx)** - 50units under your tongue each morning (from Cape Drugs 800-248-5978).

___ 108C.   **Galantamine** - 8mg a day for 1 month, then 16 mg a day for 1 month. Then you can increase to 24mg a day or stay on 16mg a day. It takes 2 months at 16mg a day to work. Made from daffodils, it helps sleep, mental clarity and energy by raising Acetylcholine levels. Available from 'Life Enhancement' at 800-543-3873. If nausea occurs - temporarily lower the dose.

___ 109. **Hypericum (St. John's Wort)** - 300 to 625 mg - 3 x a day (takes 6 weeks to see the antidepressant effect). Use one standardized to at least .3% hypericum. Can take 2/3 of the total daily dose at night to help sleep. Can take up to 2000mg Hypericum a day if not on other antidepressants (otherwise limit to 1000mg a day).

___ 110. **Parlodel (Rx, Bromocriptine)** - 2 1/2 mg - 1/2 tablet at night for 1st week, then 1 tablet at night. Lowers elevated Prolactin levels. Vitamin B6 200mg a day can also lower Prolactin.

___ 110A. **Questran Light (Rx)** - 1 packet or scoop 4 times a day mixed with fluids (e.g., water). Binds other treatments so take them at least 1 hour before or 4 hours after Questran if possible. Can cause severe and dangerous constipation. Take #111C, D, E, F and/or G as needed to have at least 1 bowel movement a day. If Questran flares your symptoms, stop it and take **Actos (Rx)** 45mg a day for 5 days first (caution - may drop blood sugar - monitor while on it) and then retry Questran (and consider adding antibiotics).

___ 111A. **Peppermint Oil** - Enteric/stomach coated (2/10 =.2cc) capsules, 1 to 2 capsules 3 times a day between meals (**not** with food) for spastic colon. Peppermint Plus from Enzymatic Therapies.

___ 111B. **Simethicone (mylicon)** - 40 to 80mg, **chew** one tablet 3 times a day as needed for abdominal gas pains.

Constipation

Can adjust these as needed for one soft bowel movement a day. Increasing your water, fiber (e.g., 1 bowl of whole grain cereal in the morning) and magnesium intake is also helpful.

___ 111C. **Artichoke Extract** - 160mg By Enzymatic Therapies. Take 2 capsules 3 times a day. It can also help spastic colon. Stimulates bile acid release and may also help gall stones.

___ 111D. **Miralax Laxative (Rx)** - 1 heaping tablespoon a day in 8 oz. Water (comes in 14 oz. and 26 oz bottles).

___ 111E. **Lactulose Liquid (Rx)** - Take as needed for constipation.

___ 111F. **Challenge Caps** - up to 2 capsules 3 times a day between meals.

___ 111G. **Prunes and/or Prune Juice**

Pain Treatments

(Antidepressants #93-99 or Lithium #51 <u>often</u> help FMS pain). **THE NATURAL TREATMENTS CAN BE SUBSTITUTED FOR OR ADDED TO THE PRESCRIPTION PAIN MEDICATIONS.**

___ 112. **Rolfing, Trager, Myofascial Release, Chiropractic & other body work**, manipulation modalities and/or acupuncture.

___ 112A. **Rhus tox (homeopathic treatment)** - dissolve under the tongue as directed on the bottle as needed for muscle pain.

___112B. **Flexagility** - From Enzymatic Therapies and PhytoPharmica. Take 1 tablet twice a day. Contains a super concentrate of Ginger and Greater Galanga. This product is excellent. It takes 2 weeks to start working and 6 weeks to see the full effects (like a natural Celebrex).

___ 112C. **Phytodolor (herbal from Phyto Pharmica)** - 30 drops, 3 times a day. Takes 1 to 2 weeks to work.

___ 112D. **Heel Lift** - _____ inches for _____ foot.

___ 112E. **John Sarno, MD's** - Approach for **localized** pain. The mind can decrease blood flow to muscles to distract us from uncomfortable emotional feelings. When you feel pain, tell your mind you will use the pain as a signal to look for and feel uncomfortable feelings for 10-15 minutes. The pain will often leave within 6 weeks.

___ 113A. **Arizona Pain Formula Cream (Rx)** - Rub a pea size amount onto painful areas 3 times a day as needed (from Ron Partam - Pharmacist 877-340-5922). You can use this on up to 3 or 4 "silver dollar" sized areas at a time.

___ 113B. **Glucosamine** <u>Sulfate</u> - 500mg, 3 times a day (for arthritis). Takes 6 weeks to see if it will help. When the maximum benefit is seen, you can decrease to the lowest dose that maintains the effect.

___ 113C. **Trauma Enzymes** - 4 capsules 3 times a day between meals for 2 bottles (do not use if gastritis or ulcers are present).

OR

___ 113D. **Megazyme** (Enzymatic Therapies) or **Biozyme** (PhytoPharmica) - Like a super Wobenzyme. Take 2-4 capsules 3 times a day between meals.

PLUS

___ 113E. **Osteo Enzymes** - 3 capsules 3 times a day between meals for 2 bottles.

___ 114. **Lidocaine 15% in PLO Gel (Rx)** - Rub on areas of nerve pain as needed. From Ron's Pharmacy (see #113A).

___ 114B. **Neurontin 10% in PLO Gel (Rx)** - Rub on areas of nerve pain as needed. From Ron's Pharmacy (see #113A).

___ 115. **Lidocaine Intravenously (I.V) (Rx)** - _____mg (_____mg 1st dose) I.V. each 3 to 20 days as needed. Can give up to 120mg per hour. Take with I.V. Myers - see #90B.

___ 116. **Robaxin (Rx, methocarbimol)** - 750mg - 1 to 2 capsules 3 to 4 times a day as needed for pain (sedating).

___ 117. **Daypro (Rx)** - 600mg - 2 each morning as needed. Aspirin family medications can cause stomach bleeding. Take with an antacid or food if it upsets your stomach. If gastritis persists, stop the medicine or lower the dose. **If you have a black stool (and are not taking iron tablets or Pepto Bismol), this may represent a life threatening stomach bleed (the stool will often have a very foul smell). If this occurs, go to the emergency room immediately.**

___ 118. **Voltaren (Rx)** - ____ mg ____ times a day as needed. Aspirin family medications can cause stomach bleeding. Take with an antacid or food if it upsets your stomach. If gastritis persists, stop the medicine or lower the dose. **If you have a black stool (and are not taking iron tablets or Pepto Bismol), this may represent a life threatening stomach bleed (the stool will often have a very foul smell). If this occurs, go to the emergency room immediately.**

___ 119. **Zanaflex (Rx, tizanidine)** - 4mg - Take with food - 1 to 3 tablets 3 times a day as needed for spasm and/or pain (sedating). Begin 4mg at night. If side effects occur raise dose more slowly. You can raise dose by 2mg each 2-3 days to a maximum of 36mg/day. May rarely cause hallucinations, delusions or liver inflammation and may lower blood pressure. Stop if causes nightmares.

___ 119A. **Catapres TTS 1 Patch (Rx)** - Wear 1-3 at a time and change patch weekly. Related to Zanaflex but cheaper and lowers blood pressure more. Helps pain and raises growth hormone.

___ 119B. **Marinol** - 5mg capsules 1-2 twice a day. As this is a THC extract it may cause sedation and increased appetite.

___ 120. **Dextromethorphan (Rx, DM)** - 25mg - 2 times a day if on narcotics (e.g., codeine/vicodin) makes the narcotic more effective. From Cape Drugs 800-248-5978.

___ 121. **Copper/Magnet Bracelet** - Use nail polish remover to remove any coating on the inside of the bracelet so the copper is in direct contact with your skin.

___ 121B. **Cetyl Myristoleate** - 385mg capsules - 3 capsules 2 times a day for 10 days. You can raise the dose to a maximum of 17gm a day. For pain - benefits often persist after the 10 days of treatment.

___ 122. **Ultram (Rx, Tramadol)** - 50mg 1 to 2 tablets up to 4 times a day as needed for pain. Caution: May rarely cause seizures or raise serotonin too high when combined with antidepressants. May cause nausea/vomiting.

___ 122A. **Dantrium (Rx)** - (25mg) For muscle spasm take 1 a day for 1 week. Then one 3 times a day for 1 week, then 2 tablets 3 times a day for 1 week then 100mg 3 times a day. Adjust to the lowest dose that feels the best. Stop or lower dose if severe diarrhea occurs. Check liver blood tests (#143) at 6, 12 and 24 weeks and then each 1 to 6 months to make sure there is no liver inflammation.

___ 123. **Skelaxin (Rx, metaxolone)** - 400mg 1-2 tablets 4 times a day as needed for pain. This is usually non-sedating.

___ 124. **Norflex Tablets (Rx)** - 1 tablet twice a day.

___ 125. **Celebrex (Rx, Celecoxib)** - 100 to 200mg 1 to 2 times a day for pain. Do not take if you're allergic to sulfa or Aspirin (e.g., hives). Do not use over the 200mg a day while on Sporanox or Diflucan. FlexAgility (#112B) is a natural form and is safer.

___ 125B. **Vioxx (Rx, Refecoxib)** - 25mg, 1/2 to 1 tablet daily. Do not use if you are aspirin allergic (e.g., hives).

___ 125C. **Bextra (Rx, Valdecoxib)** - 10-20mg once a day. Take twice a day for menstrual pain.

___ 126. **Neurontin (Rx, Gabapentin)** - ____mg ____ times a day (to a maximum of 3600mg a day). Cut back if it causes any uncomfortable or unusual neurologic symptoms or excessive sedation. Begin with 300mg at night, slowly increase to 300mg 3 times a day as is comfortable. You can go up to 3600mg a day.

___ 127. **Baclofen (Rx)** - 10 to 20mg 1 to 3 times a day (sedating).

___ 128. **Magnets** - Start with spot magnets, insoles and seat. If they help in 2 months, consider a mattress pad. Available from Bren Jacobsen (410-224-4877) or Amy Podd (410-757-7295).

__ 128A. **Flexyx or Alpha-Stim Micro Current** - Flexyx can be very effective.

___ 129. **Cod Liver Oil** - 1/2 Tablespoon (5000mg) a day. Do not use if you are about to get pregnant - it may have too much vitamin A.

___ 129A. **Risperdal (Risperidone)** - 1/4 mg to 1 1/2 mg a day (not more). Begin with 1/4 mg and increase by 1/4 mg each 6 weeks. Going above optimal dose will cancel out the effect. Takes 2 weeks to work. Blocks Serotonin (not dopamine at this low dose). Helps pain, anxiety and sleep.

Goldstein Protocol Treatments

___ 130. **Nimotop (Rx, Nimodipine)** - 30mg 1 to 4 times a day as is beneficial for symptoms.

___ 131. **Naphzoline .1% Eye Drops (Rx)** - 1 drop in each eye 3 to 4 times a day as needed for symptoms.

___ 132. **TRH Eye Drops (Rx)** - 500units in 9cc artificial tears - 1 drop in each eye 3 to 4 times a day as is helpful.

___ 133. **Tasmar (Rx, talcopone)** - 100mg twice a day. Use if it helps mental clarity and energy.

Heartburn, Indigestion or Reflux

Using chronic acid blockers (e.g., Prilosec) is a poor long-term solution for these problems, as it worsens digestion and your defense against bowel infections. Use the treatment(s) checked off below. After 1 month you can stop your prescription acid blocker and switch to Tagamet (cimetidine - over-the-counter), up to 400mg 3 times a day as needed, then taper off the Tagamet as able. Use #2 - Complete Gest Digestive Enzymes as well and sip warm liquids with meals instead of cold water (digestive enzymes work poorly at cold temperatures). Taking a minute to relax before eating and chewing your food will also help digestion.

___ 133A. **Mastic Gum** - 500mg 2 capsules twice a day for 2 months - then as needed.

___ 133B. **Heartburn Free** - by Enzymatic Therapies. 1 every other day for 20 days (may initially aggravate reflux).

___ 133C. **DGL Licorice/Rhizinase** - 380mg (not the sugar free one). Chew 2 tablets 20 minutes before meals, from Enzymatic Therapies/PhytoPharmica.

___ 133D. **Saventaro Cat's Claw** _____.

Follow Up Testing

___ 134. **Stool O&P (ova & parasite)** at The Institute Of Parisitology in Arizona in _____ week(s). Get a kit from UROKEEP (480) 545-9236.

___ 135. **Stool O&P, culture, and sensitivity** - must be sent to Great Smokey Mountain Labs (800-572-4762).

___ 136. **Sleep apnea study** (get insurance pre-authorization - it costs $2000).

___ 137. **IGE Food Allergy Blood Test** - send to Great Smokey Mountain Lab (800-572-4762). **IGNORE** the IgG Section - it is meaningless and will only make you nuts - **only** look at the IgE section.

___ 138. **DHEA - Sulphate** level in _____ weeks (**not** DHEA level).

___ 139. **Free T4 level** in _____ weeks.

___ 140. **Potassium level** in _____ weeks.

___ 141. **Lithium level.**

___ 141. **Free testosterone level** in _____ weeks.

___ 142. **Prolactin level** in _____ weeks.

___ 143. **ALT, AST** - in _____ weeks (liver tests - if taking Sporanox or Diflucan for more than 3 months, check every 6 to 12 weeks).

___ 144. **HHV-6, CMV, and EBV PCR** Testing

___ 145. **CFIDS Coagulation Blood Profile** - must send to Hemex Labs (800-999-2568) (ISAC panel for CFS/FM = FIB, F1 & 2:T/AT, SFM, PA score - $335).

___ 145A. **Hereditary Thrombotic Panel** - at Hemex Labs.

___ 146. **Blood test for Mycoplasma & Chlamydia** (General Screens) - send to The Institute For Molecular Medicine (714-903-2900).

___ 147. **Platelet Count and P.T.T. Blood Test** - each 3 days for 9 days and then each 2 weeks while on Heparin.

___ 148. **P.T./INR Blood Test** - each 2 days for the 1st 8 days on Coumadin, then every 2 weeks for 6 weeks then each 6 to 8 weeks while on Coumadin. Check 2 days after making any change to your medication and/or supplement regimen and consult your physician before making these changes. Keep the INR at the lowest level that leaves the patient feeling well, but not over 3.

___ 149. **Dexa Scan** for Osteoporosis.

___ 150. **MRI** of _____ head; _____ neck

___ 151. **Blood Test** (Elisa-Act) at Elisa/Act Biotechnologies (800-553-5472). We consider this the best lab for food allergies.

___ 152. **24 Hour Urine Kit** - Be off all non-prescription treatments for 24 hours before and the 24 hours during the urine collection. Follow directions that come with the kit. Tests to see what enzymes are most likely to help you.

___ 153. **Do vision test** at www.neurotoxins.com. - Although approximately 1/2 of CFS/FMS patients test positive on the test, I found that approximately 1/2 of the healthy people also flunk the test. If test is positive, consider Questran treatment (#110A)

REFERENCES

1. Travell, J.G., Simons, D.G. *The Trigger Point Manual*. Williams & Wilkins, 1983.
2. Teitelbaum, J., Bird, B. Effective treatment of severe chronic fatigue: a report of a series of 64 patients. *J Musculoskel Pain*, 1995; 3(4), 91-110.
3. Teitelbaum, J. *From Fatigued to Fantastic*. Avery Press, 1996. (See item 3220 on page 63-64).
4. Teitelbaum, J. *From Fatigued to Fantastic*. Newsletter, February 1997.
5. Jefferies, W. *Safe Uses of Cortisol*. Charles C. Thomas Publishing, 1996.
6. Neeck, G., Riedell, W. Thyroid function in patients with fibromyalgia syndrome. *J Rheum*, 1992; 19:1120-22.
7. Teitelbaum, J. *From Fatigued to Fantastic*. Newsletter, July 1997.
8. Teitelbaum, J. Effective treatment of severe chronic fatigue states. *J Musculoskel Pain*, 1995; 3(1):28.

Medically reviewed and edited by Jacob Teitelbaum, M.D.

Address: **Dr. Jacob Teitelbaum**
466 Forelands Road
Annapolis, MD 21401
Phone: (410) 573-5389 • Fax (410) 266-6104
Web site: www.endfatigue.com

APPENDIX

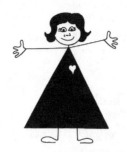

SUPPORT GROUP LEADERS

Taking Charge of your Group

Julie and Rosalie know how much work, time and energy is spent running a support group for FMS patients. We started the first FMS support group in Minneapolis, Minnesota at Abbott Northwestern Hospital in 1991 with Jenny Fransen, RN. We are trained Arthritis foundation leaders as well. Our training was helpful, but we learned most about running a group while on "the job." Even though we do not run a support group anymore, our work brings us into contact with groups we teach in our educational classes, and at work where we run groups on a variety of topics. Rosalie's past teaching experience and clinical work with psychological issues has also helped us to learn techniques for dealing with both large and small groups.

We know how easily one can become burned out by the demands of this volunteer effort. We would like to supply support group leaders with information which may help better run an effective group. Suggestions from fibromyalgia support group leaders have also been included. We also asked leaders to let us know what has not worked for them and have included those comments as well. It is important to know the good, the bad and the ugly so you will avoid making mistakes.

We also are including information on how to use this book with your group. We have taken topics from various chapters and share ideas for activities and discussion at group meetings. Topics and activities for discussion when you do not have a speaker are also included, as that seems to be an area for which leaders need additional ideas.

Important points to note for groups in general:

▲ People will relate more positively in a group setting if they feel they are part of the group. It takes time for people to feel comfortable with a group.

▲ Some people are shy and need help in meeting others and in opening up.

▲ Groups need a leader who can lead. That is: the leader must be in control in a positive way. Leaders should be able to handle difficult group members in a non- confrontive, yet assertive way.

▲ Groups need direction: always have a topic, a speaker, or an activity planned. This will keep your group from getting out of hand and will make your life easier. It will be helpful to have back-up activities planned when your speaker cancels. We offer some suggestions for you to keep in your arsenal of plans for use when speakers cancel, particularly at the last minute.

▲ Allowing group members to be a part of the group by giving them defined jobs that they enjoy performing will make your group more cohesive and will also remove some of the pressure from the leader by delegating tasks.

▲ Allow group members to determine topics they would like to hear or activities they would enjoy doing. You will never know unless you ask members what their preferences are. Hand out surveys or suggestion cards for topics. See if members will help set up speakers or activities they would enjoy.

▲ The more people you can get to help you, the less pressured the leader will feel. Remember that 10% of the people in any group do 90% of the work.

▲ Your group should have a focus, mission and goal. Remember that these can change and will as the needs of the group change. You must be able to bend with the changes, too. Staying stuck in a rut will not benefit your members or your group's purpose. Change with the times.

▲ Nancy Groth of Terre Haute, Indiana, offers some good suggestions for groups:

Have guest speakers only once every three months so there is plenty of sharing time.

Try to have someone on the steering committee who is a service provider and cares about the illness so they can keep things going well when the rest of you have run out of steam.

Don't try to remind members via e-mail or phone more than a week in advance of the meeting: they may not remember due to fibro-fog.

Leaders should keep their own problems to the steering committee. Your group members are dependent on you and may see you as needy.

▲ Sue Nelson, a personal trainer who works with patients in the water states that she "creates ripples" of education, compassion and encouragement. You never know where the ripples will lead or when they might turn into a wave.

How to Make your Group Positive

Many leaders and members of groups complain that too often, support group meetings turn into pity sessions with a lot of negativity being expressed by group members. This can cause frustration for leaders as well as group members. In fact, it is one of the most often mentioned problems facing fibromyalgia support groups. We know that people with fibromyalgia may be frustrated due to a variety of reasons including; lack of adequate health care, high pain and fatigue levels, loss of jobs, friends, and numerous other reasons we may not even begin to ascertain. These people may feel a need to vent their feelings and have no other place to do this. Some people who are constantly irritable and complaining, may be in need of psychological help or anti-depressants. One of the hallmarks of depression is irritability. Many of us think that crying, or feelings of sadness are the main symptoms of depression, but in reality, irritability and feelings of hopelessness are oftentimes just as present in depression as that of sadness. Some of the dysregulation in body chemistry is actually causing FMS patients to feel irritable. We should not be judgmental as we are not standing in their shoes, so to speak. Have compassion and remember that each person is affected differently by this illness. Those who whine may be lonely and have no one else to talk to. Of course, there are some people who are just plain irritable and would be like that even if they didn't have fibromyalgia! Dealing with these individuals can be difficult and challenging, to say the least. The leader, or your co-leaders, should be able to confront those people who present with the most negativity in a non-critical, compassionate, yet assertive way. If you or someone in your group cannot, it could cause difficulties for the group.

Why it is important to keep your group focused on the positive.

One of the more important reasons for keeping a group focused on positive issues is that by doing this, you will decrease their anxiety and stress, enhance their feelings of hope and increase their ability to handle the problems that occur when living with fibromyalgia. Research shows that without hope, people have difficulty improving. Negative thoughts fuel the fire of depressive thoughts, increase sadness and make us feel that we should not even try because things won't or can't get better.

Here are some ideas for keeping meetings positive:

▲ One of the most effective means to deter complaining is one of the most obvious: leaders need to announce at the beginning of each meeting that complaining is not allowed. This may be difficult for some leaders to do as it is often difficult to confront those issues that bother us the most. Also, you may just forget to mention it at each meeting (we can blame this on fibro-fog). As a leader, you will have to take the initiative to bring this problem to the forefront of discussion. If you don't, members will talk about their dissatisfaction with the group anyway; either behind your back, or during breaks. So you might as well talk about it openly. Members may not come back if you cannot stop the negativity from spreading. It might help if you make up a speech beforehand, one about being positive and the necessity for being positive, so that when negativity shows up, you will feel confident in handling it. Announcing it at all meetings will also help new members understand what your group expects and allows.

▲ Make a large poster that is visible at all meetings with a reminder to keep the group positive. A number of leaders have mentioned that when they developed guidelines for keeping a group positive, they had better success. This can be an activity for the group to perform. Have the group members decide what to put on the poster. This will allow them to discuss their feelings regarding negativity in the group and will allow for some ventilation of their own feelings. It is also a nice group activity to help set the direction of the group.

▲ Decide in advance how you will handle a negative member. Will one of the group's co-leaders take that negative person aside privately, will you point to your poster which clearly states the meetings are positive, or will you just announce to the group *" I feel our discussion is getting too negative and we must remember to stay positive."*

▲ Announce that members will be allowed 15 minutes (or whatever length of time you decide) of total complaining time after which complaints will no longer be allowed. It is important to mention that each individual person who wants to complain will only be give a few minutes to do so. Use a timer, if necessary: an ordinary kitchen timer will do nicely. Then another person can complain. Those who continue to complain after the 15 minutes, will be reminded that the time is up and be redirected to a more positive topic. One way to do this is to say to the member who is the complainer, *"I hear you are feeling very frustrated about ...... Is there anyone in the group who has some way of coping with this particular problem?"* After the allotted time is up for complaining, you will then discuss positive ways of coping with the complaints!

▲ Assign a buddy to new members. A buddy is someone who will talk privately to the new member either at the meeting, on the phone, or who might meet with them after the meeting. They can explain the group's goals and focus to the new member and provide one-to-one support which will also assist the new member in feeling like a part of the group.

▲ There is an effective way of communicating with difficult people that works very well. It is a simple technique, called active listening, which takes a little practice, but once you get the hang of it, you can utilize it not only for problem support group members, but also with your children, spouse, significant other, friends, and family. It is so effective you will be amazed! When someone is complaining you only need to reflect back what they have said to you in such a way as to make them feel you sympathize with them, but you change their words. For instance:

Complainer says: *"My doctor does not help me at all, he just spends 2 seconds with me and then pushes me out the door!"*

Leader says very simply: *"Your doctor doesn't take time with you"* (this is a very simple reply which validates the complainer's statements and makes them feel that they have been heard)

Complainer might then say: *"Right, how can he help me if he doesn't take the time to listen to me?"*

Leader reflects back this statement by saying something like: *"It takes longer to help a fibro patient than other patients he/she usually sees"* or *"You feel like he doesn't help you?"*

Complainer says: *"Yes, he doesn't help me. I am still in pain."*

Leader asks the group: *"What would anyone else do in this situation?"* to deflect the conversation to a more positive focus.

This way you can move the conversation to the positive ways of coping with a doctor who spends little time with a patient. This will set up a good topic to discuss with the group. You should then get responses such as: *"My doctor spends a lot of time with me and her name is….."* or *"I think I would find a new doctor."* Another response could be: *"I take in a list of topics I want to cover during my appointment and that seems to help."* This can lead to a good discussion with some useful tips which will actually aid people in dealing with their doctors rather than setting up a "doctor bashing" session. If other members begin joining in on the complaining, continue deflecting their negative responses to positive and constructive ideas.

This would be a good time then to get out our chapter on dealing with doctors and go over some points addressed in it.

▲ Place the serenity prayer in an obvious location. Read it out loud to the group.

▲ Be reminded that no matter how much you try to keep your group from becoming negative, there may be someone you just cannot keep from whining. Say the serenity prayer yourself, often!

▲ Occasionally, you may have a member who is suffering from a mental illness, or who becomes extremely emotional during the meeting. This has happened to Julie and I. Although it is a difficult thing to do, you may have to call the police or security if things get out of hand if you are holding meetings in a health facility. If this happens, do not attempt to confront the person, as one can not know what a person in a highly agitated state might do. Get help. Speak in a low, soft voice, as this will calm them down. If you raise your voice to their pitch, they will just escalate. Remain calm, it will help them calm down.

▲ One leader encourages members to "sandwich" negative thoughts between positive thoughts.

▲ Include a regular time at each meeting when members are allowed to share a positive thought for coping, or provide a new resource or information. This will encourage members to look for positive news to report.

▲ Diane Spizzirri, of Schaumberg, Illinois, starts out every meeting with a joke. You may have to write down the joke if you have a bad case of fibro-fog. Group members could be encouraged to provide their own jokes. Have a joke box!! Let everyone put a joke in it and pick one at each meeting. Have members read it out loud.

Topics for Discussion and Activities

Many leaders have requested ideas for topics to discuss when speakers are not available. We have come up with a variety of discussion questions for you to use at meetings and also provide ways to use our book in your group to help you facilitate meetings.

▲ One activity to utilize which is easy to do and group members love, is to divide the group up into small groups with 3- 5 people in the smaller groups. Have members count off from 1-5 and all the 1's get together in one area of the room. Other numbers get together in another area. This way people will get to know each other personally and you will keep people from engaging in "clique" activity. Have a topic for each small group to discuss for a time - maybe 20 minutes. One person in each group will be the spokesperson for that group whose duty it is to take down notes and report to the larger group. You then come together as a large group and discuss the topic. Allow each group to report with time limits.

Topics for Discussion

What local resources are available?

Tips for pacing.

Tips for coping.

How to expand your support network.

What are the most difficult things you experience due to FMS?

Discussions on effective exercise.

What helps you sleep?

How does your family help?

How do you get your family to help?

What to say to people when they ask you about your illness.

How do people cope with holidays?

Suggestions for traveling on planes and by car.

Suggested Activities

▲ Carol Johnson, from Red Oak, Iowa, had her group participate in two surveys from universities.

▲ Some leaders make packets of information and send them to local doctors. It would also be nice to have the group put these packets together at a meeting and take or send them out. This would encourage group sharing and facilitate personal connections between people.

▲ Ask the local mall if you could have a booth there and hand out fliers about FMS and/or your group. This will get members active and will also help spread the word. FM awareness day, May 12, might be a great time for this activity.

▲ If you live in a smaller community, you may be able to get on the local news broadcast. Call them, you may be surprised as they are always on the lookout for news. If you are feeling uncomfortable about calling, delegate this activity to someone who does.

▲ Show videos to the group and discuss afterwards. These do no necessarily have to be on FMS, but could be on a topic related such as t'ai chi or easy yoga. Everyone can have fun while trying out the best relaxation and movement activities there are.

▲ Potlucks are always fun and encourage socialization.

▲ Your group could meet at a local warm water pool or health club to encourage socialization as well as participating in exercise. One of the health club trainers could explain techniques helpful for FMS. This activity could encourage members to exercise as well as finding a buddy to exercise with.

▲ Try to vary your activities and programs to provide a variety of events. This will help your group stay interested instead of becoming dull or boring.

It is important to have fun as well as be well-educated!

Members often need to know about local or national resources. Keeping a resource list which is updated regularly will allow your group to be informed and up-to-date.

How to Use our Book in a Group Setting

Encourage members to read a specific chapter from our book before the meeting. Or in desperation, read it out loud at the meeting. This may sound grade schoolish- but some people have fibro-fog quite badly and may have a difficult time reading and remembering.

Leaders have permission to use our worksheets (journal pages) from any of the sections we have provided worksheets for. Have members get together in the small group settings to fill them out. Then come together as a large group after about 30-45 minutes of discussion time to share with the larger group.

Specific suggestions for worksheets:

▲ Support Ring Page: the worksheet with the support ring from the coping chapter would be a good one to use. Each member can fill it out individually then share their responses with the larger group. This way you may find out which members have little support or friends and could use some from your group. Discussion questions could be: How can you find or put together a "family" if you have few family members living near you? Other members might provide local resources that your community offers.

▲ Exercise sheet: have members share which exercises work for them. Members could discuss local resources. Go over the exercise chapter and discuss our exercise program. Encourage members to bring in their sheets at meetings and share their experiences.

▲ Stress management: Beg, borrow or buy a stress relaxation tape and use our information on deep breathing to practice relaxation exercises with the group. It is nice if everyone can lie down in the room, and listen to the tape you provide. Ask members to practice daily and report back at the next meeting. Your group could practice abdominal breathing and then try meditating as a group. Have the group focus on one word or on their breathing when meditating, as it helps facilitate positive results from the practice of meditation. Discuss ways in which people use relaxation to help their symptoms. Have them share what works and what doesn't. Use the daily stress management chart and fill it out in small groups. Or you could use it for a large group discussion.

▲ Go over our "Most important daily affirmations list." Make up your own.

▲ Negative self talk journal page: discuss negative thoughts and negative talk in general. Have members fill out our worksheet and discuss their answers. Have them write down how many times a day their thoughts are negative. Work on ways to counteract this. Members will have some good ideas.

▲ Discuss positive uplifts. This concept is found in the chapter on "Coping with Psychological Aspects" and is also included in the support ring diagram. Have people write ideas and share them out loud. A list of possibilities is found in the same section of the book. It would be nice to have someone compile all the results and have it available at meetings. This is something that could be added to at every meeting. People need to be encouraged to provide themselves with a daily uplift, or at least a few times a week. The uplifts need not be expensive or lengthy, but can be free and take only 5-15 minutes.

▲ Everyone likes to talk about their medication. Have people bring in their pill bottles. They can fill out our medication diary which may best be done in small groups. They could also work on the journal page "Questions to ask your Physician." You could then use our medication section to talk about and answer questions they might have.

▲ Use a poster board, large paper or blackboard and have everyone list their symptoms. Or use our symptom check list. Discussion could be: which are the most difficult to cope with? Which are FMS related or could be related to another illness? Which are the hardest for family or friends to understand? Use our symptom and diagnosis section for this topic.

▲ You could have a similar discussion using the feelings journal from the book, found in the "Psychological Aspects" of our book, as well. List feelings members experience and how they cope with them.

▲ Have a family night. Encourage family members to attend and share experiences on how FMS affects families. Use our family section in the psychological coping area as a framework for discussion. It may be interesting to separate family members from patients and allow them to have their own discussion. This may allow them to share experiences and learn from each other.

▲ Discuss alternative therapies they have used. What worked, what didn't and local resources.

▲ Have a computer night. Share internet resources. Discuss which are the best and make up a list for members. You can use our list as a resource. A group member could bring in a laptop computer to access specific sites for the entire group to share. Going to the local library to meet and have lessons from the computer person there would help members become familiar with using computers. Group members could also assist other members who are inexperienced with computers.

These are only some suggestions, certainly not everything that could be discussed. Ask members what they would like to hear about as well. Remember, that if your group can get to know each other personally, they are more likely to attend. Also, we think you can see from this list, that you do not always need a speaker or a video. People need support as well as education. Letting group members become involved during group meetings will help provide group synergy and allow your group to get to know each other better.

Contact national organizations listed in our resource section for more information about support groups.

Remember, Have Fun!!

INDEX

INDEX

INDEX

INDEX

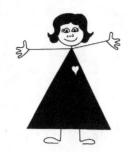

ORDERING INFORMATION

Fibromyalgia Educational Systems, Inc.
326 Broadway Avenue South #206
Wayzata, MN 55391-1712

Phone: 847-480-7479 or 952-224-4413

www.fibrobook.com or *www.fmsedsys.com*

Please call or check the Web site for ordering information.
The Web site has prices for bulk quantities, shipping rates,
and instructions for orders outside of the U.S.

NOTES

NOTES